Updates in Pharmacologic Strategies in ADHD

Editors

JEFFREY H. NEWCORN
TIMOTHY E. WILENS

CHILD AND ADOLESCENT PSYCHIATRIC CLINICS OF NORTH AMERICA

www.childpsych.theclinics.com

Consulting Editor
JUSTINE LARSON

July 2022 • Volume 31 • Number 3

ELSEVIER

1600 John F. Kennedy Boulevard • Suite 1800 • Philadelphia, Pennsylvania, 19103-2899

http://www.theclinics.com

CHILD AND ADOLESCENT PSYCHIATRIC CLINICS OF NORTH AMERICA Volume 31, Number 3
July 2022 ISSN 1056–4993, ISBN-13: 978-0-323-91991-3

Editor: Megan Ashdown
Developmental Editor: Arlene Campos

Child and Adolescent Psychiatric Clinics of North America (ISSN 1056-4993) is published quarterly by Elsevier Inc., 360 Park Avenue South, New York, NY 10010-1710. Months of issue are January, April, July, and October. Business and Editorial Offices: 1600 John F. Kennedy Boulevard, Suite 1800, Philadelphia, PA 19103-2899. Periodicals postage paid at New York, NY and additional mailing offices. Subscription prices are $358.00 per year (US individuals), $869.00 per year (US institutions), $100.00 per year (US & Canadian students), $399.00 per year (Canadian individuals), $895.00 per year (Canadian institutions), $459.00 per year (international individuals), $895.00 per year (international institutions), and $200.00 per year (international students). International air speed delivery is included in all *Clinics* subscription prices. All prices are subject to change without notice. **POSTMASTER:** Send address changes to *Child and Adolescent Psychiatric Clinics of North America*, Elsevier Health Sciences Division, Subscription Customer Service, 3251 Riverport Lane, Maryland Heights, MO 63043. **Customer Service: 1-800-654-2452 (U.S. and Canada); 314-447-8871 (outside U.S. and Canada). Fax: 314-447-8029. E-mail:** JournalsCustomer Service-usa@elsevier.com **(for print support) or** journalsonlinesupport-usa@elsevier.com **(for online support).**

Reprints. For copies of 100 or more of articles in this publication, please contact the Commercial Reprints Department, Elsevier Inc., 360 Park Avenue South, New York, New York 10010-1710 Tel.: 212-633-3874; Fax: 212-633-3820, E-mail: reprints@elsevier.com.

Child and Adolescent Psychiatric Clinics of North America is covered in *MEDLINE/PubMed (Index Medicus), ISI, SSCI, Research Alert, Social Search, Current Contents,* and *EMBASE/Excerpta Medica.*

Contributors

CONSULTING EDITOR

JUSTINE LARSON, MD, MPH, DFAACAP
Medical Director, Schools and Residential Treatment, Consulting Editor, Child and
Adolescent Psychiatric Clinics of North America, Sheppard Pratt, Rockville, Maryland,
USA

EDITORS

JEFFREY H. NEWCORN, MD
Professor of Psychiatry and Pediatrics, Director, Division of ADHD, Learning Disabilities,
and Related Disorders, Icahn School of Medicine at Mount Sinai, Director, Pediatric
Psychopharmacology, Mount Sinai Health System, New York, New York, USA

TIMOTHY E. WILENS, MD
Chief, Division of Child and Adolescent Psychiatry, Child Psychiatry Service, Co-Director,
Center for Addiction Medicine, Clinical and Research Program in Pediatric
Psychopharmacology, Massachusetts General Hospital, Professor of Psychiatry, Harvard
Medical School, Boston, Massachusetts, USA

AUTHORS

MIGUEL ÁNGEL ÁLVAREZ-MON, PhD, MD
Psychiatry and Mental Health Department, Hospital U. Infanta Leonor, Department of
Legal Medicine and Psychiatry, Complutense University, Madrid, Spain; Department of
Psychiatry, Cooper Medical School of Rowan University, Camden, New Jersey, USA

LENARD A. ADLER, MD
Professor, Departments of Psychiatry and Child and Adolescent Psychiatry, NYU
Grossman School of Medicine, New York, New York, USA

AVERY B. ALBERT, BA
Clinical Psychology, Syracuse University, Syracuse, New York, USA

DEEPTI ANBARASAN, MD
Associate Professor, Departments of Neurology and Psychiatry, NYU Grossman School of
Medicine, New York, New York, USA

MICHAEL C. ANGELINI, MA, PharmD
Professor, Massachusetts College of Pharmacy and Health Sciences University, Boston,
Massachusetts, USA

RAMAN BAWEJA, MD, MS
Associate Professor, Department of Psychiatry and Behavioral Health and Public Health,
Associate Vice Chair for Faculty Development, Department of Psychiatry and Behavioral
Health, Penn State College of Medicine, Hershey, Pennsylvania, USA

AMY BERGER, BS
Child and Adolescent Psychiatry, Massachusetts General Hospital, Boston, Massachusetts, USA

ANN C. CHILDRESS, MD
Center for Psychiatry and Behavioral Medicine, Inc., Las Vegas, Nevada, USA

BARBARA J. COFFEY, MD, MS
Professor and Chairman, Department of Psychiatry and Behavioral Sciences, Division Chief, Child and Adolescent Psychiatry, Director, Tourette Association Center of Excellence, University of Miami Miller School of Medicine, Miami, Florida, USA

LOURDES M. DELROSSO, MD, PhD
Associate Professor of Pediatrics, University of Washington, Seattle, Washington, USA

RALF W. DITTMANN, MSc, MD, PhD
Pediatric Psychopharmacology, Department of Child and Adolescent Psychiatry, Central Institute of Mental Health, University of Heidelberg, Mannheim, Germany

STEPHEN V. FARAONE, PhD
Departments of Psychiatry and Behavioral Science and Neuroscience and Physiology, SUNY Upstate Medical University, Institute for Human Performance, Syracuse, New York, USA

PAUL HAMMERNESS, MD
Chair, Psychiatry Services, Southcoast Health, New Bedford, Massachusetts, USA

ROBERT J. JAFFE, MD
Training Director, Child and Adolescent Psychiatry Fellowship, Director, Assistant Professor, Departments of Psychiatry and Pediatrics, Icahn School of Medicine at Mount Sinai, New York, New York, USA

GAGAN JOSHI, MD
The Alan and Lorraine Bressler Clinical and Research Program for Autism Spectrum Disorder, Clinical and Research Program in Pediatric Psychopharmacology, Massachusetts General Hospital, Department of Psychiatry, Harvard Medical School, Boston, Massachusetts, USA

NAYLA M. KHOURY, MD
Department of Psychiatry and Behavioral Sciences, Upstate Medical University, Syracuse, New York, USA

BETH KRONE, PhD
Assistant Professor, Department of Psychiatry, Division of ADHD, Learning Disabilities, and Related Disorders, Icahn School of Medicine at Mount Sinai, New York, New York, USA

JOHN S. MARKOWITZ, PharmD
Department of Pharmacotherapy and Translational Research, Center for Pharmacogenomics and Precision Medicine, College of Pharmacy, University of Florida, Gainesville, Florida, USA

PHILIP W. MELCHERT, PharmD
Department of Pharmacotherapy and Translational Research, College of Pharmacy, University of Florida, Gainesville, Florida, USA

FERNANDO MORA, MD, PhD
Psychiatry and Mental Health Department, Hospital U. Infanta Leonor, Department of Legal Medicine and Psychiatry, Complutense University, Madrid, Spain; Department of Psychiatry, Cooper Medical School of Rowan University, Camden, New Jersey, USA

JEFFREY H. NEWCORN, MD
Professor of Psychiatry and Pediatrics, Director, Division of ADHD, Learning Disabilities, and Related Disorders, Icahn School of Medicine at Mount Sinai, Director, Pediatric Psychopharmacology, Mount Sinai Health System, New York, New York, USA

VICTOR PEREIRA-SANCHEZ, MD, PhD
Clinical Assistant Professor, Department of Child and Adolescent Psychiatry, NYU Grossman School of Medicine

STEVEN R. PLISZKA, MD
Dielmann Distinguished Professor and Chair, Department of Psychiatry and Behavioral Sciences, The University of Texas Health Science Center at San Antonio

JAVIER QUINTERO, MD, PhD, HEAD OF SERVICE
Psychiatry and Mental Health Department, Hospital U. Infanta Leonor, Department of Legal Medicine and Psychiatry, Complutense University, Madrid, Spain; Department of Psychiatry, Cooper Medical School of Rowan University, Camden, New Jersey, USA

NEVENA V. RADONJIĆ, MD, PhD
Department of Psychiatry and Behavioral Sciences, Upstate Medical University, Syracuse, New York, USA

BARBARA ROBLES-RAMAMURTHY, MD
Assistant Professor of Psychiatry, Department of Psychiatry and Behavioral Sciences, The University of Texas Health Science Center at San Antonio

ALBERTO RODRíGUEZ-QUIROGA, MD, PhD
Psychiatry and Mental Health Department, Hospital U. Infanta Leonor, Department of Legal Medicine and Psychiatry, Complutense University, Madrid, Spain; Department of Psychiatry, Cooper Medical School of Rowan University, Camden, New Jersey, USA

ANTHONY L. ROSTAIN, MD, MA
Psychiatry and Mental Health Department, Hospital U. Infanta Leonor, Department of Legal Medicine and Psychiatry, Complutense University, Madrid, Spain; Department of Psychiatry, Cooper Medical School of Rowan University, Camden, New Jersey, USA

GABRIELLA SAFYER, MD
Clinical Instructor, Department of Psychiatry, NYU Grossman School of Medicine, New York, New York, USA

MARK A. STEIN, PhD
Professor of Psychiatry and Behavioral Sciences, Pediatrics, University of Washington, Seattle, Washington, USA

DARIA TAUBIN, BA
Clinical Research Coordinator, Pediatric Psychopharmacology Program, Division of Child and Adolescent Psychiatry, Massachusetts General Hospital, Boston, Massachusetts, USA

JAMES G. WAXMONSKY, MD
Professor, Department of Psychiatry and Behavioral Health, University Chair in Child Psychiatry, Penn State University, Division Chief, Child and Adolescent Psychiatry, Penn State College of Medicine, Hershey, Pennsylvania, USA

MARGARET DANIELLE WEISS, MD, PhD
Director of Clinical Research, Department of Child Psychiatry, Cambridge Health Alliance, Cambridge, Massachusetts, USA

TIMOTHY E. WILENS, MD
Chief, Division of Child and Adolescent Psychiatry, Child Psychiatry Service, Co-Director, Center for Addiction Medicine, Clinical and Research Program in Pediatric Psychopharmacology, Massachusetts General Hospital, Professor of Psychiatry, Harvard Medical School, Boston, Massachusetts, USA

JULIA C. WILSON, BA
Clinical Research Intern, Pediatric Psychopharmacology Program, Division of Child and Adolescent Psychiatry, Massachusetts General Hospital, Boston, Massachusetts, USA

COURTNEY ZULAUF-MCCURDY, PhD
Institute of Education Sciences Post-Doctoral Fellow, University of Washington, Seattle, Washington, USA

Contents

> Adult attention-deficit/hyperactivity disorder (ADHD) is an early-onset dis-
> order with many functional impairments and psychiatric comorbidities.
> Although no treatment fully mitigates impairments associated with
> ADHD, effective management is possible with pharmacologic and non-
> pharmacologic treatments. The etiology and pathophysiology of ADHD
> are remarkably complex and the disorder is continuously distributed in
> the population. While these findings have been well documented in studies
> with predominantly white samples, ADHD may affect racial and ethnic mi-
> norities differentially, given diagnostic and treatment disparities. This re-
> view provides an updated overview of the epidemiology, etiology,
> neurobiology, and neuropharmacology of ADHD, addressing racial and
> ethnic disparities whereby data are available.

> Measurement informed care is a cornerstone of evidence-based practice
> and shared decision-making. A structured diagnostic interview specific to
> ADHD provides a globally agreed-on standard of evaluation. These inter-
> views are accessible in the public domain in multiple languages and are
> helpful to clinicians new to the diagnosis of ADHD. Broad-based rating
> scales looking at multiple domains of psychopathology are critical to as-
> suring recognition of comorbid diagnoses, which might otherwise be
> missed, differential diagnoses, and identification of the most prominent
> or treatable diagnosis. Recent innovations in computerized adaptive
> testing have improved the efficiency and accuracy of diagnostic
> screening. Rating scales specific to ADHD and disruptive behavior disor-
> ders establish the severity of the disorder and response to intervention.
> Age- and gender-normed symptom rating scales for ADHD capture clini-
> cally salient differences between what is normative in different demo-
> graphic groups. An evaluation of functional impairment in ADHD has
> been critical to understanding the patient's perspective of the presenting
> problem. Best practice care for ADHD treatment goes beyond improve-
> ment to well-defined standards for both symptom and functional remis-
> sion. Studies of executive function, emotional regulation, mind-
> wandering, and sluggish cognitive tempo have led to a richer understand-
> ing of the breadth and depth of associated deficits commonly experienced
> by ADHD patients. Psychometrically validated tools are available to com-
> plement every aspect of ADHD care and provide global standards for
> research.

Paul Hammerness, Amy Berger, Michael C. Angelini, and Timothy E. Wilens

> The cardiovascular (CV) impact of stimulants has been examined for decades, with investigations ranging from small sample targeted studies of heart rate (HR) and blood pressure (BP), to large scale epidemiologic investigations. The preponderance of evidence is reassuring, albeit generally based on healthy samples using variable methodology, excluding those at theoretic high risk (eg, comorbid cardiac illness). Screening for theoretically vulnerable patients are recommended, as well as monitoring for CV symptoms and BP/HR, with shared inquiry/further evaluation if concerned. Future investigations to support the identification of risk are needed, while attention to stimulant-associated CV risk is an opportunity for clinicians to engage in general CV risk identification and intervention.

Gagan Joshi and Timothy E. Wilens

> Attention-deficit/hyperactivity disorder (ADHD) is the most frequent comorbid disorder that is observed at a higher rate and with greater morbidity in higher intellectually functioning populations with autism. Up to 85% of the populations with autism and 15% of individuals with ADHD suffer from a reciprocal comorbidity that is highly under-recognized in intellectually capable populations. Limited empirical evidence is available on the response of anti-ADHD agents in autism populations with ADHD. In autism spectrum disorder (ASD) populations, response to methylphenidate for the treatment of hyperactivity is worse than typically expected in the presence of the intellectual disability. The anti-ADHD response to atomoxetine in autism populations is worse than typically expected although tolerability is similar to that observed in the typicals. The hyperactivity response to guanfacine treatment in predominantly intellectually impaired populations with ASD is as robust as observed in the typicals although tolerability was worse than typically expected. Further trials are warranted to document the extent of atypical anti-ADHD response in intellectually capable populations with autism.

Robert J. Jaffe and Barbara J. Coffey

> A complete and comprehensive medical and psychiatric evaluation is necessary to delineate tic symptoms from attention-deficit/hyperactivity disorder, and to prioritize the most problematic symptoms for intervention. Stimulants are the recommended first-line pharmacotherapy to treat attention-deficit/hyperactivity disorder symptoms in patients with tic disorders. Comprehensive behavioral intervention for tics is an effective behavioral therapy that is generally considered the first-line treatment of persistent tic disorders. α-Agonists can be added to stimulants if tics increase or be used as monotherapy to target attention-deficit/hyperactivity disorder and tics. Atomoxetine is also an excellent option to treat attention-deficit/hyperactivity disorder and tics.

social relations). This stage is especially difficult for adolescents suffering from attention deficit hyperactivity disorder (ADHD), who have to move on from child and adolescent mental health services to adult mental health services. This review analyzes developmental and environmental risk and protective factors as well as critical variables such as executive functioning and self-monitoring that influence the course of ADHD in transitional age youth and guide the priorities for an optimal transition of care. The influence of the COVID-19 pandemic is also discussed. We reflect on the unmet needs for an optimal transition of care and propose practice and policy recommendations to achieve this goal.

Attention-deficit/hyperactivity disorder (ADHD) significantly worsens quality of life and long-term functional outcomes in adults. Individual impairments in adults with ADHD can be further contextualized within considerable costs to society at large. Food and Drug Administration (FDA) approved stimulants and nonstimulant medications can significantly improve ADHD symptoms in adults. In the past 2 decades, the United States FDA has expanded approval of pharmacotherapeutic options for adult ADHD. However, limitations still persist in available psychotropics for certain patient populations such as those with comorbid substance use or cardiovascular illness. Clinicians therefore must appreciate several ongoing investigations into medications with unique mechanisms of action. This article reviews the current FDA approved and emerging medication options while providing guidelines for pharmacologic management of adult ADHD.

Clinical practice guidelines (CPGs) are systematically developed statements to assist practitioner and patient decisions about appropriate health care for specific clinical circumstances. CPGs have evolved during the last 2 decades from general consensus statements by prominent practitioners in the field to highly structured instruments. The Institute of Medicine has laid out specific standards for selecting the experts who develop a CPG and the process by which CPGs are developed. Attention-deficit/hyperactivity disorder (ADHD) has been the focus of more than 20 CPGs created by governments and professional societies, both in the United States and internationally. There is a good deal of consensus across these CPGs regarding the principles of the diagnosis and treatment of ADHD. Drawing on the rich research base in ADHD, all CPGs emphasize the need for screening, a diagnosis based on history and standardized rating scales, as well as the use of evidence-based psychosocial and pharmacologic treatments. They vary in terms of their emphasis on the role of psychosocial treatment and the degree to which they address comorbid disorders in ADHD. Although limited research has shown ADHG CPGs do change provider practice, there is no research examining if the changes in practice brought about by CPGs impact patient outcomes.

CHILD AND ADOLESCENT PSYCHIATRIC CLINICS

SERIES OF RELATED INTEREST
Psychiatric Clinics of North America
https://www.psych.theclinics.com/
Pediatric Clinics of North America
https://www.pediatric.theclinics.com/

AACAP Members: Please go to www.jaacap.org for information on access to the Child and Adolescent Psychiatric Clinics. *Resident* Members of AACAP: Special access information is available at www.childpsych.theclinics.com.

THE CLINICS ARE AVAILABLE ONLINE!
Access your subscription at:
www.theclinics.com

Preface

So What Really Is New in the Pharmacotherapy of Attention-Deficit/Hyperactivity Disorder?

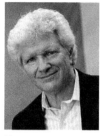
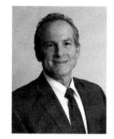

Jeffrey H. Newcorn, MD   Timothy E. Wilens, MD
Editors

Over the past three decades, there have been tremendous efforts to better understand the cause or causes, course, comorbid presentations, and treatment of attention-deficit/hyperactivity disorder (ADHD) across the lifespan. ADHD remains one of the most common neurobehavioral disorders presenting for treatment in childhood, with estimates demonstrating a prevalence in children and adolescents of 6% to 9%. Data derived from cross-cultural studies also show a similar prevalence of ADHD throughout the world, with moderate to severe impairments in academic and/or occupational outcomes, interpersonal functioning, and self-esteem. Risks for physical injuries, motor vehicle accidents, and even premature death from a variety of causes are also elevated. Moreover, there are higher rates of numerous Axis I and Axis II psychiatric disorders across the lifespan (for the most current evidence-based international perspective, see Faraone and colleagues[1]).

Recent research in large registry and insurance data sets highlights the amelioration of many of the symptomatic and functional outcomes seen in ADHD with pharmacologic treatment (not only pharmacologic treatment, of course, but that is the focus of this issue). Hence, there is a great need for practitioners, researchers, and public health officials to understand the contemporary literature on pharmacologic treatment of ADHD.

This issue of the *Child and Adolescent Psychiatric Clinics of North America*, "Updates in the Pharmacologic Strategies of ADHD," presents the most current information on existing and new medication treatments for ADHD and how to best use them. Detailed descriptions by many of the investigators who have conceptualized and completed the cited research are provided for both the stimulant and the nonstimulant classes of medication. Recent work on the pharmacokinetics,

Child Adolesc Psychiatric Clin N Am 31 (2022) xiii–xiv
https://doi.org/10.1016/j.chc.2022.03.011
1056-4993/22/© 2022 Published by Elsevier Inc.

childpsych.theclinics.com

pharmacogenomics, and safety considerations of medications used in ADHD has been highlighted throughout. Since many special groups of individuals are affected by ADHD, an emphasis has been made to highlight the diagnosis and treatment of these complex presentations. Cooccurring autism, mood/anxiety, tics/Tourette, sleep, and substance use disorders each have dedicated sections discussing the most current diagnostic and treatment considerations. While the majority of the articles focus on the pediatric age group, we highlight the importance of considering a lifespan perspective. Consequently, evaluation and treatment of adults are also covered. Finally, to aid practitioners in the clinical care of individuals with ADHD, sections addressing both clinical guidelines and measurement instruments that can be used to track ADHD symptoms and functional status and to monitor the progress of treatment over time are included.

We sincerely hope that you will find "Updates in the Pharmacologic Strategies of ADHD" to be a comprehensive and up-to-date text on ADHD, that is both intellectually stimulating and clinically pragmatic and relevant. We believe that the research data, clinical vignettes, treatment recommendations, and algorithms presented herein will provide empirically based information, written by world experts, that is directly applicable to your daily clinical care of patients with ADHD. We trust that you will have as much satisfaction reading this "Update" as we did in inviting, contributing to, and editing this collective work.

Jeffrey H. Newcorn, MD
Division of ADHD and Learning Disorders
Icahn School of Medicine at Mount Sinai
Pediatric Psychopharmacology
Mount Sinai Health System
New York, NY 10029, USA

Timothy E. Wilens, MD
Division of Child and Adolescent Psychiatry
Center for Addiction Medicine
Massachusetts General Hospital
Harvard Medical School
Boston, MA 02114, USA

E-mail addresses:
jeffrey.newcorn@mssm.edu (J.H. Newcorn)
TWILENS@mgh.harvard.edu (T.E. Wilens)

REFERENCE

1.. Faraone, et al. The World Federation of ADHD International Consensus Statement: 208 Evidence-based conclusions about the disorder. Neurosci Biobehav Rev 2021 Sep;128:789–818. https://doi.org/10.1016/j.neubiorev.2021.01.022.

From Structural Disparities to Neuropharmacology

A Review of Adult Attention-Deficit/Hyperactivity Disorder Medication Treatment

Nayla M. Khoury, MD[a], Nevena V. Radonjić, MD, PhD[a], Avery B. Albert, B.A.[b], Stephen V. Faraone, PhD[c,d],*

KEYWORDS

- ADHD epidemiology • ADHD racial and ethnic disparities
- ADHD etiology and neurobiology

KEY POINTS

- Despite great strides in understanding adult attention-deficit/hyperactivity disorder (ADHD) and neurobiology, there is much to learn regarding disparities with regard to diagnosis, treatment, and outcome based on structural, socioeconomic, and cultural factors.
- Given continuous distribution in the population, viewing ADHD on a continuum may increase our understanding of how ADHD symptoms may be adaptive up to a certain point and highlights the contextual specificity of when symptoms are relevant.
- While consensus holds that medication effectiveness does not differ based on race and ethnicity, there is a multitude of reasons why minority youth may be less likely to receive the diagnosis and appropriate treatment.
- Reducing disparities in ADHD diagnosis and treatment may benefit from increasing psychoeducational assessment access, policies to improve mental health care access, anti-bias and cultural sensitivity training, psychoeducation regarding medications, and a focus on maternal mental health for prevention.

[a] Department of Psychiatry and Behavioral Sciences, Upstate Medical University, Syracuse, NY, USA; [b] Clinical Psychology, Syracuse University, Syracuse, NY, USA; [c] Department of Psychiatry and Behavioral Science, SUNY Upstate Medical University, Institute for Human Performance, Room 3707, 505 Irving Avenue, Syracuse, NY 13210, USA; [d] Department of Neuroscience and Physiology, SUNY Upstate Medical University, Institute for Human Performance, Room 3707, 505 Irving Avenue, Syracuse, NY 13210, USA
* Corresponding author. Department of Psychiatry and Behavioral Science, SUNY Upstate Medical University, Institute for Human Performance, Room 3707, 505 Irving Avenue, Syracuse, NY 13210.
E-mail address: sfaraone@childpsychresearch.org

Child Adolesc Psychiatric Clin N Am 31 (2022) 343–361
https://doi.org/10.1016/j.chc.2022.03.002
1056-4993/22/© 2022 Elsevier Inc. All rights reserved.

EPIDEMIOLOGY

Adult attention-deficit/hyperactivity disorder (ADHD) is a common disorder with a prevalence estimate of 5.9% and a 2 to 1 ratio of affected boys to girls.[1] ADHD prevalence has not been found to differ across cultures[2] and the prevalence rate has remained stable over the past 3 decades.[2] Although ADHD as a disorder is a binary concept, population data consistently show that the symptoms of ADHD occur as traits in the population with no clear demarcation separating those with and without the disorder.[3] Epidemiologic and clinical studies indicate that ADHD frequently co-occurs with disruptive behavior, mood, anxiety and substance use disorders.[4,5]

Some patients with ADHD improve symptomatically with increasing age and prefrontal cortex development; however, two-thirds have persistent symptoms and significant functional impairments well into adulthood.[6,7] These impairments include increased risk of premature death and suicide, substance abuse, incarceration, academic and vocational challenges and difficulties with peers.[8] Risk factors for symptom persistence include the severity of childhood ADHD symptoms, parental mental health disorder, and environmental factors such as toxicants, nutrient deficiencies, perinatal events, stress and social determinants of health.[9-13] Protective factors include the utilization of ADHD support services, improved executive function skills and reduced depressive symptoms.[14] According to a meta-analysis of population studies, the prevalence of ADHD in adults is estimated to be 2.8%,[15] while the prevalence in adults over 50 ranges between 0.2% and 1.5%.[16]

There is limited epidemiologic research examining ADHD in racial and ethnic minority populations. However, racial and ethnic disparities in ADHD diagnosis and treatment have been documented. Several studies with nationally representative samples report lower rates of diagnosis and treatment of ADHD among African American and Latinx youth compared with white youth.[17-19] This disparity persists even among children displaying significant ADHD symptoms, per parent and teacher reports.[17] Racial and ethnic disparities have been documented outside of the US as well, with lower rates of ADHD diagnosis and treatment reported in European studies comparing immigrant and nonimmigrant youth, and in studies of minority youth in Israel.[20] However, recent studies, one using a nationally representative US sample and one conducting a metanalysis of samples from the US and other black minority countries, have suggested that the racial gap in ADHD diagnosis may be shrinking, or even that black youth are now at greater risk of receiving an ADHD diagnosis.[21-23] Despite mixed findings, this research highlights the need for more culturally responsive assessment and treatment of ADHD for racial/ethnic minority populations.

Other factors shown to differentially impact ADHD diagnosis include gender, economics, family status, non-English language in the home, and neighborhood safety. Females are less likely to be diagnosed than their male peers, in part because inattentive symptoms, which are often more prominent in female presentations of ADHD, are not as disruptive to others as the hyperactive and impulsive symptoms more common to male presentations of the disorder. Thus, ADHD symptoms in females may be overlooked or mistaken for anxiety or depression.[24,25] Diagnostic uncertainty also exists in the case of children exposed to abuse and neglect, given the potential for overlapping symptoms and associated risks. For example, an American population-based study found an increased risk of inattentive-type ADHD in children exposed to sexual abuse and neglect, when controlling for other factors.[26] Socioeconomic status (SES) also contributes to risk, given the known association between family income and risk of ADHD, as well as low social class, Rutter's indicator of adversity, and paternal criminality, maternal mental disorder, and severe marital discord.[8] Although the mechanisms may be complex, SES and related factors are important environmental risk factors for ADHD.[27–29]

Factors affecting ADHD helpseeking and diagnosis include social and structural determinants of health, and cultural differences which might delay diagnosis and treatment.[30–32] A recent review of socio-cultural factors contributing to diagnostic and treatment disparities identified the following: differential problem identification and knowledge about ADHD, fear of stigmatization, access to mental health services, shortage of culturally appropriate services, inaccurate diagnosis, and treatment adherence.[20] The persistence of racial and ethnic disparities even when controlling for SES and other access-based barriers suggests a need to increase assessment and monitoring among minority youth.

ETIOLOGY

ADHD is most commonly caused by the cumulative effects of many genetic and environmental risks, each of which usually exerts a small individual effect. Exceptions include specific rare genetic abnormalities associated with ADHD, such as Turner syndrome, Fragile X, or Tuberous Sclerosis[33]; additionally, extreme environmental deprivation[34] and traumatic brain injury early in life[35,36] have been documented as sufficient causes of ADHD.

Environmental risk factors

Many environmental events have been found to increase the risk for ADHD or ADHD symptoms. As reviewed by Faraone and colleagues,[37] the strongest evidence is for:

- Exposure during the fetal period to maternal smoking, acetaminophen, valproate, maternal hypertension, high maternal phthalate levels, maternal obesity, maternal thyroid dysfunction, prior maternal miscarriage, maternal grief, and complications of pregnancy and delivery.
- Exposure during childhood to out of home care, poverty, sexual abuse, physical neglect, death in the family, low family cohesion, absence of community supports, enterovirus infection, lead, cigarette smoke, food dyes, organophosphate pesticides, nitrogen dioxide, sulfur dioxide, particulate matter, and perfluoroalkyl substances.

Genetic risk factors

A review of 37 twin studies from the United States, Europe, Scandinavia, and Australia shows that ADHD is highly heritable (76%), indicating that genes and gene–environment interaction play a substantial role in causing ADHD.[33] The heritability of the disorder is similar in children and adults but both twin and molecular genetic data suggest that different genomic loci may account for onset and persistence of the disorder.[38–40]

Twin studies show a strong genetic link between extreme and subthreshold ADHD symptoms.[41] This suggests that ADHD is the extreme expression of a continuous distribution of symptoms in the population and that the genetic factors that cause ADHD also account for the full range of symptoms in the population. Through development, genetic risk influences both stable and dynamic processes.[42,43] The stable component comprises genomic loci common to persistent ADHD and its pediatric form. The dynamic component suggests that the set of genetic variants accounting for the onset of ADHD differs from those accounting for the persistence and remission of the disorder.

Family studies and subsequent twin studies confirm that ADHD may share genetic risks with disruptive behavior, anxiety, mood, and substance use disorders[33,44–46]. These studies also support spectrum-specific genetic factors, such as genetic factors that load specifically on externalizing disorders.[47]

One of the key breakthroughs for the genetics of ADHD was the completion of a genome-wide association study (GWAS) comprising 20,183 people with ADHD and 35,191 controls. Twelve loci achieved genome-wide significance, which means they could be unequivocally declared as playing a role in causing ADHD. The GWAS analyses also showed that about one-third of ADHD's heritability is due to the polygenic effects of many common variants, each having very small effects. These small effects suggest that thousands or even tens of thousands of genomic loci may be involved in the disorder. These loci also contribute to the expression of the full range of ADHD symptoms in the population. Moreover, part of the polygenic risk for ADHD is shared with other disorders.[48,49]

PATHOPHYSIOLOGY

Multiple brain regions and networks are implicated in the pathophysiology of ADHD by neuropsychology and neuroimaging studies. Neuropsychology studies show that people with ADHD are at increased risk of having cognitive deficits in at least one of several domains, although it is unclear whether the deficits themselves cause ADHD or reflect pleiotropic outcomes of risk factors. The domains implicated in ADHD include visuospatial processing, verbal working memory, inhibitory control, vigilance, temporal processing, emotional regulation, and planning. Reward processing is frequently dysregulated in ADHD, such that individuals with ADHD tend to prefer immediate rather than delayed rewards or overestimate the magnitude of proximal versus distal rewards.[6] Deficient reward processing likely explains why youth with ADHD are at high risk for substance use disorders.

Cortical regions of the brain affected include those linked to working memory (dorsolateral prefrontal cortex), complex decision making and strategic planning (ventromedial prefrontal cortex), and orientation of attention (parietal cortex). The brain changes associated with ADHD are small and not useful for diagnosis. They do, however, implicate regions of the brain responsible for regulating attention, behavior, and executive functions and are consistent with the symptoms of ADHD.

Structural and functional brain imaging of individuals with ADHD demonstrate altered brain networks compared with those without ADHD. Orbito-temporal-occipital networks related to inattentive symptoms and frontal–amygdala–occipital networks related to hyperactive/impulsivity networks are altered compared with healthy controls on functional imaging.[50]

Brain imaging studies implicate under-activation of areas of the brain which mediate goal-directed executive function, such as in frontostriatal and frontoparietal networks. Additionally, individuals with ADHD demonstrate an over-active default mode network (DMN) which requires an increased threshold to de-activate during specific tasks and stimuli; stimulant medications have been shown in small studies to normalize this threshold.[51–53]

Brain maturation delay is implicated as a potential mechanism for ADHD, given delayed peaks of subcortical maturation in patients with ADHD. Mega and meta-analysis of structural magnetic resonance imaging (MRI) demonstrate small volume differences in intracranial and subcortical structures that vary with age. While differences in basal ganglia, amygdala, and hippocampus volume were found in children, only hippocampus volume differed for adolescents, and no volume differences were found for adults.[54] Decreased total cortical surface area and decreased cortical thickness in specific parts of the brain have also been observed in children with ADHD compared with control children, most prominently in young children (under 9 years of age) and are no longer significant in adolescents and adults.[55]

However, developmental catch-up is not universal and significant differences in structure and connectivity remain for many adults with ADHD. Smaller basal ganglia volumes and reduced dorsal surface area in adolescents with ADHD persisted in longitudinal MRI studies. Cortical thinning in specific brain regions implicated in executive function persists as well as cortical thickening in other brain regions. Meta-analysis of imaging data from ADHD individuals across all age groups demonstrates altered white matter integrity in the striatum, frontal, temporal, and parietal lobes.

Multiple neurotransmitter pathways have been implicated in the etiology and pathophysiology of ADHD. These affect brain structures mediating executive function, working memory, emotion regulation, and reward processing.[6] The dopamine system, involved in the planning and initiation of motor response, activation, switching, reaction to novelty, and processing of reward, has been implicated in the neurobiology of ADHD via its pharmacologic treatment. A positron emission tomography (PET) study of young males with ADHD reported dysfunctional dopamine (DA) metabolism in the putamen, amygdala, and dorsal midbrain relative to healthy controls, regardless of treatment status. Among treatment-naive adolescents with ADHD, dopamine transporter (DAT) density was found to have an inverse relationship with blood flow to areas of the brain involved in modulating attention, such as the cingulate cortex, frontal and temporal lobes, and cerebellum.[56] Additionally, observed changes exist in noradrenergic (NE) system as well as glutamatergic (GLU), serotoninergic (5-HT), cholinergic (ACH), and opioid systems.

More recent data have implicated mitochondrial dysfunction in the pathophysiology of ADHD; for example, Chang and colleagues demonstrated an increased risk of ADHD with mitochondrial DNA (mtDNA) haplogroups.[57] in European Americans. Similarly, in Turkey, an association was found between mtDNA copy number and ADHD such that children with ADHD had 1.3-times higher mtDNA copy number than children without ADHD.[58] As the major source of reactive oxygen species, mitochondrial dysfunction has been linked to neurodegenerative disorders. Some evidence suggesting a role for inflammation in the pathogenesis of ADHD is consistent with a meta-analysis finding elevated levels of oxidative stress in patients diagnosed with ADHD.[59] Oxidative stress has also been implicated in the lower brain volumes seen in patients with ADHD.[60] Correlations between mitochondria-associated proteins and ADHD were found among girls with ADHD but not boys in Taiwan, suggesting a potential gender-specific mitochondrial pathway involved in the pathophysiology of ADHD.[61]

NEUROPHARMACOLOGY

Pharmacologic treatments for ADHD mimic or enhance the beneficial effects of DA and NE on the prefrontal cortex (PFC).[56,62,63] Available FDA-approved pharmacologic treatments are classified into stimulants (amphetamine (AMP) and methylphenidate (MPH)) and nonstimulants (atomoxetine, extended-release viloxazine, extended-release clonidine, and extended-release guanfacine). Omega 3 fatty acid supplementation is the only well-studied nutrient treatment. We do not discuss other nonpharmacologic treatments as they have no known implications for pathophysiology. Less is known about nonapproved traditional alternative treatments such as acupuncture,[64] yoga,[65,66] and mindfulness therapies.[67,68]

Stimulants

Stimulants are the first-line treatment of ADHD in professional guidelines, except for preschool children for whom a trial of family behavior therapy is recommended.[69,70] Although stimulants are safe and used in preschool children with severe ADHD symptoms,[71–75] they are less effective and have increased side effects in children under 5 years of age. Meta-analysis of their efficacy/tolerability tradeoff suggests that methylphenidate is the best first choice for youth, but amphetamine is a better first choice for adults assuming that it is consistent with patient or parent preferences[28,76,77]. Insomnia and weight loss are side effects more common among individuals treated with AMP compared with MPH. Nevertheless, adverse effects found in both classes of stimulants include reduced total sleep time, delayed onset sleep, and decreased sleep efficiency.[78–80] Abdominal pain, decreased appetite and growth are also common side effects that require monitoring.[81]

In addition to reducing symptoms of ADHD, meta-analyses report that stimulants modestly reduce symptoms of emotional dysregulation,[82] which are common in ADHD.[83] They also have modest effects in reducing anxiety,[84] aggression, oppositional behavior, and conduct problems.[85,86] Naturalistic studies in very large samples suggest that stimulant treatment reduces accidental injuries, traumatic brain injury, substance abuse, cigarette smoking, educational underachievement, bone fractures, sexually transmitted infections, depression, suicide, criminal activity, and teenage pregnancy. For reviews please see the following references.[6,87,88]

There has been limited research and mixed evidence regarding differences in ADHD treatment outcomes by race and ethnicity. An older study found that a sample of African American patients with ADHD who were homozygous for the 10-repeat allele of the dopamine transporter gene was nonresponsive to methylphenidate; however, the study was limited due to the lack of a white comparison group.[89] The more recent consensus is that stimulants work equally well regardless of race and ethnicity. The Multimodal Treatment of ADHD (MTA) study found no significant difference in medication treatment outcome by ethnicity after controlling for public assistance. Compared with nonminority youth, ethnic minority youth responded more favorably when MPH treatment was supplemented by behavioral therapy, and treatment × ethnicity interactions were noted for comorbidities such as oppositional defiant disorder (ODD) and anxiety. However, after controlling for public assistance, these findings became nonsignificant, suggesting that SES influences which families are more likely to benefit from combined treatment regardless of ethnicity. A more recent study [90] did not find a correlation between ethnic differences and ADHD treatment benefits as measured by parent and child behavior.[90] Moreover, parent training for ADHD in a study using the Incredible Years program had nonsignificant differences across ethno-racial groups.[20,91]

Multiple factors affect treatment disparities for racial and ethnic minorities. Among these, diagnostic disparities are especially relevant for clinicians. For example, Blum's ethnography shows that, compared with white youth, boys and young men of color are more likely to be referred to special education and less likely to be treated with stimulant medication. A recent review reports that the odds of taking a medication for ADHD in African American children compared with white children range from 0.35 to 0.65, with lower treatment adherence and higher rates of discontinuation for African American children.[92] Other factors include increased likelihood of nonmedical explanatory models for ADHD-like behaviors among African American caregivers and differences in willingness to consider medication treatment. ADHD diagnosis and medications are also sometimes seen as a form of social control among African

American caregivers, which makes sense given a documented history of over-pathologizing African American behaviors in ways that promoted racist policies and practices.[92]

Additionally, race and ethnicity may influence medication titration and ADHD symptom ratings by parents and teachers. In the MTA study, parents of Hispanic children reported less improvement after treatment than white and African American parents and this affected titration dose with Hispanic children titrated to lower doses of medication than non-Hispanic children by study completion. This difference by race-ethnicity was not seen in teacher ratings for Hispanic children but was seen in African American children compared with white children, with a bias toward reporting increased symptoms of ADHD and conduct disorder for African American children.[20] Other studies, similarly, have found teachers to rate black children as displaying greater ADHD symptoms and externalizing behaviors compared with white children. Negative racial attitudes among teachers were found to contribute to these higher symptom ratings for black children, suggesting racial biases may interfere with a valid assessment of ADHD in racial and ethnic minority youth.[93,94]

DISCUSSION

Decades of epidemiologic, clinical, and basic research have taught us much about ADHD. This early-onset disorder frequently persists and augurs many functional impairments and psychiatric comorbidities. Although we have no treatment that fully mitigates impairments associated with ADHD, its symptoms and impairments can be managed very effectively with pharmacologic and nonpharmacologic treatments. The etiology and pathophysiology of ADHD are remarkably complex. Many genetic and environmental risk factors, each with a small effect, combine to cause small changes in the brain which are believed to mediate the symptoms of the disorder. ADHD and its genetic risk are continuously distributed in the population. While these findings have been well-documented in studies with predominantly white samples, ADHD may affect racial and ethnic minorities differentially, given diagnostic and treatment disparities. This is an especially vexing issue for genetic studies whereby it has been well documented that genetic prediction models created using data from white samples do not generalize well to other ancestry groups.[95–98] More studies are needed on the epidemiology, etiology, pathophysiology, neuropharmacology, and treatment effectiveness in minority populations.

Existing data about the etiology and pathophysiology of ADHD have implications for clinical practice. Because many of the environmental causes of ADHD are exposures during fetal development, improved care for pregnant women is essential, especially for those living in poverty. **Fig. 1** depicts maternal factors that increase the risk for ADHD in offspring. Maternal adverse childhood experiences and early life pregnancies significantly increase the risk for ADHD, as do peripartum mental health stress and challenged interactions of the dyad. Upstream social and structural efforts to buffer the effects of adverse childhood experiences, including poverty, and prevent unwanted or unplanned pregnancies in young teens are needed.

Indeed, the impact of maternal mental health on the risk of ADHD symptoms in offspring is an area that requires greater focus given the potential for prevention efforts. Stress,[99–101] death in family,[102] depression,[103] use of antidepressants[104] and anxiety[105,106] during pregnancy all increase risk of ADHD. Additionally, children of mothers who are experiencing depression and anxiety in the postnatal period demonstrate increased ADHD symptoms.[107–111] Proposed pathways for how maternal postnatal depression impacts psychosocial adjustment of the child include shared genetic

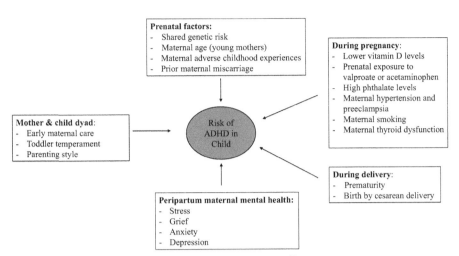

Prenatal factors:
- Shared genetic risk
- Maternal age (young mothers)
- Maternal adverse childhood experiences
- Prior maternal miscarriage

During pregnancy:
- Lower vitamin D levels
- Prenatal exposure to valproate or acetaminophen
- High phthalate levels
- Maternal hypertension and preeclampsia
- Maternal smoking
- Maternal thyroid dysfunction

Mother & child dyad:
- Early maternal care
- Toddler temperament
- Parenting style

Risk of ADHD in Child

During delivery:
- Prematurity
- Birth by cesarean delivery

Peripartum maternal mental health:
- Stress
- Grief
- Anxiety
- Depression

Fig. 1. Maternal factors increasing the risk of ADHD in offspring.

risk, parenting, and stressful environmental context, with parenting being the domain we can clinically impact the most.[112] This further justifies the need for combined behavioral treatments (eg, behavioral parent training). The negative impact of adverse parenting behaviors such as corporal punishment highlights the importance of working with families to improve outcomes, particularly in families with parental ADHD[113] or other comorbidities.

The limited data on treatment outcomes by race and ethnicity underscore the critical role poverty plays in affecting outcomes. While stimulants alone are highly effective, vulnerable communities may benefit from combined behavioral treatments that offer critical support to parents. Discrepancies in access to mental health services and the disproportionate number of minority youth with ADHD sent to correctional facilities mean tragically that youth who could benefit the most from combined treatments often do not receive the most effective treatment.

Fig. 2 highlights some of the known disparities in ADHD diagnosis and treatment of racial and ethnic minorities and includes areas of ongoing and potential future research. Although consensus holds that medication effectiveness does not differ based on race and ethnicity, there are a multitude of reasons why minority youth may be less likely to receive appropriate diagnoses and treatment. Some issues include bias and differential ratings of clinicians, teachers, and caregivers, as well as differential caregiver knowledge and beliefs regarding ADHD.

Additionally, increased rates of comorbid diagnosis in racial and ethnic minorities can complicate the clinical assessment of ADHD and contribute to treatment disparities. For example, higher rates of comorbid anxiety and trauma-related disorders among racial and ethnic minorities may make clinicians hesitant to offer first-line treatment of ADHD, given concerns for worsening comorbid symptoms. Moreover, overlapping symptoms of anxiety and ADHD can complicate the assessment of ADHD, which may delay diagnosis and treatment.

Suggestions for reducing disparities include (1) increasing access to psychoeducational assessments, which can aid with ADHD diagnosis, (2) improving policies that impact access to mental health care, (3) mandating antibias training for health care providers and educators to reduce differential ratings and treatment approaches, and (4) increasing research into the complicated relationship between trauma/anxiety

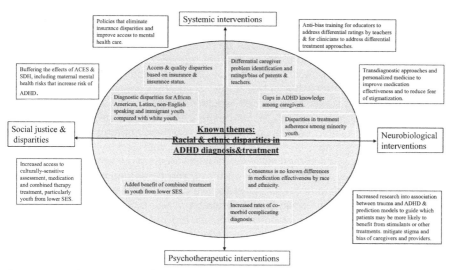

Fig. 2. Areas of ongoing and future research.

and ADHD to help target which individuals may benefit from stimulants and which may not. Current evidence suggests a reciprocal relationship whereby those with trauma histories may be at increased risk of ADHD and those with ADHD may be at increased risk of experiencing trauma.[114,115] In addition, more efforts are needed to increase access to culturally responsive care among racial and ethnic minority communities. Increased psychoeducation regarding the relative safety of stimulant medication, even among individuals with anxiety, may be beneficial for practitioners working with minority populations. Cultural adaptations of behavioral treatment of ADHD (eg, behavioral parent training) may help increase treatment acceptability and adherence among racial and ethnic minority families.[116]

Ideally, neuroscience studies would lead to new targets for pharmacologic treatment or prediction models that could be used for personalized medicine. While that hope remains, much more work is needed to achieve this goal. Currently, no neuropsychological, neuroimaging, or genomic test is useful for diagnosing or ruling out ADHD although, for some cases, neuropsychological testing can be used for planning remediation and for optimizing cognitive behavior therapy.

Neuropsychological models provide some guidance as to what treatment targets may be most effective for treating ADHD. In addition, these models provide useful heuristics that can help clinicians formulate treatment plans for patients with ADHD. Barkley's theory[117,118] assumes that the symptoms of ADHD derive from a core deficit in self-regulation. He posits that our executive functions evolved to shift the control of behavior from external circumstances, such as immediate rewards and punishments, to internal representations of future outcomes. When a biological vulnerability or external stressors prevent these internal representations from guiding our emotions, behaviors, and cognitions, the symptoms of ADHD emerge. This model suggests that external social and emotional scaffolding, as described by Faraone and Biederman,[119] can delay the onset of ADHD and mitigate its symptoms.

For clinicians, this theory has important implications for improving external social and emotional scaffolding as it relates to training with parents and support within the school setting. More recent approaches to adopt universal social-emotional curriculums in schools may be particularly beneficial for youth at risk for ADHD. Parenting programs may also help parents improve their own organization and regulation and learn how to adapt parenting behaviors for youth with ADHD. As child development progresses, the social and emotional supports provided by parents diminish, which challenges the child's executive functions to exchange parent-regulation with self-regulation. Additionally, while the symptoms of ADHD may be effectively addressed with medication, deficits may require either behavior therapy (for children) or cognitive behavior therapy (for adolescents and adults) to teach self-regulation skills.

Sonuga-Barke's triple pathway model posits that temporal processing, inhibitory control, and delay-related deficits combine to cause the symptoms of ADHD.[120] His work provides 3 treatment targets and is consistent with Barkley's theory as each target can be seen as a self-regulatory mechanism. Much of our behavior is regulated by our knowledge of whereby we are on the space-time continuum. If we cannot localize ourselves in time or predict whereby we will be in the future, self-regulation collapses. Inhibition is an obvious self-regulator. When patients with ADHD fail to "apply the brakes," attention wanders, impulses are not controlled and activity becomes excessive. Sonuga-Barke's "delay-related" deficits refer to the dysregulation of reward mechanisms and motivation experienced by many people with ADHD. Treatment development targeting poor self-regulation of reward and motivation will likely lead to better therapies.

Genomic studies are beginning to point to biological pathways that may eventually yield useful pharmacologic targets for ADHD. Recent studies on mitochondrial dysfunction, oxidative stress, and the significant, albeit small, efficacy of omega-3 fatty acid treatment suggests that additional searches for treatment targets in the area of oxidative stress and inflammation might be successful. Perhaps the most important contribution of genomic studies, however, is the confirmation that genetic vulnerability to ADHD is a continuous trait in the population that is partly shared with other disorders.

The continuous nature of ADHD suggests we reconceptualize the use of diagnostic thresholds. Currently, children can achieve the symptom threshold for ADHD with only 6 inattentive symptoms or 6 hyperactive-impulsive symptoms. A child with 5 symptoms from each class, that is, a total of 10 symptoms, does not meet the symptom criterion. *Prima facie*, that does not make sense. We now know that current thresholds are not consistent with the disorder's genomic vulnerability and or the epidemiology of symptoms in the population. It seems that the diagnosis of ADHD should be seen in the same light as we view hypertension and obesity. These traits vary in the population and a threshold is applied to maximize outcomes for those at the high end of the continuum. Social and structural determinants of health affect diagnosis, treatment, and outcome of ADHD, as they do other chronic diseases. The spectrum view of ADHD may decrease the stigma of the disorder, which in itself would significantly reduce ADHD disparities. This aligns with newer transdiagnostic perspectives on psychiatric disorders. Additionally, viewing ADHD on a continuum may increase our understanding of how ADHD symptoms can be adaptive up to a certain point and highlight the contextual specificity of when symptoms are relevant and for whom.

The science and practice of ADHD have made great strides since Wiekard and Crichton first described the syndrome in the 18th century. Yet, despite many breakthroughs in diagnosis, treatment, and neurobiology we still have much more to learn to completely understand etiology and pathophysiology and find treatments that can fully mitigate impairments associated with ADHD. We also have much work to do to better delineate and address disparities in diagnosis, treatment and outcome based on structural, socioeconomic, and cultural factors.

CLINICS CARE POINTS

- To improve functional impairment for individuals with ADHD, ADHD support services, family and social supports and reduction in ADHD severity with evidence-based treatments are critical.

- To improve ADHD prevention efforts, attention should be given to programs that can improve external social and emotional scaffolding for youth and their parents, such as parenting programs, school-based curriculums as well as improved care for pregnant women and maternal mental health.

- To reduce disparities in ADHD diagnosis and treatment, increase access to mental health services, psychoeducational assessments, antibias training, and increase research in racial and ethnic minority populations are needed.

- Attention-deficit/hyperactivity disorder (ADHD) is a neurodevelopmental disorder characterized by inattention, hyperactivity, and impulsivity that onsets in childhood. The syndrome we call ADHD today was first described in medical textbooks published in Germany in 1775 and Scotland in 1798. Thus, ADHD has been with us for a long time. For an overview of its history see.[6] This review provides an updated overview of the epidemiology, etiology, neurobiology, and neuropharmacology of ADHD, addressing racial and ethnic disparities whereby data are available. It adds to prior reviews of these topics by integrating more recent studies on mitochondrial dysfunction and newer medications. We end with a discussion of clinical implications and future directions.

FINANCIAL DISCLOSURES

In the past year, Dr S.V. Faraone received income, potential income, travel expenses continuing education support, and/or research support from, Akili, Arbor, Genomind, Ironshore, KemPharm/Corium, Ondosis, Otsuka, Rhodes, Shire/Takeda, Supernus, and Tris. With his institution, he has US patent US20130217707 A1 for the use of sodium–hydrogen exchange inhibitors in the treatment of ADHD. In previous years, he received support from: Alcobra, Aveksham, CogCubed, Eli Lilly & Co, Enzymotec, Impact, Janssen, Lundbeck/Takeda, McNeil, NeuroLifeSciences, Neurovance, Novartis, Pfizer, Sunovion, and Vallon. He also receives royalties from books published by Guilford Press: Straight Talk about Your Child's Mental Health; Oxford University Press: Schizophrenia: The Facts; and Elsevier: ADHD: Non-Pharmacologic Interventions. He is also the Program Director of www.adhdinadults.com. Dr N.M. Khoury, Dr N.V. Radonjić, and A.B. Albert have no financial disclosures.

FUNDING ACKNOWLEDGEMENTS

Dr S.V. Faraone is supported by the European Union's Horizon 2020 research and innovation program under grant agreement No 667302 and 965,381; NIMH grants U01MH109536-01, U01AR076092-01A1, R0MH116037, and 5R01AG06495502; Oregon Health and Science University, Otsuka Pharmaceuticals and Supernus Pharmaceutical Company.
  Dr N.M. Khoury, Dr N.V. Radonjić, and A.B. Albert have no funding to disclose.

REFERENCES

1. Willcutt EG. The prevalence of DSM-IV attention-deficit/hyperactivity disorder: a meta-analytic review. Neurotherapeutics 2012;9(3):490–9.

2. Polanczyk GV, Willcutt EG, Salum GA, et al. ADHD prevalence estimates across three decades: an updated systematic review and meta-regression analysis. Int J Epidemiol 2014;43(2):434–42.

3. Asherson P, Trzaskowski M. Attention-deficit/hyperactivity disorder is the extreme and impairing tail of a continuum. J Am Acad Child Adolesc Psychiatry 2015;54(4):249–50.

4. Biederman J, Faraone SV, Spencer T, et al. Patterns of psychiatric comorbidity, cognition, and psychosocial functioning in adults with attention deficit hyperactivity disorder. Am J Psychiatry 1993;150(12):1792–8.

5. Biederman J, Newcorn J, Sprich S. Comorbidity of attention-deficit hyperactivity disorder (ADHD). In: Association AP, editor. DSM-IV sourcebook, 3. Washington: American Psychiatric Association; 1997.

6. Faraone SV, Asherson P, Banaschewski T, et al. Attention-deficit/hyperactivity disorder. Nat Rev Dis Primers 2015;1:15020.

7. Faraone SV, Biederman J, Mick E. The age-dependent decline of attention deficit hyperactivity disorder: a meta-analysis of follow-up studies. Psychol Med 2006;36(2):159–65.

8. Faraone, S. V., & Radonjić, N. V. (In print). Neurobiology of attention-deficit/ hyperactivity disorder. In R. M. B. In: Tasman A., Schulze T.G., et al (Eds) (Ed.), Tasman's psychiatry 5th edition: SpringerNature, Switzerland.

9. Bijlenga D, Vollebregt MA, Kooij JJS, et al. The role of the circadian system in the etiology and pathophysiology of ADHD: time to redefine ADHD? Atten Defic Hyperact Disord 2019;11(1):5–19.

10. Bloch MH, Qawasmi A. Omega-3 fatty acid supplementation for the treatment of children with attention-deficit/hyperactivity disorder symptomatology: systematic review and meta-analysis. J Am Acad Child Adolesc Psychiatry 2011; 50(10):991–1000.

11. Bonvicini C, Faraone SV, Scassellati C. Attention-deficit hyperactivity disorder in adults: a systematic review and meta-analysis of genetic, pharmacogenetic and biochemical studies. Mol Psychiatry 2016;21(11):1643.

12. Bymaster FP, Katner JS, Nelson DL, et al. Atomoxetine increases extracellular levels of norepinephrine and dopamine in prefrontal cortex of rat: a potential mechanism for efficacy in attention deficit/hyperactivity disorder. Neuropsychopharmacology 2002;27(5):699–711.

13. Millichap JG, Yee MM. The diet factor in attention-deficit/hyperactivity disorder. Pediatrics 2012;129(2):330–7.

14. DuPaul GJ, Gormley MJ, Anastopoulos AD, et al. Academic trajectories of college students with and without ADHD: predictors of four-year outcomes. J Clin Child Adolesc Psychol 2021;1–16.

15. Fayyad J, Sampson NA, Hwang I, et al. The descriptive epidemiology of DSM-IV adult ADHD in the world health organization world mental health surveys. Atten Defic Hyperact Disord 2017;9(1):47–65.

16. Dobrosavljevic M, Solares C, Cortese S, et al. Prevalence of attention-deficit/ hyperactivity disorder in older adults: a systematic review and meta-analysis. Neurosci Biobehav Rev 2020;118:282–9.

17. Coker TR, Elliott MN, Toomey SL, et al. Racial and ethnic disparities in ADHD diagnosis and treatment. Pediatrics 2016;138(3). https://doi.org/10.1542/peds.2016-0407.

18. Miller TW, Nigg JT, Miller RL. Attention deficit hyperactivity disorder in African American children: what can be concluded from the past ten years? Clin Psychol Rev 2009;29(1):77–86.

19. Shi Y, Hunter Guevara LR, Dykhoff HJ, et al. Racial disparities in diagnosis of attention-deficit/hyperactivity disorder in a us national birth cohort. JAMA Netw Open 2021;4(3):e210321.
20. Slobodin O, Masalha R. Challenges in ADHD care for ethnic minority children: a review of the current literature. Transcult Psychiatry 2020;57(3):468–83.
21. Cénat JM, Blais-Rochette C, Morse C, et al. Prevalence and risk factors associated with attention-deficit/hyperactivity disorder among us black individuals: a systematic review and meta-analysis (Online ahead of print). JAMA Psychiatry 2020. https://doi.org/10.1001/jamapsychiatry.2020.2788.
22. Chang JP, Su KP, Mondelli V, et al. Omega-3 polyunsaturated fatty acids in youths with attention deficit hyperactivity disorder: a systematic review and meta-analysis of clinical trials and biological studies. Neuropsychopharmacology 2018;43(3):534–45.
23. Fairman KA, Peckham AM, Sclar DA. Diagnosis and treatment of ADHD in the United States: update by gender and race. J Atten Disord 2020;24(1):10–9.
24. Thompson M, Wilkinson L, Hyeyoung W. Social characteristics as predictors of ADHD labeling across the life course. Soc Ment Health 2021;11(2):91–112.
25. Trzepacz PT, Williams DW, Feldman PD, et al. CYP2D6 metabolizer status and atomoxetine dosing in children and adolescents with ADHD. Eur Neuropsychopharmacol 2008;18(2):79–86.
26. Ouyang L, Fang X, Mercy J, et al. Attention-deficit/hyperactivity disorder symptoms and child maltreatment: a population-based study. J Pediatr 2008;153(6):851–6.
27. Choi Y, Shin J, Cho KH, et al. Change in household income and risk for attention deficit hyperactivity disorder during childhood: a nationwide population-based cohort study. J Epidemiol 2017;27(2):56–62.
28. Cinnamon Bidwell L, Dew RE, Kollins SH. Alpha-2 adrenergic receptors and attention-deficit/hyperactivity disorder. Curr Psychiatry Rep 2010;12(5):366–73.
29. Larsson H, Asherson P, Chang Z, et al. Genetic and environmental influences on adult attention deficit hyperactivity disorder symptoms: a large Swedish population-based study of twins. Psychol Med 2013;43(1):197–207.
30. Haack LM, Meza J, Jiang Y, et al. Influences to ADHD problem recognition: mixed-method investigation and recommendations to reduce disparities for latino youth. Adm Policy Ment Health 2018;45(6):958–77.
31. Hawkey E, Nigg JT. Omega-3 fatty acid and ADHD: blood level analysis and meta-analytic extension of supplementation trials. Clin Psychol Rev 2014;34(6):496–505.
32. Herbst EA, Paglialunga S, Gerling C, et al. Omega-3 supplementation alters mitochondrial membrane composition and respiration kinetics in human skeletal muscle. J Physiol 2014;592(6):1341–52.
33. Faraone SV, Larsson H. Genetics of attention deficit hyperactivity disorder. Mol Psychiatry 2018;24(4):562–75.
34. Kennedy M, Kreppner J, Knights N, et al. Early severe institutional deprivation is associated with a persistent variant of adult attention-deficit/hyperactivity disorder: clinical presentation, developmental continuities and life circumstances in the English and Romanian Adoptees study. J Child Psychol Psychiatry 2016;57(10):1113–25.
35. Stojanovski S, Felsky D, Viviano JD, et al. Polygenic risk and neural substrates of attention-deficit/hyperactivity disorder symptoms in youths with a history of mild traumatic brain injury. Biol Psychiatry 2019;85(5):408–16.

36. Surette ME. The science behind dietary omega-3 fatty acids. CMAJ 2008; 178(2):177–80.

37. Faraone SV, Banaschewski T, Coghill D, et al. The world federation of ADHD international consensus statement: 208 evidence-based conclusions about the disorder. Neurosci Biobehav Rev 2021;128:789–818.

38. Franke B, Faraone SV, Asherson P, et al. The genetics of attention deficit/hyperactivity disorder in adults, a review. Mol Psychiatry 2011;17(10):960–87.

39. Froehlich TE, McGough JJ, Stein MA. Progress and promise of attention-deficit hyperactivity disorder pharmacogenetics. CNS Drugs 2010;24(2):99–117.

40. Fusar-Poli P, Rubia K, Rossi G, et al. Striatal dopamine transporter alterations in ADHD: pathophysiology or adaptation to psychostimulants? a meta-analysis. Am J Psychiatry 2012;169(3):264–72.

41. Larsson H, Anckarsater H, Rastam M, et al. Childhood attention-deficit hyperactivity disorder as an extreme of a continuous trait: a quantitative genetic study of 8,500 twin pairs. J Child Psychol Psychiatry 2012;53(1):73–80.

42. Chang Z, Lichtenstein P, Asherson PJ, et al. Developmental twin study of attention problems: high heritabilities throughout development. JAMA Psychiatry 2013;70(3):311–8.

43. Kuntsi J, Rijsdijk F, Ronald A, et al. Genetic influences on the stability of attention-deficit/hyperactivity disorder symptoms from early to middle childhood. Biol Psychiatry 2005;57(6):647–54.

44. Biederman J, Faraone SV, Keenan K, et al. Further evidence for family-genetic risk factors in attention deficit hyperactivity disorder. Patterns of comorbidity in probands and relatives in psychiatrically and pediatrically referred samples. Arch Gen Psychiatry 1992;49(9):728–38.

45. Faraone SV, Biederman J, Mick E, et al. A family study of psychiatric comorbidity in girls and boys with attention deficit hyperactivity disorder. Biol Psychiatry 2001;50:586–92.

46. Faraone SV, Glatt SJ. A comparison of the efficacy of medications for adult attention-deficit/hyperactivity disorder using meta-analysis of effect sizes. J Clin Psychiatry 2010;71:754–63.

47. Lahey BB, Van Hulle CA, Singh AL, et al. Higher-order genetic and environmental structure of prevalent forms of child and adolescent psychopathology. Arch Gen Psychiatry 2011;68(2):181–9.

48. Lee PH AV, Won H, Feng YA, et al. Genomic relationships, novel loci, and pleiotropic mechanisms across eight psychiatric disorders. Cell 2019;179(7): 1469–82.e1411.

49. Smoller JW, Andreassen OA, Edenberg HJ, et al. Psychiatric genetics and the structure of psychopathology. Mol Psychiatry 2019;24(3):409–20.

50. Cocchi L, Bramati IE, Zalesky A, et al. Altered functional brain connectivity in a non-clinical sample of young adults with attention-deficit/hyperactivity disorder. J Neurosci 2012;32(49):17753–61.

51. Liddle EB, Hollis C, Batty MJ, et al. Task-related default mode network modulation and inhibitory control in ADHD: effects of motivation and methylphenidate. J Child Psychol Psychiatry 2011;52(7):761–71.

52. Lin HY, Gau SS. Atomoxetine treatment strengthens an anti-correlated relationship between functional brain networks in medication-naïve adults with attention-deficit hyperactivity disorder: a randomized double-blind placebo-controlled clinical trial. Int J Neuropsychopharmacol 2015;19(3):pyv094.

53. McGough JJ, Sturm A, Cowen J, et al. Double-blind, sham-controlled, pilot study of trigeminal nerve stimulation for attention-deficit/hyperactivity disorder. J Am Acad Child Adolesc Psychiatry 2019;58(4):403–11.e403.

54. Hoogman M, Bralten J, Hibar DP, et al. Subcortical brain volume differences in participants with attention deficit hyperactivity disorder in children and adults: a cross-sectional mega-analysis. Lancet Psychiatry 2017;4(4):310–9.

55. Hoogman M, Muetzel R, Guimaraes JP, et al. Brain imaging of the cortex in ADHD: a coordinated analysis of large-scale clinical and population-based samples. Am J Psychiatry 2019;176(7):531–42.

56. Faraone SV. The pharmacology of amphetamine and methylphenidate: relevance to the neurobiology of attention-deficit/hyperactivity disorder and other psychiatric comorbidities. Neurosci Biobehav Rev 2018;87:255–70.

57. Chang X, Liu Y, Mentch F, et al. Mitochondrial DNA haplogroups and risk of attention deficit and hyperactivity disorder in European Americans. Transl Psychiatry 2020;10(1):370.

58. Öğütlü H, Esin İ S, Erdem HB, et al. Mitochondrial DNA copy number may be associated with attention deficit/hyperactivity disorder severity in treatment: a one-year follow-up study. Int J Psychiatry Clin Pract 2021;25(1):37–42.

59. Joseph N, Zhang-James Y, Perl A, et al. Oxidative stress and attention deficit hyperactivity disorder: a meta-analysis. J Atten Disord 2015;19(11):915–24.

60. Hess JL, Akutagava-Martins GC, Patak JD, et al. Why is there selective subcortical vulnerability in ADHD? Clues from postmortem brain gene expression data. Mol Psychiatry 2017;23(8):1787–93.

61. Lee CJ, Wu CC, Chou WJ, et al. Mitochondrial-associated protein biomarkers in patients with attention-deficit/hyperactivity disorder. Mitochondrion 2019; 49:83–8.

62. Warikoo N, Faraone SV. Background, clinical features and treatment of attention deficit hyperactivity disorder in children. Expert Opin Pharmacother 2013.

63. Wigal SB, Wigal T, Hobart M, et al. Safety and efficacy of centanafadine sustained-release in adults with attention-deficit hyperactivity disorder: results of phase 2 studies. Neuropsychiatr Dis Treat 2020;16:1411–26.

64. Chen YC, Wu LK, Lee MS, et al. The efficacy of acupuncture treatment for attention deficit hyperactivity disorder: a systematic review and meta-analysis. Complement Med Res 2021;1–11.

65. Balasubramaniam M, Telles S, Doraiswamy PM. Yoga on our minds: a systematic review of yoga for neuropsychiatric disorders. Front Psychiatry 2012;3:117.

66. Barbosa DJ, Capela JP, Feio-Azevedo R, et al. Mitochondria: key players in the neurotoxic effects of amphetamines. Arch Toxicol 2015;89(10):1695–725.

67. Xue J, Zhang Y, Huang Y. A meta-analytic investigation of the impact of mindfulness-based interventions on ADHD symptoms. Medicine (Baltimore) 2019;98(23):e15957.

68. Zhu M, Tian Y, Zhang H, et al. Methylphenidate ameliorates hypoxia-induced mitochondrial damage in human neuroblastoma SH-SY5Y cells through inhibition of oxidative stress. Life Sci 2018;197:40–5.

69. National Institute for Health Care and Excellence. Attention defificit hyperactivity disorder: diagnosis and management. 2018. Available at: https://www.nice.org.uk/guidance/ng87.

70. Nigg JT, Lewis K, Edinger T, et al. Meta-analysis of attention-deficit/hyperactivity disorder or attention-deficit/hyperactivity disorder symptoms, restriction diet, and synthetic food color additives. J Am Acad Child Adolesc Psychiatry 2012;51(1):86–97, e88.

71. Childress AC, Foehl HC, Newcorn JH, et al. Long-Term treatment with extended-release methylphenidate treatment in children aged 4 to < 6 Years [online ahead of print]. J Am Acad Child Adolesc Psychiatry 2021. https://doi.org/10.1016/j.jaac.2021.03.019.

72. Vitiello B, Abikoff HB, Chuang SZ, et al. Effectiveness of methylphenidate in the 10-month continuation phase of the preschoolers with attention-deficit/hyperactivity disorder treatment study (PATS). J Child Adolesc Psychopharmacol 2007;17(5):593–604.

73. Volkow ND, Fowler JS, Gatley SJ, et al. PET evaluation of the dopamine system of the human brain. J Nucl Med 1996;37(7):1242–56.

74. Wall SC, Gu H, Rudnick G. Biogenic amine flux mediated by cloned transporters stably expressed in cultured cell lines: amphetamine specificity for inhibition and efflux. Mol Pharmacol 1995;47(3):544–50.

75. Wang M, Ramos BP, Paspalas CD, et al. Alpha2A-adrenoceptors strengthen working memory networks by inhibiting cAMP-HCN channel signaling in prefrontal cortex. Cell 2007;129(2):397–410. Available at: http://www.ncbi.nlm.nih.gov/entrez/query.fcgi?cmd=Retrieve&db=PubMed&dopt= Citation&list_uids= 17448997.

76. Cortese S, Adamo N, Del Giovane C, et al. Comparative efficacy and tolerability of medications for attention-deficit hyperactivity disorder in children, adolescents, and adults: a systematic review and network meta-analysis. Lancet Psychiatry 2018;5(9):727–38.

77. Costa A, Riedel M, Pogarell O, et al. Methylphenidate effects on neural activity during response inhibition in healthy humans. Cereb Cortex 2013;23(5):1179–89.

78. Kidwell KM, Van Dyk TR, Lundahl A, et al. Stimulant medications and sleep for youth with ADHD: a meta-analysis. Pediatrics 2015;136(6):1144–53.

79. Kollins SH, DeLoss DJ, Cañadas E, et al. A novel digital intervention for actively reducing severity of paediatric ADHD (STARS-ADHD): a randomised controlled trial. Lancet Digital Health 2020;2(4):e168–78.

80. Kowalczyk OS, Cubillo AI, Smith A, et al. Methylphenidate and atomoxetine normalise fronto-parietal underactivation during sustained attention in ADHD adolescents. Eur Neuropsychopharmacol 2019;29(10):1102–16.

81. Holmskov M, Storebo OJ, Moreira-Maia CR, et al. Gastrointestinal adverse events during methylphenidate treatment of children and adolescents with attention deficit hyperactivity disorder: a systematic review with meta-analysis and Trial Sequential Analysis of randomised clinical trials. PLoS One 2017;12(6):e0178187.

82. Lenzi F, Cortese S, Harris J, et al. Pharmacotherapy of emotional dysregulation in adults with ADHD: a systematic review and meta-analysis. Neurosci Biobehavioral Rev 2018;84:359–67.

83. Faraone SV, Rostain AL, Blader J, et al. Practitioner review: emotional dysregulation in attention-deficit/hyperactivity disorder - implications for clinical recognition and intervention. J Child Psychol Psychiatry 2019;60(2):133–50.

84. Coughlin CG, Cohen SC, Mulqueen JM, et al. Meta-analysis: reduced risk of anxiety with psychostimulant treatment in children with attention-deficit/hyperactivity disorder. J Child Adolesc Psychopharmacol 2015;25(8):611–7.

85. Pringsheim T, Hirsch L, Gardner D, et al. The pharmacological management of oppositional behaviour, conduct problems, and aggression in children and adolescents with attention-deficit hyperactivity disorder, oppositional defiant disorder, and conduct disorder: a systematic review and meta-analysis. Part 1:

psychostimulants, alpha-2 agonists, and atomoxetine. Can J Psychiatry 2015; 60(2):42–51.

86. Puri BK, Martins JG. Which polyunsaturated fatty acids are active in children with attention-deficit hyperactivity disorder receiving PUFA supplementation? A fatty acid validated meta-regression analysis of randomized controlled trials. Prostaglandins Leukot Essent Fatty Acids 2014;90(5):179–89.

87. Biederman J, DiSalvo M, Fried R, et al. Quantifying the protective effects of stimulants on functional outcomes in attention-deficit/hyperactivity disorder: a focus on number needed to treat statistic and sex effects. J Adolesc Health 2019; 65(6):784–9.

88. Faraone SV, Gomeni R, Hull JT, et al. Early response to SPN-812 (viloxazine extended-release) can predict efficacy outcome in pediatric subjects with ADHD: a machine learning post-hoc analysis of four randomized clinical trials. Psychiatry Res 2021;296:113664 [Online ahead of print].

89. Winsberg BG, Comings DE. Association of the dopamine transporter gene (DAT1) with poor methylphenidate response. J Am Acad Child Adolesc Psychiatry 1999;38(12):1474–7.

90. Jones HA, Epstein JN, Hinshaw SP, et al. Ethnicity as a moderator of treatment effects on parent–child interaction for children with ADHD. J Atten Disord 2010; 13(6):592–600.

91. Reid MJ, Webster-Stratton C, Beauchaine TP. Parent training in head start: a comparison of program response among African American, Asian American, Caucasian, and Hispanic mothers. Prev Sci 2001;2(4):209–27.

92. Glasofer A, Dingley C, Reyes AT. Medication decision making among african American caregivers of children with ADHD: a review of the literature. J Atten Disord 2021;25(12):1687–98.

93. Kang S, Harvey EA. Racial differences between black parents' and white teachers' perceptions of attention-deficit/hyperactivity disorder behavior. J Abnorm Child Psychol 2020;48(5):661–72.

94. Laswson GM, Nissley-Tsiopinis J, Nahmias A, et al. Do parent and teacher report of ADHD symptoms in children differ by SES and racial status? J Psychopathol Behav Assess 2017;39:426–40.

95. Mostafavi H, Harpak A, Agarwal I, et al. Variable prediction accuracy of polygenic scores within an ancestry group. Elife 2020;9. https://doi.org/10.7554/eLife.48376.

96. Mueller S, Costa A, Keeser D, et al. The effects of methylphenidate on whole brain intrinsic functional connectivity. Hum Brain Mapp 2014;35(11):5379–88.

97. Myer NM, Boland JR, Faraone SV. Pharmacogenetics predictors of methylphenidate efficacy in childhood ADHD. Mol Psychiatry 2018;23(9):1929–36.

98. Nasser A, Liranso T, Adewole T, et al. A phase III, randomized, placebo-controlled trial to assess the efficacy and safety of once-daily SPN-812 (Viloxazine Extended-release) in the treatment of attention-deficit/hyperactivity disorder in school-age children. Clin Ther 2020;42(8):1452–66.

99. Grizenko N, Shayan YR, Polotskaia A, et al. Relation of maternal stress during pregnancy to symptom severity and response to treatment in children with ADHD. J Psychiatry Neurosci 2008;33(1):10–6.

100. Rodriguez A, Bohlin G. Are maternal smoking and stress during pregnancy related to ADHD symptoms in children? J Child Psychol Psychiatry 2005; 46(3):246–54.

101. Talge NM, Neal C, Glover V. Antenatal maternal stress and long-term effects on child neurodevelopment: how and why? J Child Psychol Psychiatry 2007; 48(3–4):245–61.

102. Li J, Olsen J, Vestergaard M, et al. Attention-deficit/hyperactivity disorder in the offspring following prenatal maternal bereavement: a nationwide follow-up study in Denmark. Eur Child Adolesc Psychiatry 2010;19(10):747–53.

103. Wolford E, Lahti M, Tuovinen S, et al. Maternal depressive symptoms during and after pregnancy are associated with attention-deficit/hyperactivity disorder symptoms in their 3- to 6-year-old children. PLoS One 2017;12(12):e0190248.

104. Clements CC, Castro VM, Blumenthal SR, et al. Prenatal antidepressant exposure is associated with risk for attention-deficit hyperactivity disorder but not autism spectrum disorder in a large health system. Mol Psychiatry 2015;20(6): 727–34.

105. Van den Bergh BR, Marcoen A. High antenatal maternal anxiety is related to ADHD symptoms, externalizing problems, and anxiety in 8- and 9-year-olds. Child Dev 2004;75(4):1085–97.

106. Van Doren J, Arns M, Heinrich H, et al. Sustained effects of neurofeedback in ADHD: a systematic review and meta-analysis. Eur Child Adolesc Psychiatry 2019;28(3):293–305.

107. Elgar FJ, Curtis LJ, McGrath PJ, et al. Antecedent-consequence conditions in maternal mood and child adjustment: a four-year cross-lagged study. J Clin Child Adolesc Psychol 2003;32(3):362–74.

108. Fagundes AO, Scaini G, Santos PM, et al. Inhibition of mitochondrial respiratory chain in the brain of adult rats after acute and chronic administration of methylphenidate. Neurochem Res 2010;35(3):405–11.

109. Romano E, Tremblay RE, Farhat A, et al. Development and prediction of hyperactive symptoms from 2 to 7 years in a population-based sample. Pediatrics 2006;117(6):2101–10.

110. Schlösser RG, Nenadic I, Wagner G, et al. Dopaminergic modulation of brain systems subserving decision making under uncertainty: a study with fMRI and methylphenidate challenge. Synapse 2009;63(5):429–42.

111. Schwartz S, Correll CU. Efficacy and safety of atomoxetine in children and adolescents with attention-deficit/hyperactivity disorder: results from a comprehensive meta-analysis and metaregression. J Am Acad Child Adolesc Psychiatry 2014;53(2):174–87.

112. Goodman SH, Gotlib IH. Risk for psychopathology in the children of depressed mothers: a developmental model for understanding mechanisms of transmission. Psychol Rev 1999;106(3):458–90.

113. Tung I, Brammer WA, Li JJ, et al. Parenting behavior mediates the intergenerational association of parent and child offspring ADHD symptoms. J Clin Child Adolesc Psychol 2015;44(5):787–99.

114. Spencer AE, Faraone SV, Bogucki OE, et al. Examining the association between posttraumatic stress disorder and attention-deficit/hyperactivity disorder: a systematic review and meta-analysis. J Clin Psychiatry 2016;77(1):72–83. https://doi.org/10.4088/JCP.14r09479.

115. Stern A, Agnew-Blais J, Danese A, et al. Associations between abuse/neglect and ADHD from childhood to young adulthood: a prospective nationally-representative twin study. Child Abuse Negl 2018;81:274–85.

116. Lau AS. Making the case for selective and directed cultural adaptations of evidence-based treatments: examples from parent training. Clin Psychol Sci Prac 2006;13(4):295–310. https://doi.org/10.1111/j.1468-2850.2006.00042.x.

117. Barkley RA. Emotional dysregulation is a core component of ADHD. In: Barkley RA, editor. Attention-deficit hyperactivity disorder: a handbook for diagnosis and treatment. 4th ed. New York: Guilford Press; 2015.
118. Bédard AC, Schulz KP, Krone B, et al. Neural mechanisms underlying the therapeutic actions of guanfacine treatment in youth with ADHD: a pilot fMRI study. Psychiatry Res 2015;231(3):353–6.
119. Faraone SV, Biederman J. Can attention-deficit/hyperactivity disorder onset occur in adulthood? JAMA Psychiatry 2016;73(7):655–6.
120. Sonuga-Barke E, Bitsakou P, Thompson M. Beyond the dual pathway model: evidence for the dissociation of timing, inhibitory, and delay-related impairments in attention-deficit/hyperactivity disorder. J Am Acad Child Adolesc Psychiatry 2010;49(4):345–55.

Measurement Informed Care in Attention-Deficit/ Hyperactivity Disorder (ADHD)

Margaret Danielle Weiss, MD PhD[a],*, Mark A. Stein, PhD[b]

KEYWORDS

- ADHD • Measurement • Outcome • Scales • Symptoms • Function • Improvement
- Remission

KEY POINTS

- Best practice in management of ADHD requires measurement informed care with standardized rating scales.
- Outcome in ADHD must capture core ADHD symptoms, comorbid conditions, and associated impairments.
- An evaluation of functional impairment is essential to establish targeted interventions and c to identify continued difficulty despite ADHD symptom response.
- Optimal treatment goes beyond improvement to remission of both symptoms and symptom-driven functional impairment.
- Outcome in ADHD is dynamic and fluctuates with the patient's current challenges. Repeated use of a systematic assessment battery over time identifies those environmental challenges and patient strengths that may be critical to long-term outcome.

INTRODUCTION

A landmark in this history of our understanding of optimizing outcome in ADHD was the MTA finding that expert medication management was superior to community-based care. The take-home message of this finding was that systematic evaluation, gathering of collateral information, individualized and systematic titration, and careful follow-up were critical to optimizing drug outcome. Measurement informed care (MIC) is now a cornerstone of both shared decision-making and evidence-based practice. This article reviews current best practice in use of diagnostic interviews and rating scales in assessment and follow-up evaluation. This includes MIC for diagnostic evaluation, broad-based symptom screening, diagnosis-specific symptom screening, and

[a] Department of Child Psychiatry, Cambridge Health Alliance, 1493 Cambridge Street, Cambridge, MA 02139, USA; [b] Departments of Psychiatry and Behavioral Sciences, and Pediatrics, University of Washington School of Medicine, 1959 NE Pacific Street, Box 356560, Seattle, WA 98195-6560, USA
* Corresponding author.
E-mail address: Margaret.weiss@icloud.com

Child Adolesc Psychiatric Clin N Am 31 (2022) 363–372
https://doi.org/10.1016/j.chc.2022.03.010
childpsych.theclinics.com

assessment of health quality outcomes such as functional impairment. MIS is also always personalized to address-specific, patient-targeted challenges such as executive function or emotional dysregulation.

ADHD INTERVIEWS

The cornerstone of assessment is the clinical interview. Several structured interview tools specific to ADHD have been developed to assist clinicians in conducting and documenting a diagnostic evaluation. These interviews provide clinicians with a structured format to assure that they cover the most salient aspects of a psychiatric interview in general, as well screening for issues specific to an ADHD evaluation of comorbid conditions, the developmental history and family history, the severity of symptoms, and patient examples and screening for the presence of symptoms in childhood or earlier in life.

The first such diagnostic interview to come to prominent attention was the Conners' Adult ADHD Diagnostic Interview for DSM-IV (https://storefront.mhs.com/collections/caadid).

The Diagnostic Interview for ADHD in Adults (DIVA) (www.divacenter.eu) has now been translated into more than 25 languages and has greatly facilitated clinician acceptance and comfort with diagnostic assessment for ADHD.[1] DIVA-5 [2] asks about the presence of ADHD symptoms in adulthood as well as childhood, the chronicity of these symptoms, and significant lifetime impairments due to these symptoms. DIVA-5 has been adjusted for children age 5 to 17 (Young DIVA-5) and for people with intellectual disability (DIVA-5-ID). The DIVA can be downloaded for a fee to offset the cost of development. The interview can be scored for DSM-5 diagnoses.

The ADHD Child Evaluation (ACE) and the adult version (ACE +) are comprehensive interviews in the public domain (https://www.psychology-services.uk.com/ACE-and-ACE-plus/). These interviews have been translated into 22 languages, and online training is available to support their use. The interviews include a guide to scoring per DSM-5 and ICD-10.

The ACE rating scales are preassessment tools that can be completed in advance of the ACE clinical interview, with either self-report or informant report. The scales differ from other rating scales because the rater is asked to provide specific examples of how each endorsed symptom impacts on the person's behavior when they were (a) a child (by the age of 12 years old) and/or (b) in the last 6 months (the self-report version only enquires about behavior over the last 6 months). With the addition of this qualitative information, the scales are useful tools to gain preassessment and follow-up information on the person's functioning across settings.

BROAD-BASED SYMPTOM SCREENING

Most patients with ADHD present with comorbid diagnoses that may drive outcome as much as the core symptoms of ADHD. This is particularly true in tertiary referral settings. An evaluation of symptoms requires systematic empirical assessment for multiple conditions to establish the most prominent or treatable disorder, the comorbid dia diagnoses, and differential diagnosis before establishing targeted treatment for one condition.

Although this seems self-evident, broad based symptom screening is not always routine practice. This is most evident in looking at some key Web sites, which provide clinicians with assessment tools such as the AACAP Toolbox for Clinical Practice and Outcomes (https://www.aacap.org/AACAP/Member_Resources/AACAP_Toolbox_for_Clinical_Practice_and_Outcomes/Home.aspx) or the NIH Toolbox (https://www.

healthmeasures.net/explore-measurement-systems/nih-toolbox/obtain-and-administer-measures), neither of which include a broad-based diagnostic symptom screen. The systematic clinical use of a broad based symptom measure to augment the assessment interview would significantly improve the identification of disorders that would otherwise be missed, assist in differential diagnosis and a primary diagnosis.

The Strengths and Difficulties Questionnaire (SDQ) (www.sdqinfo.org) is the most widely used broad-based screening tool. The SDQ is remarkable in its scope and design. The advantages of the SDQ include:

- Validation and widespread use in clinical, population, and research settings.
- Extensive population norms from different geographic regions that include age and gender norms.
- Availability of comparative forms for self-report and collateral including parents and teachers.
- An 'impact' module to look at the impact of symptoms.
- Translation into more than 75 languages.
- Use in more than 5000 publications and more than 100 countries in a wide range of studies.
- Short, easy to use and patient friendly.
- Five key domain outcomes of clinical interest are emotional problems, conduct problems, hyperactivity, peer problems, and a positive prosocial scale. The hyperactive domain consists of two attention items, two hyperactive items, and one impulsive item.
- Electronic or paper scoring.

There are several, commercially available broad-based scales that provide both dimensional ratings of various domains and DSM-5 screening. These are also age and gender normed and available in paper and pencil format and electronically, with online assessment able to provide both scoring and a report. Different forms for these measures have also been developed for different ages and informants. Some of the best known such measures are the Behavior Assessment System for Children (up to age 21 years),[3] the Achenbach (https://aseba.org), and the Conners (https://mhs.com/info/conners3).

The American Psychiatric Association now offers 'emerging' measures designed to address the need for broad-based DSM-5 screening (https://www.psychiatry.org/psychiatrists/practice/dsm/educational-resources/assessment-measures): one for children (The DSM-5 Parent/Guardian-Rated Level 1 Cross-Cutting Symptom Measure—Child Age 6–17) and another for adults (DSM-5 Self-Rated Level 1 Cross-Cutting Symptom Measure—Adult). These tools screen for depression, anger, irritability, mania, anxiety, somatic symptoms, inattention, suicidal ideation/attempt, psychosis, sleep disturbance, repetitive thoughts and behaviors, and substance use. These scales are limited by the absence of large psychometric validation studies, age and gender norms, translations, and difficulty of scoring and interpretation. Similar limitations apply to the Weiss Symptom Record–II (WSR-II) developed in Canada over the last 15 years (https://www.caddra.ca/wp-content/uploads/WSR-II.pdf). The WSR-II group items by diagnostic domain with a built in calculator are simplifying the clinicians' ability to immediately compare and contrast the severity of different disorders.

A revolution in broad-based assessment occurred with the development of computerized adaptive testing (CAT). It may be said that one of the reasons for the sluggish growth of broad-based screening is that to cover every possible condition for every individual, measures were both lengthy and contained an excess of items that were irrelevant. Adaptive testing is the personalized medicine of rating scales.

CAT uses artificial intelligence, so that as the subject answers questions, the test selects from a large data bank of questions those items that are most relevant to that patient. As a result, a full assessment for a wide variety of conditions can be completed in minutes with a much higher level of detail and accuracy for the areas that relevant for that individual. Increasing the relevance of items also increases the subject's interest, motivation, and completion.[4]

Since CAT responses can be stored electronically, it becomes possible to collect a large amount of information that can contribute to population norming, validation and evaluation of sensitivity, and specificity of outcomes against clinical diagnostic assessment. Limitations of adaptive testing may be cost and need for a digital interface. Several private adaptive testing companies such as Adaptive Testing Technologies (https://adaptivetestingtechnologies.com/team) and Assessment Systems Corporation (https://assess.com/about-assessment-systems) continue to pioneer these methods globally and in many large behavioral health systems.

The Patient-Reported Outcomes Measurement Information Systems (PROMIS) program has evolved over the last 10 years to generate a well-organized and effective assessment system in clinical research in a wide variety of chronic diseases. The second phase of PROMIS studies (PROMIS II), funded from 2009 to 2014, incorporated novel features that included longitudinal analyses and more sociodemographically diverse samples. PROMIS includes broad-based, quality of life, and targeted assessments as well as adaptive testing.

Whether a clinician elects to use an older and simpler broad-based screening tool such as the SDQ, an electronic measure or to invest in adaptive testing, an initial broad-based screening improves the accuracy and efficiency of an initial assessment.

TARGETED ADHD SYMPTOM ASSESSMENT

The broad-based screening tools described above will include some type of assessment of attention and disruptive behavior, but once this has been identified as a target of intervention a measure specific to ADHD with or without disruptive behavior is needed to assess severity and to allow easy, sequential administration to track change over time. ADHD outcome measures exist in the public domain, for purchase with age and gender norms, on paper, and electronically.

ADHD diagnosis in adults presents the unique challenge of demonstrating the presence of ADHD in childhood. The Wender Utah Rating Scale (WURS) has demonstrated good sensitivity and specificity as a measure that can increase the reliability of a retrospective childhood diagnosis[5,6] Notably, the WURS expands on DSM symptom lists and includes broader symptom clusters.

Ideally, a targeted follow-up outcome measure should include the ability to generate a comparison with pretreatment baseline. Treatment outcome measures should be evaluated to determine a psychometrically validated standard for the minimally important clinical difference (MICD). There are various ways to do this, such as patient report of a visible difference or a psychometric standard of ½ SD.[7]

The MICD can be used to define the percent of patients who have 'improved.' Improvement is an evaluation of change. Equally important is determining whether the patient is 'well' or in 'remission' at end point. A patient who is severely ill may improve significantly and still be severely ill. By contrast, for a patient who has mild difficulties only slight degree of improvement may result in an end score that meets the criteria for remission.

For many disorders such as depression,[8] remission is predictive of a better outcome. For ADHD, this is more complex, and a status of 'remission' may change over time as the balance between symptom control and shifts in environmental supports and demands.[9] The classical definition of remission in ADHD is a mean score of 1 or less on any measure based on a 4-point Likert-type scale of the 18 items of ADHD.[10] Improvement in functioning can also be defined as meeting the threshold for a 40% decrease in functional impairment or a change consistent with the MICD. Alternatively, functional remission can be understood as any patient who falls below the receiver operating characteristic (ROC) cutoff that distinguishes the clinical population from the normative population.[11]

Two of the earliest and most commonly used ADHD symptom outcome measures are the Swanson, Nolan and Pelham (SNAP) and the National Institute for Children's Health Quality Vanderbilt forms (https://www.aap.org/en/publications/caring-for-children-with-adhd-2nd-ed/adhd2/). These measures were developed for children and youth. The advantage of these measures is that they are free, short, and the SNAP is one of the few measures in the public domain that has norms.[12] This is particularly important in ADHD where there are such wide discrepancies between age and genders : a level of hyperactive behavior that is appropriate for a male toddler would be a clinical concern in a female adolescent. One of the important and often unrecognized limitations in how these measures are used in clinical practice is that they are scored categorically, with ratings or often or very often for more than 6/9 items being considered 'diagnostic.' The wide disparity in the cutoff between what is normative or at risk when one evaluates age and gender norms means that categorical use of scales as positive or negative for 6/9 items or either domain will lead systematic over and under identification of ADHD.

Like the SDQ, the SNAP has been translated into many languages and used in many studies. Both SNAP and Vanderbilt also attempt to capture to a limited degree the most common and concerning aspects of comorbidity, such as opposition or conduct externalizing symptoms (SNAP) and depressive or anxiety internalizing symptoms (Vanderbilt). These forms are widely available as PDF files for printing or online self-scoring electronic platforms. Electronic, self-scoring measures in the public domain are particularly useful in telehealth settings where there is no direct access to giving the patient a form. The clinician can send the link to such a scale in the virtual chat and then 'share screen' to review the results in a future meeting.

In 2012, Swanson and colleagues recognized that using statistical cutoffs in a population in which scores are highly skewed toward pathology was problematic. He created the Strengths and Weaknesses of ADHD Symptoms and Normal Behavior Rating Scale (SWAN), so that the measure might be informative of both skills and deficits. The SWAN consists of 30 items measuring the full range of behavior, instead of only the pathologic signs and symptoms of ADHD. The psychometric properties of the scale have been demonstrated to be excellent.[13,14] The paradigm shift from the SNAP, which is pathology oriented to the dimensional approach of the SWAN, supports the clinician who wishes to take a strength-based approach to treatment.

The World Health Organization developed, normed, and validated a measure of ADHD in adults, the Adult Self-Report Rating Scale (ASRS) for use in the National Comorbidity Survey. This is available free of charge in more than 20 languages (https://www.hcp.med.harvard.edu/ncs/asrs.php). This work has had a major impact in improving access and care for ADHD in adults and providing an international standard for measurement of severity and population screening. The ASRS consists of 6 quick screening questions, which are also used to establish the sensitivity/specificity of the scoring paradigm. The other core symptoms of ADHD are included in Part B for clinical reference. The format of the ASRS does not group symptoms by inattentive/hyperactive-impulsive domains making it somewhat more cumbersome to easily iden visualize domain-specific scores.

There are several ADHD-specific scales available for purchase either electronically or in paper and pencil format. These are popular and widely used despite the cost because they offer age and gender norms, age-specific formats, informant-specific formats and provide considerably more information regarding where the individual is in the normal range, at clinical risk or above 1.5 SD from the norm. The electronic version of such measures may generate a report, which is very useful as a tool to provide students with support for a 504 or an Individual Education Plan. The Conners 3[15] includes a short and a long form for this purpose and is currently under revision for a fourth edition. The Conners 4 will be released Fall 2021.

FUNCTIONAL OUTCOME

Diagnostic evaluation is a reflection of the clinician perspective: "What disorder(s) am I treating?" The patient perspective is typically based on functional impairment: "I have a problem with…". For example, a parent comes in complaining that her son has no friends, an adolescent girl complains her parents nag her, or a college student complains that he has partied away the semester and is now going to 'flunk out.' A 2012 study compared measured outcome in ADHD studies and found that 95% of studies included symptom outcomes and less than half of studies looked at quality outcomes such as functional impairment.[16] This is changing with growing appreciation for the importance of looking beyond core symptoms.[17,18]

In most of the cases, there is a strong overlap and a moderate correlation between symptoms and functioning, but the clinician is particularly interested in the way in which identified symptoms of emotional or behavior problems are driving the patient's perceived functional impairment. From a clinical perspective, it is those instances in which symptoms and function are *not* correlated that may be of interest. If treatment leads to symptom improvement and remission but the patient-identified target or functioning has not changed, additional intervention is needed. For example, a parent may present complaining that her daughter is not doing as well in school as expected and the clinician successfully treats the child for attention deficits, but there is no improvement in academic outcome. Further assessment identifies a learning disability, which responds to an individualized education program. Without an evaluation of both symptoms and functional impairment, the patient's difficulty would not have been addressed.

The converse is also possible. Some patients may describe significant symptoms, without complaints of functional impairment. Screening may identify that a young woman describes herself as a disruptive child and still describes residual difficulty with ADHD symptoms. However, she notes that this does not cause her any distress, impact her relationships, academic or social functioning, or cause any other difficulty that might be a concern. Her perception is that she has 'channeled her ADHD into being more productive at work.' Symptoms in the absence of impairment do not necessarily warrant treatment.

Early global assessment measures such as the Children's Global Assessment Scale[19] have been used as a marker of severity to complement any diagnosis and included items relevant to functioning. The Brief Impairment Scale[20] and the Impairment Rating Scale (IRS)[21] have been widely used in ADHD populations as short, reliable measures of function sensitive to change with treatment. The IRS is one of the few ADHD function scales that offers a version specifically for teachers. The scale has limitations as a measure of domain-specific impairment since there are a small number of items in each domain and the scale loads as a single factor.

The Barkley Functional Impairment Scale[22] is an age- and gender-normed measure of function in ADHD populations. The measure provides an opportunity for standardized and systematic evaluation of how an individual is functioning as compared with peers. The BFIS looks at functioning over the last 6 months, independent of whether impairment is secondary to mental health, so that it is an excellent measure of function as a trait in ADHD populations rather than a state sensitive to brief changes driven by improvement in symptoms.

The Weiss Functional Impairment Rating Scale (WFIRS) is a parent (WFIRS-P) or self-report (WFIRS-S) survey of impairment in several distinct domains: school (learning and behavior) or work, self-concept, social, life skills, family, and high-risk activities. Identification of domain-specific scores allows the clinician to identify functional strengths and weaknesses to assist with developing targeted treatment plans for specific areas of impairment. The measure is individualized in that only items relevant to the patient are scored. Population norms for ADHD and clinical controls generated T scores, which provide estimations of clinical concern (1–1.5 SD) or ROC cutoff scores (>1.5 SD) for each domain and the total score. The WFIRS measures functional impairment *secondary* to symptoms and is highly sensitive to change, making it particularly useful as an outcome in ADHD treatment trials. The WFIRS is translated in more than 20 languages and validated in research, population, and clinical populations in 7 different countries with robust cross setting, cross informant, and cross-cultural validity.[23]

MEASUREMENT INFORMED CARE WITH ADHD-RELATED DIMENSIONS OF OUTCOME

Other domains of outcome have been found to be closely related to ADHD and patient outcomes, including executive function, emotional regulation, sluggish cognitive tempo, and mind-wandering. Specific measures to evaluate these outcomes include the Behavior Rating Inventory of Executive Function,[24] the Barkley Deficits in Executive Function Scale,[25] the Sluggish Cognitive Tempo Scale,[26] and the Mind Wandering Scale.[27] These scales are clinically relevant in providing a personalized assessment where these concerns are central in the patient's presentation and have also enabled research into the relationship between each of these domains and ADHD as a diagnosis.

Two ADHD symptom scales are particularly popular in that they give greater prominence to some of these important areas of disability critical to understanding the ADHD patient. The Wender Rheimherr [28,29] is a broad-based symptom rating scale that reflects the important role Paul Wender originally placed on emotional dysregulation as a core construct in ADHD. Tom Brown has conceptualized a model of ADHD with six domains: activation, focus, effort, emotion, memory, and action, which are in turn captured in the Brown scales for measurement of ADHD.[30] Historically, these were some of the earliest broad-based measures for clinical assessment of ADHD, which have now taken on new interest as the field has embraced moving beyond the core 18 symptoms to embrace the breadth of difficulties experienced by patients with ADHD.

SUMMARY

MIC is an essential component of best practice. This includes use of appropriate diagnostic interviews and rating scales in

- Evaluation
- Establishing a childhood history in adults

- Differential diagnosis and identification of comorbid conditions
- Obtaining collateral information from different informants and settings
- Improvement and remission of ADHD symptoms
- Improvement and remission of functional impairment secondary to symptoms
- Identification of strengths and weakness in particular domains of functional impairment
- Identification of deficits in associated domains such as executive function, emotional dysregulation, sluggish cognitive tempo, and mind-wandering

In all these areas, MIC is critical to the therapeutic alliance, patient education, efficiency and accuracy of evaluation, documentation of results, and establishment of treatment response. This review has identified some of the strengths and weakness of the tools available to assist ADHD clinicians in each of these areas. Clinicians have access to psychometrically validated, user-friendly tools to assist with all aspects of ADHD care. This has been a remarkable clinical and research achievement, which has historically done a great deal to establish confidence in the diagnosis and global access to the best standard of care.

CLINICS CARE POINTS

- ADHD-specific assessment with a child or adult begins with a diagnostic interview.
- Baseline assessment should include screening for a broad range of comorbid conditions, in addition to targeted diagnosis-specific symptom severity scales.
- Measurement of functional impairment is critical; typically, this is the chief complaint.
- MIC is the key to patient understanding of the diagnosis, shared decision-making, psychoeducation, and global initiatives to establish core global standards for clinical care, training, and research.
- Outcome measures allows the clinician to push beyond improvement in core symptoms to achieving optimal functioning and symptom remission.
- Evaluations are needed pre and post treatment, following major life changes, and at least annually to assure continued response and need for additional interventions.
- Clinicians are now able to access associated deficits such as emotional regulation and executive function, which has enriched the depth of our understanding of the patient experience and our ability to establish personalized care for their unique challenges.

DISCLOSURE

M.D. Weiss has received consulting fees/honoraria from Tris, Purdue, Adlon, Takeda, Huron, Mundipharma, MHS Assessment, Rhodes, CBPartners and Idorsia; support for travel to meetings, manuscript preparation, or other purposes from World Federation of ADHD, Eunethydis, Canadian Attention Deficit Disorder Resource Alliance (CADDRA), Children and Adults with Attention Deficit Disorder (CHADD), American Professional Society for ADHD and Related Disorders (APSARD), Israeli Federation of ADHD, Purdue CA, Purdue US, Rhodes Pharmaceutical, Akili. Takeda, Global Medical Education, and Boston Children's Hospital; payment for lectures from Global Medical Education, Center for ADHD Awareness Canada (CADDAC), and CADDRA; and has received royalties from Multi Health Systems, Johns Hopkins University Press.

REFERENCES

1. Pettersson R, Söderström S, Nilsson KW. Diagnosing ADHD in adults: an examination of the discriminative validity of neuropsychological tests and diagnostic assessment instruments. J Atten Disord 2018;22(11):1019–31.

2. Hong M, JJS K, Kim B, et al. Validity of the Korean version of DIVA-5: a semistructured diagnostic interview for adult ADHD. Neuropsychiatr Dis Treat 2020; 16:2371–6.

3. Reynolds CR, Kamphaus RW, Vannest KJ. Behavior assessment system for children (BASC). In: Kreutzer JS, DeLuca J, Caplan B, editors. Encyclopedia of clinical neuropsychology. New York: Springer; 2011. p. 366–71.

4. Gibbons RD, Weiss DJ, Frank E, et al. Computerized adaptive diagnosis and testing of mental health disorders. Annu Rev Clin Psychol 2016;12:83–104.

5. Lundervold AJ, Vartiainen H, Jensen D, et al. Test-retest reliability of the 25-item version of wender Utah rating scale. impact of current adhd severity on retrospectively assessed childhood symptoms. J Atten Disord 2021;25(7):1001–9.

6. Stein MA, Sandoval R, Szumowski E, et al. Psychometric characteristics of the Wender Utah Rating Scale (WURS): reliability and factor structure for men and women. Psychopharmacol Bull 1995;31(2):425–33.

7. Hodgkins P, Lloyd A, Erder MH, et al. Estimating minimal important differences for several scales assessing function and quality of life in patients with attention-deficit/hyperactivity disorder. CNS Spectr 2016;22:1–10. FirstView.

8. Quitkin FM, McGrath PJ, Stewart JW, et al. Chronological milestones to guide drug change. When should clinicians switch antidepressants? Arch Gesamte Psychol 1996;53(9):785–92. NOT IN FILE.

9. Sibley MH, Arnold LE, Swanson JM, et al. Variable patterns of remission from ADHD in the multimodal treatment study of ADHD. Am J Psychiatry 2021;0(0). https://doi.org/10.1176/appi.ajp.2021.21010032.

10. Swanson JM, Kraemer HC, Hinshaw SP, et al. Clinical relevance of the primary findings of the MTA: success rates based on severity of ADHD and ODD symptoms at the end of treatment. J Am Acad Child Adolesc Psychiatry 2001;40(2): 168–79. https://doi.org/10.1097/00004583-200102000-00011.

11. Weiss M, Childress A, Nordbrock E, et al. Characteristics of ADHD symptom response/remission in a clinical trial of methylphenidate extended release. J Clin Med 2019;8(4). https://doi.org/10.3390/jcm8040461.

12. Bussing R, Fernandez M, Harwood M, et al. Parent and teacher SNAP-IV ratings of attention deficit hyperactivity disorder symptoms: psychometric properties and normative ratings from a school district sample. Assessment 2008;15(3):317–28.

13. Brites C, Salgado-Azoni CA, Ferreira TL, et al. Development and applications of the SWAN rating scale for assessment of attention deficit hyperactivity disorder: a literature review. Braz J Med Biol Res 2015;48(11):965–72.

14. Lai KY, Leung PW, Luk ES, et al. Validation of the Chinese strengths and weaknesses of ADHD-symptoms and normal-behaviors questionnaire in Hong Kong. J Atten Disord 2013;17(3):194–202.

15. Izzo VA, Donati MA, Novello F, et al. The Conners 3-short forms: evaluating the adequacy of brief versions to assess ADHD symptoms and related problems. Clin Child Psychol Psychiatry 2019;24(4):791–808.

16. Hoagwood KE, Jensen PS, Acri MC, et al. Outcome domains in child mental health research since 1996: have they changed and why does it matter? J Am Acad Child Adolesc Psychiatry 2012;51(12):1241–1260 e2.

17. Coghill DR, Werner-Kiechle T, Farahbakhshian S, et al. Functional impairment outcomes in clinical trials of different ADHD medications: post hoc responder analyses and baseline subgroup analyses. Eur Child Adolesc Psychiatry 2021; 30(5):809–21.
18. Coghill DR, Joseph A, Sikirica V, et al. Correlations between clinical trial outcomes based on symptoms, functional impairments, and quality of life in children and adolescents with ADHD. J Atten Disord 2019;23(13):1578–91.
19. Bird HR, Canino G, Rubio-Stipec M, et al. Further measures of the psychometric properties of the children's global assessment scale. Arch Gen Psychiatry Sep 1987;44(9):821–4.
20. Bird HR, Canino GJ, Davies M, et al. The Brief Impairment Scale (BIS): a multidimensional scale of functional impairment for children and adolescents. J Am Acad Child Adolesc Psychiatry 2005;44(7):699–707.
21. Fabiano GA, Pelham WE Jr, Waschbusch DA, et al. A practical measure of impairment: psychometric properties of the impairment rating scale in samples of children with attention deficit hyperactivity disorder and two school-based samples. J Clin Child Adolesc Psychol 2006;35(3):369–85.
22. Barkley RA. Barkley functional impairment scale. Guilford; 2011.
23. Weiss MD, McBride NM, Craig S, et al. Conceptual review of measuring functional impairment: findings from the Weiss functional impairment rating scale. Evid Based Ment Health 2018;21(4):155–64.
24. Peters C, Algina J, Smith SW, et al. Factorial validity of the behavior rating inventory of executive function (BRIEF)-Teacher form. Child Neuropsychology 2012; 18(2):168–81.
25. Barkley RA. Deficits in executive function scale. Guilford; 2011.
26. Jacobson LA, Murphy-Bowman SC, Pritchard AE, et al. Factor structure of a sluggish cognitive tempo scale in clinically-referred children. J abnormal child Psychol 2012;40(8):1327–37.
27. Mowlem FD, Skirrow C, Reid P, et al. Validation of the mind excessively wandering scale and the relationship of mind wandering to impairment in adult ADHD. J Atten Disord 2019;23(6):624–34.
28. Marchant BK, Reimherr FW, Robison D, et al. Psychometric properties of the wender-reimherr adult attention deficit disorder scale. Psychol Assess 2013; 25(3):942–50.
29. Weibel S, Bicego F, Muller S, et al. Two facets of emotion dysregulation are core symptomatic domains in adult ADHD: results from the SR-WRAADDS, a broad symptom self-report questionnaire. J Attention Disord 2022. https://doi.org/10.1177/10870547211027647.
30. Brown T. Brown attention deficit disorder scales. Rucklidge; 2001.

Stimulants

Ann C. Childress, MD

KEYWORDS

- Stimulants • Amphetamine • Methylphenidate
- Attention-deficit/hyperactivity disorder • ADHD

KEY POINTS

- Stimulants which include methylphenidate (MPH) and amphetamine (AMPH) are the most effective treatments for attention-deficit/hyperactivity disorder (ADHD.)
- Multiple immediate-release (IR) and extended-release (ER) stimulant formulations are available.
- AMPH and MPH are both very effective.
- Patients may have a better response or tolerability to one class (AMPH or MPH) or formulation.
- A patient's individual needs should be taken into account when prescribing a stimulant.

INTRODUCTION

Attention-deficit/hyperactivity disorder (ADHD) is the most common neurobehavioral disorder in childhood with an estimated prevalence in children aged 2 to 17 years of 6.1 million in 2016.[1,2] Symptoms of ADHD consist of inattention and/or hyperactivity-impulsivity that are present on or before age 12 years, are excessive for developmental level, and impair social and academic or occupational functioning.[3] A history of ADHD in childhood is associated with lower educational achievement, lower income, risky sexual behavior, and occupational problems as adults compared to peers who did not have the disorder.[4] Treatment of ADHD may improve symptoms and associated functional impairments.[5] Medication treatment may improve academic outcome, decrease accidents and injuries, and reduce the risk of developing mood disorders.[6]

Of all available ADHD treatments, central nervous system stimulants including methylphenidate (MPH) and amphetamine (AMPH) are the most effective, with AMPH being slightly more efficacious than MPH.[7,8] Stimulants are more effective than nonstimulants (atomoxetine, guanfacine extended-release and clonidine extended-release.)[7,9]

Center for Psychiatry and Behavioral Medicine, Inc., 7351 Prairie Falcon Road, Suite 160, Las Vegas, NV 89128, USA
E-mail address: drann87@aol.com

Child Adolesc Psychiatric Clin N Am 31 (2022) 373–392
https://doi.org/10.1016/j.chc.2022.03.001
childpsych.theclinics.com

AMPH competes with endogenous monoamines (dopamine, norepinephrine, and serotonin) for transport into the nerve cells by binding to reuptake transporters, and once inside the nerve cell, it displaces monoamines from the cytosolic pool.[10] AMPH also prevents monoamine uptake into intraneuronal storage vesicles. The result is the transport of endogenous monoamines from the nerve cells into the nerve terminal.[10] MPH also binds to norepinephrine and dopamine transporters, resulting in an increase of norepinephrine and dopamine in the nerve terminal but does not cause the release of intracellular monoamines.[11]

HISTORY

AMPH was first marketed in 1935 under the brand name Benzedrine,[10] a racemic mixture (RA-AMPH), consisting of the dextro (*d*-) and levo (*l*-) isomers in an equal ratio. RA-AMPH is currently marketed in the United States (US) under different brand and generic names. In 1937, *d*-AMPH was marketed under the brand name Dexedrine.[10] RA-AMPH was not used to treat symptoms consistent with ADHD until Bradley used it for children with behavior problems in 1937 and saw rapid improvement during the first day after drug administration.[12] The *L*-isomer of AMPH alone (Cydril) was also shown to be effective in the treatment of ADHD.[10,13] It is not currently marketed in the US. MPH was first marketed in the US as Ritalin in 1955.[14]

The products initially marketed were all immediate-release (IR) compounds that must be dosed multiple times daily. For example, the duration of effect for MPH-IR is up to 4 hours and it is usually dosed three times daily.[15] Multiple daily dosing is inconvenient, doses may be forgotten and patient privacy may be impacted. Extended-release (ER) products were developed to obviate the need to take medication more than once a day. The first long-acting MPH product developed was Ritalin-SR (MPH-SR), which was approved in 1982 but has since been discontinued.[16] Although it was supposed to be equivalent to MPH-IR dosed twice daily, MPH-SR was less effective than MPH-IR.[17]

The maximum duration of effect of AMPH-IR is approximately 5.4 hours, and it also is frequently dosed three times daily.[18] A longer acting formulation, d-AMPH-SR (Dextroamphetamine Spansules) was developed for once or twice daily use. However, when d-AMPH-SR was compared with AMPH-IR, it was significantly less effective.[19]

Since 2000, advancements in technology have led to the development of multiple ER AMPH and ER MPH formulations. Some drugs have an onset of effect as early as 30 minutes after dosing, while others may take up to 2 hours to start working. Duration of efficacy also varies significantly among formulations. Some are designed to last approximately 8 hours while others may last up to 16 hours. Additionally, one formulation is designed to have an approximately 10-h delay. The percentage of IR and ER components, onset and duration of effect, specific details about each formulation's technology, adverse effects, and considerations for use will be discussed. MPH products will be presented first, then AMPH compounds. For each class, formulations will be discussed in the order that they were approved by the United States Food and Drug Administration (FDA). Brand names are listed to avoid confusion. MPH formulations are listed in **Table 1** and AMPH formulations are listed in **Table 2**.

METHYLPHENIDATE EXTENDED-RELEASE

All MPH products have similar side effects. They have a boxed warning for a "high potential for abuse and dependence."[20] In clinical trials, the most common (>5% and twice the rate of placebo) MPH adverse reactions were decreased appetite, insomnia, nausea, vomiting, dyspepsia, abdominal pain, weight decreased, anxiety, dizziness,

Table 1
Methylphenidate formulations approved since 2000

Drug	Dose Form	Effect Onset[a]	Effect Max Duration[a]	Dosing
Adhansia XR™ (MPH-MLR-XR)	25, 35, 45, 55, 70, 85 mg caps	1.0 h	16 h	25–85 mg Increase 10–15 mg q 5 d
Aptensio XR® (MPH-MLR)	10, 15, 20, 30, 40, 50, 60 mg caps	1.0 h	12 h	10–60 mg Increase by 10 mg q 7 d
Azstarys® (SDX/d-MPH)	26.1/5.2, 39.2/7.8, 52.3/10.4 mg caps	0.5 h	12 h	Start with 39.2/7.8 mg cap & increase or decrease to optimal dose
Concerta® (OROS-MPH)	18, 27, 36, 54 mg tabs	1.0 h	12.5 h	18–54 mg children 18–72 mg adolescents and adults (Not to exceed 2 mg/kg/d)
Cotempla XR-ODT® (MPH-ER ODT)	8.6, 17.3, 25.9 mg tabs	1.0 h	12 h	17.3–51.8 mg Increase 8.6–17.3 mg/ d q 7 d
Daytrana® (MTS)	10, 15, 20, 30 mg patch	2 h	12 h (when worn for 9 h)	10–30 mg
Focalin® (d-MPH)	2.5, 5, 10 mg tabs	not reported	6.3–7.5 h	5–20 mg New patients-start at 5 mg Patients on MPH, start at ½ MPH dose Titrate weekly 2.5–5 mg
Focalin XR® (d-MPH-ER)	5, 10, 15, 20, 25, 30, 35, 40 mg caps	0.5 h	12 h	5–30 mg children 10–40 mg adults
Jornay PM® (DR/ER-MPH)	20, 40, 60, 80, 100 mg caps	10 h after dosing	23 h after dosing	20–100 mg Increase 20 mg weekly
Metadate CD® (MPH-CD)	10, 20, 30, 40, 50, 60 mg caps	1.5 h	7.5–12 h (depending on dose)	10–60 mg
Quillivant XR® (MEROS)	ER suspension 25 mg/5 mL	0.75 h	12 h	20–60 mg Increase 10–20 mg q 7 d
QuilliChew ER ® (MPH-ER-CT)	20, 30, 40 mg tabs	2.0 h	8 h	20–60 mg Increase 10–20 mg q 7 d
Ritalin LA® (MPH-LA)	10,20,30, 40 mg caps	0.5 h	10–12 h (depending on dose)	10–60 mg

Abbreviations: caps, capsules; CD, controlled delivery; CT, chewable tablet; DR/ER, delayed-release/extended-release; ER, extended-release; h, hour; LA, long-acting; MEROS, methylphenidate extended-release oral suspension; mg, milligram; MLR, multi-layer release; MPH, methylphenidate; MTS, methylphenidate transdermal system; ODT, oral disintegrating tablet; OROS, osmotic release oral system; SDX, serdexmethylphenidate; tabs, tablets; XR, extended-release.

[a] Data for onset and duration of effect may not be in the Food and Drug Administration approved label.

irritability, affect lability, tachycardia and increased blood pressure.[21] Other reported adverse events include: crying, daydreams, anxiety, emotional disturbances, social withdrawal, fingernail biting, headaches, tics, somnolence, mood alteration, night-mares, unusually happy, fatigue, dry mouth, nervousness, changes in heart rate, abnormal behavior and depression.[22] The MPH label also contains warnings regarding serious cardiovascular reactions, blood pressure and heart rate increases, psychiatric adverse reactions, priapism, peripheral vasculopathy and long term suppression of growth.[20] Some formulations have unique side effects because of the technology used or the route of administration and these adverse effects will be discussed with individual products.

Concerta

Concerta (Osmotic-Release Oral System, or OROS MPH) was approved by the FDA to treat children and adolescents in 2000 and is currently indicated for patients aged 6 to 65 years with ADHD.[23] It was designed to mimic MPH-IR dosing three times daily. The OROS MPH tablet is comprised of an IR MPH overcoat containing 22% of the total MPH designed to dissolve within 1 hour and a tri-layer core that is osmotically active.[23] The core contains a semipermeable membrane with 2 drug layers and a push layer. The end of the tablet contains a laser-drilled hole that allows fluid into the inner layers. Drug is then pushed out of the tablet as osmotically active excipients expand. OROS has an initial peak MPH concentration at 1 hour, then a gently ascending subsequent peak during the next 5 to 9 hours followed by a gradual decrease in MPH concentration. The drug label indicates that the onset of effect is at 2 hours after dosing and continues through 12 hours.[23] However, a laboratory classroom trial demonstrated efficacy from 1 hour through 12.5 hours after dosing.[24]

Because of the unique technology used, the OROS MPH tablet does not dissolve. There is the potential for gastrointestinal (GI) obstruction because the tablet does not change shape in the GI tract.[23] It also must be swallowed whole and cannot be cut, crushed, or chewed.

Metadate CD

Metadate CD (MPH-CD) is approved by the FDA for the treatment of ADHD in children and adolescents aged 6 to 15 years.[25] The formulation is composed of 30% MPH-IR beads and 70% MPH-ER beads. After dosing, MPH-CD has an initial maximum concentration (Cmax) at about 1.5 hours. A second peak occurs at approximately 4.5 hours after dosing.[25] In a clinical trial comparing MPH-CD with OROS-MPH, MPH-CD demonstrated an onset of effect at 1.5 hours after dosing and efficacy waned after 7.5 hours.[26]

Focalin

Focalin (dexmethylphenidate, or d-MPH) is the active D-isomer of d,l-MPH and is administered at half the dose of d,l-MPH.[27] For MPH, the D-isomer is the more physiologically active of the 2 isomers.[28] Efficacy of d-MPH was established in a 4-week, double-blind, placebo-controlled trial that enrolled subjects aged 6 to 17 years.[27] Median duration of effect is estimated to be 6.3 to 7.5 hours.[29]

Ritalin LA

Ritalin LA (MPH-LA) is approved for the treatment of ADHD in patients aged 6 to 12 years.[30] The formulation uses the SODAS (Spheroidal Oral Drug Absorption System) technology.[31] Each capsule of MPH-LA contains half as IR beads and half as enteric-coated, delayed-release beads. After dosing, MPH-LA has a bi-modal plasma

Table 2
Amphetamine formulations approved since 2000

Drug	Dose Form	Effect Onset [a]	Max Effect Duration [a]	FDA Approved Dosing
Adderall XR® (MAS-XR)	5, 10, 15, 20, 25, 30 mg caps	1.5 h	12.5 h	5–30 mg (aged 6–12y) 5–20 mg (aged 13–17y) 20 mg adults
Adzenys XR- ODT® (AMPH-XR-ODT)	3.1, 6.3, 9.4, 12.5, 15.7, 18.8 mg tabs	Bioequivalent to MAS-XR	Bioequivalent to MAS-XR	6.3–18.8 mg (aged 6–12y) 6.3–12.5 mg (aged 13–17y) 12.5 mg adults
Adzenys ER® SUSPENSION (AMPH-ER-SUSP)	1.25 mg/mL ER suspension	Bioequivalent to MAS-XR	Bioequivalent to MAS-XR	6.3–18.8 mg (aged 6–12y) 6.3–12.5 mg (aged 13–17y) 12.5 mg adults
Dyanavel® XR (AMPH-EROS& AMPH-ER-CT)	2.5 mg/mL ER suspension 5, 10, 15, 20 mg tabs	0.5 h	13 h	2.5–20 mg (aged 6y and older) Increase 2.5–5 mg q 4–7 d
Evekeo® (RA-AMPH)	5 and 10 mg tablets	0.75 h	10 h	5–40 mg divided daily or twice daily (aged 6y and older)
Evekeo ODT® (RA-AMPH-ODT)	5, 10, 15, 20 mg tabs	Bioequivalent to RA-AMPH	Bioequivalent to RA-AMPH	Aged 6–17y Start 5 mg once or twice daily Increase 5 mg weekly Maximum dose not listed in label
Mydayis® (SHP465-MAS)	12.5, 25, 37.5, 50 mg caps	2.0 h	16 h	12.5–25 mg (aged 13–17y) 12.5–50 mg adults
Vyvanse® (LDX)	10, 20, 30, 40, 50, 60, 70 mg caps 10, 20, 30, 40, 50, 60 mg chewable tabs	1.5 h	14 h in adults 13 h in children	30–70 mg Increase 10–20 mg weekly

Abbreviations: AMPH, amphetamine; caps, capsules; CT, chewable tablet; ER, extended-release; EROS, extended-release oral suspension; h, hours; LDX, lisdexamfetamine.MAS, mixed amphetamine salts; mg, milligram; ODT, oral disintegrating tablet; RA, racemic amphetamine; SUSP, suspension; tabs, tablets; XR, extended-release; y, year.

[a] Data for onset and duration of effect may not be in the Food and Drug Administration approved label.

concentration–time profile with 2 peaks about 4 hours apart.[30] Duration of effect ranges from 10 to 12 hours depending on dose.[32]

Focalin XR

Focalin XR (*d*-MPH-ER) is an ER formulation of *d*-MPH developed using the SODAS technology and is indicated for the treatment of patients aged 6 years and older.[33,34] It has a bimodal plasma concentration-time pharmacokinetic curve with 2 peaks that occur approximately 4 hours apart.[33]

In laboratory classroom studies, the onset of effect was seen as early as 30 minutes after dosing and lasted through 12 hours.[34,35] Duration of effect depends on dose, with 30 mg showing significant improvement at 12 hours after dosing compared with 20 mg.[36] Additionally, d-MPH-ER 20 mg and 30 mg were compared with OROS MPH 36 mg and 54 mg and to placebo in a laboratory classroom trial.[37] The d-MPH-ER doses had a faster onset of efficacy while OROS MPH showed greater effect at the end of a 12-h classroom day.

Daytrana

Daytrana, an MPH transdermal patch (MTS), is approved for the treatment of ADHD in patients aged 6 to 17 years.[38] The patch contains MPH in a multipolymeric adhesive that is dispersed in a silicon adhesive.[38] The dose of MPH delivered is a function of wear time and patch size. MTS sizes describe the amount of MPH delivered during a 9-h wear time. Instructions in the drug label state that the MTS should be applied to alternating hips approximately 2 hours before the time that an effect is required, and it should be removed by 9 hours after application.[38] With a 9-h wear time, efficacy was seen in a laboratory classroom from 2 through 12 hours.[39] In another trial, a 4-h wear time was efficacious through 6 hours after application, while a 6-h wear time was efficacious through 8 hours.[40]

In addition to the usual MPH adverse events, mild to moderate skin erythema and irritant contact dermatitis are frequent side effects.[41] Rare MTS side effects include allergic contact dermatitis, allergic contact urticaria and chemical leukoderma. Furthermore, direct heat should not be applied to the application site as it will increase the rate and amount of MPH absorption.[38]

Quillivant XR

Quillivant XR (MPH-ER Oral Suspension, or MEROS) is approved for the treatment of ADHD in patients aged 6 years and older.[20] The formulation consists of a MPH- polistirex polymeric resin complex. Polistirex carries a negative charge and MPH HCl dissolved in water carries a positive charge. MPH molecules bind to polistirex in solution via ion exchange and form drug/polymer particles.[42] Some of the particles are coated with a permeable water-insoluble ER coating of varying thicknesses. MPH release is determined by the thickness of the ER coating via diffusion and ion exchange in the gut.[43] MEROS is bioequivalent to 2 doses of MPH-IR liquid dosed 6 hours apart.[44]

In a laboratory classroom study, the onset of drug effect occurred at 45 minutes after dosing and therapeutic effect lasted through 12 hours.[42] MEROS is available in a tropical fruit flavored suspension containing 25 mg of MPH HCl per 5 mL.[20] It is delivered to the pharmacy in glass bottles as a powder and is reconstituted before dispensing.[45]

QuilliChew ER

QuilliChew ER (MPH-ER Chewable Tablets, or MPH-ERCT) is approved for patients aged 6 years and older.[46] MPH-ERCT consists of the same ion exchange resin (sodium polystyrene sulfonate) MPH complex technology used in the MEROS but is compressed into tablets.[47] The tablets contain both IR and ER MPH components. Early exposure area under the curve from 0 to 4 hours of MPH-ERCT (AUC_{0-4}) is approximately 15% lower than for MEROS.[48] MPH-ERCT chewed or swallowed whole is bioequivalent.

In a laboratory classroom study, MPH-ERCT significantly improved ADHD symptoms in comparison to placebo from 0.75 through 8 hours after dosing.[49]

Aptensio XR

Aptensio XR (MPH-MLR) is modified-release ER MPH approved for patients aged 6 years and older.[50] Each capsule contains multi-layer beads composed of an IR and ER layer. Approximately 40% of the formulation is IR MPH and 60% is contained in a controlled-release layer. This composition results in a biphasic pharmacokinetic profile with an initial Cmax occurring at approximately 2 hours and a second Cmax at approximately 7 hours postdose.[51] In a laboratory classroom study, efficacy was seen at 1 through 12 hours after dosing in children aged 6 to 12 years.[52]

Although MPH-MLR is not approved in children younger than 6 years of age, it has been studied and was shown to be effective in pediatric patients aged 4 to 5 years.[53] The MPH-MLR label contains a limitation of use and states that patients in this age group "experienced higher plasma exposure than patients aged 6 years and older at the same dose and high rates of adverse reactions, most notably weight loss."[50]

Cotempla XR-ODT

Cotempla XR (MPH-XR) ODT is an Oral Disintegrating Tablet (ODT) approved for children and adolescents aged 6 to 17 years.[54] MPH-XR ODT is also a formulation produced using ion exchange technology similar to that of MPH-ERCT and MEROS.[55] The tablets disintegrate in the mouth without the need for water. About 75% of the MPH-resin particles are coated. In a laboratory classroom trial, drug efficacy was seen from 1 through 12 hours after dosing.[56]

MPH-XR ODT is available in 8.6 mg, 17.3 mg, and 25.9 mg strengths. These doses are equivalent to MPH HCl 10, 20 and 30 mg. Stimulant dosing has traditionally used the amount of the drug in the salt form.[57] However, MPH-XR ODTs do not contain MPH HCl–only the MPH base. In May 2013, the FDA enacted the U. S. Pharmacopeia Salt Policy rule which required that new medication dosing be based on the active moiety and not the salt form to clarify the relationship between AMPH/MPH base and salt forms of different products to help avoid medication errors.[58]

Jornay PM

Jornay PM (delayed-release and extended-release MPH, or DR/ER-MPH) is approved for patients aged 6 years and older.[59] It consists of beaded capsules. Each bead contains an outer DR and inner ER functional film coating that surround a drug core coated with MPH. The outer coating delays the initial release of MPH by about 10 hours while the inner ER coating controls drug release throughout the day. After taking the drug the evening before, in a 12-h laboratory classroom, a significant improvement compared to placebo was seen the next day at all time points from 10 AM to 7 PM.[60]

Adhansia XR

Adhansia XR (MPH-MLR-XR) is an ER MPH that is indicated for the treatment of ADHD for patients aged 6 years and older.[61] MPH-MLR-XR produces 2 concentration peaks. The first occurs at approximately 1.5 hours and the second occurs at approximately 12 hours after dosing. In a laboratory classroom study in children, the onset of efficacy was seen at 1 hour postdose and duration of effect through 13 hours (the last time point measured.)[62] For adults, effects lasted from 1 through 16 hours.[63] Despite the long duration of effect, insomnia was reported by 10.3% of child participants during open-label dose-optimization and 16.1% of adults in trials.[62,63]

Azstarys

Azstarys (dexmethylphenidate HCl/serdexmethylphenidate HCl, or SDX/d-MPH) is a combination of d-MPH and d-MPH prodrug approved in March 2021.[64,65] The drug is available in 26.1/5.2, 39.2/7.8 and 52.3/10.4 mg capsules (equivalent to 28/6, 42/9 and 56/12 mg of SDX HCl/d-MPH HCl, respectively.) These doses correspond to 20, 30 and 40 mg of d-MPH HCl.[64] After a single dose of SDX/d-MPH, the median time to Cmax is about 2 hours, and after administration of SDX alone the Cmax occurs at 8 hours after dosing. Although the combination product is a Schedule II drug, the Drug Enforcement Administration recommended that SDX receive a Schedule IV designation.[66] Efficacy of SDX/d-MPH in a laboratory classroom study was seen from 0.5 through 13 hours postdose.[64]

AMPHETAMINE EXTENDED-RELEASE

All AMPH formulations have similar side effects, and many are comparable to those of MPH products. The most common adverse events seen in clinical trials with AMPH products include dry mouth, anorexia, weight loss, abdominal pain, nausea, insomnia, restlessness, emotional lability, dizziness and tachycardia.[67] Other reported effects in clinical trials include: irritability, crying, daydreams, anxiety, emotional disturbances, social withdrawal, fingernail biting, stomachaches, headaches, tics, somnolence, dizziness, nightmares, unusually happy, fatigue, nervousness, vomiting and fever.[22,68]

All AMPH products carry a boxed warning for the risk of abuse and dependence.[68] Contraindications in the drug prescribing information include advanced arteriosclerosis, symptomatic cardiovascular disease, moderate to severe hypertension, hyperthyroidism, allergy to AMPH, glaucoma, agitated states, history of drug abuse and use within 14 days of administration of a monoamine oxidase inhibitor. Warnings and precautions in the drug labels include serious cardiovascular reactions, increase in blood pressure, psychiatric adverse events, long-term suppression of growth, seizures, peripheral vasculopathy, serotonin syndrome, visual disturbances and tics.

Adderall XR

Adderall XR (mixed AMPH salts ER, or MAS-XR) is comprised of a combination of 4 AMPH salts: AMPH aspartate, AMPH sulfate, d-AMPH saccharate and d-AMPH sulfate.[68] The compound has a 3:1 ratio of d-AMPH to l-AMPH. The maximum dose approved for children aged 6 to 12 years is 30 mg, while in adults, the dose is 20 mg.[68]

In a laboratory classroom study, MAS-XR 10, 20 and 30 mg were all efficacious beginning at 2 hours after dosing.[69] MAS-XR 10, 20, 30 and 40 mg were also evaluated in adolescents aged 13 to 17 years in a double-blind, forced-dose, parallel-group study.[70] The greatest decrease in ADHD symptoms occurred in the MAS-XR 20 mg group. The maximum dose approved for children aged 13 to 17 years is not explicitly stated in the drug label, although doses greater than 20 mg are not discussed.[68]

Vyvanse

Vyvanse (lisdexamfetamine dimesylate, or LDX) is a prodrug formulation containing d-AMPH and lysine that is approved for the treatment of ADHD in patients aged 6 years and older.[71] Initial approval for children aged 6 to 12 years was received in 2007. LDX is currently available in capsules and chewable tablets.[71] LDX is converted to d-AMPH and L-lysine via peptidase mediated hydrolysis by red blood cells after it is absorbed from the GI tract.[72] The Tmax of LDX is achieved at about 1 hour after dosing, and the Tmax of d-AMPH is reached at 3.5 hours after dosing.

The onset and duration of effect of LDX were evaluated in multiple laboratory classroom studies. In children, the onset of LDX effect occurred by 1.5 hours and lasted through 13 hours after dosing.[73] For adults aged 18 to 55 years, efficacy was observed from 2 to 14 hours after dosing.[74]

Although not approved in children aged 4 to 5 years, LDX effects at doses of 5 to 30 mg were studied and found to be effective.[75] The label for the drug contains a limitation of use in preschoolers because of long-term weight loss.[71]

Adzenys XR-ODT

Adzenys XR-ODT (AMPH extended-release orally disintegrating tablet, or AMPH-XR-ODT) contains a 3:1 ratio of d-to L-AMPH.[76] AMPH-XR-ODT was developed using a similar technology to MPH-XR-ODT, a cation exchange-resin.[77] The positively charged sodium ion from the exchange resin is replaced by the positively charged AMPH. Some of the ensuing microparticles are left uncoated (50%) and the other 50% are covered with an ER coating. The AMPH-XR-ODT formulation is bioequivalent to MAS-XR, meaning that Tmax, Cmax and total drug exposure are similar for both compounds.[77] The dose strengths are listed as AMPH base only, as there is no salt in the formulation.[57]

Adzenys ER

Adzenys ER (AMPH extended-release oral suspension, or AMPH-ER SUSP) uses the same technology and 3:1 ratio of d-to l AMPH as AMPH-XR-ODT, but instead of being pressed into a capsule, the formulation was manufactured as an oral suspension containing 1.25 mg AMPH per mL.[78] It is also bioequivalent to MAS-XR. The Drugs@FDA website notes that the marketing status is "discontinued."[79]

Evekeo and Evekeo ODT

Evekeo (racemic AMPH, or RA-AMPH) is an IR formulation that contains an equal amount of d- and l-AMPH.[80] It is approved for the treatment of ADHD in patients aged 3 years and older. The efficacy of RA-AMPH was evaluated in a double-blind, placebo-controlled, crossover laboratory classroom study.[81] Onset of effect was seen at 45 minutes after ingestion and lasted through 10 hours after a single morning dose.

Evekeo ODT (RA-AMPH-ODT) was approved by the FDA in January 2019.[82] It is bioequivalent to RA-AMPH and is indicated for the treatment of patients with ADHD aged 3 to 17 years.[83]

Zenzedi

Zenzedi (d-AMPH IR) is indicated as a treatment of ADHD in patients aged 3 to 16 years. It is available in dose strengths that are not available for generic d-AMPH IR. After administration of 15 mg of d-AMPH-IR, Cmax occurred at about 3 hours after dosing. The half-life was approximately 12 hours.[84]

Dyanavel XR

Dyanavel XR (AMPH extended-release oral suspension, or AMPH-EROS and AMPH-ER-CT) are ER formulations of d- and l-AMPH in a 3.2:1 ratio approved for the treatment of ADHD in patients aged 6 years and older.[67] The suspension is available in a concentration of 2.5 mg AMPH base per 1 mL of liquid, and the tablet is FDA approved in dosage strengths from 5 to 20 mg but not yet available. Similar to AMPH-ER SUSP, AMPH-ER-ODT and MPH-ER-ODT, AMPH positively charged ions are mixed with sodium polystyrene sulfonate resin, and the drug–resin complex forms micron-sized particles.[85] AMPH-EROS contains both IR and ER AMPH components. To make the ER component, an aqueous, pH-independent polymer coating of varying thickness is added to some of the IR particles. For AMPH-EROS, 1 mL containing 2.5 mg of AMPH-ER is equivalent to 4 mg of MAS.[67]

The efficacy of AMPH-EROS was evaluated in a children's laboratory classroom.[86] Onset of effect was seen at 1 hour after dosing and lasted through 13 hours after dosing. In another classroom trial, the onset of efficacy was seen at 30 minutes after dosing.[87]

Mydayis

Mydayis (SHP465 mixed AMPH salts, or SHP465 MAS) is approved by the FDA for the treatment of ADHD in patients aged 12 years and older.[88] In a laboratory classroom study in adolescents, onset of efficacy was observed at 2 hours and continued through 16 hours.[89] The SHP465 MAS prescribing information contains a limitation of use for patients aged 12 years and younger because of higher drug plasma levels than older patients at the same dose and "higher rates of adverse reactions, mainly insomnia and decreased appetite."[88]

DISCUSSION
Considerations When Choosing a Medication

With all of the available formulations, it might seem to be a daunting task to decide which medication to prescribe. The first task is to decide whether to prescribe MPH or AMPH. Cortese and colleagues[9] recently conducted a meta-analysis of 81 double-blind, randomized trials in children and adolescents and found that AMPH was slightly more effective but not tolerated as well as MPH. In an earlier review of crossover trials that compared AMPH with MPH, 68% to 97% of subjects responded to at least one class of medications.[90] Stein and colleagues[91] compared d-MPH-ER and MAS-XR and found that about 43% of subjects were preferential responders to only one of the formulations. So, it is reasonable to start with an MPH product in a stimulant naïve patient. If the patient has only a partial response or is unable to tolerate MPH, they can switch to an AMPH product.

Can the Patient Swallow a Tablet or Capsule?

Next, consider whether the patient is able to swallow a tablet or capsule. Oral suspensions, chewable tablets and ODTs are available for both MPH and AMPH. The MTS should also be considered for patients who may be unable or unwilling to take an oral formulation. Furthermore, most oral formulations are available as capsules that can be opened and the contents sprinkled on applesauce. The contents must be consumed immediately and should not be chewed to avoid dose-dumping. OROS MPH must be swallowed whole. LDX capsules' contents can also be sprinkled onto yogurt or dissolved in a small amount of water or orange juice.[71] MPH-MLR-XR capsules can also be sprinkled on yogurt.[61]

Targeting Specific Times of Day

Other factors should be considered when choosing a product. For example, what time of day is the patient having the most difficulty? For patients who have significant early morning problems, DR/ER-MPH may be a good choice. EROS, d-MPH-ER, and SDX/

d-MPH have demonstrated 30-minute onset of effect, and MPH-ER-CT and RA-AMPH have demonstrated 45-minute onset.[35,47,81,86]

Most of the compounds approved to treat ADHD since 2000 are ER products and have at least a 12-h duration of effect after dose optimization in a controlled laboratory classroom.

For patients who require efficacy later in the day, LDX, EROS and SDX/d-MPH demonstrated effect through 13 hours after dosing.[73,86] Two compounds (MPH-MLR-XR and SHP465 MAS) have an effect through 16 hours after dosing; however, only MPH-MLR-XR is FDA approved for the treatment of children younger than 13 years of age.[61,88]

Sometimes a patient may have a good response to a particular formulation, but it is not lasting long enough. Rather than switching to another product, the duration of effect may be extended by simply increasing the dose.[36,92] When increasing the dose to extend duration, side effects should be monitored. Peak drug concentrations will increase with a higher dose and patients may have tolerability issues earlier in the day.

Converting from One Formulation to Another

It is important to remember that one cannot compare different formulations on a mg per mg basis. The U. S. Pharmacopeia Salt Policy rule was discussed earlier. The doses of AMPH and MPH base do not consist of round numbers for most formulations and are difficult to remember. Some handy conversions include multiplying the MPH HCl strength by 0.8647 to obtain the MPH-XR ODT equivalent dose and the RA-AMPH dose by 0.7340 to obtain the equivalent AMPH-XR ODT dose.[57]

It is advisable to keep dosing instructions from the manufacturer handy or bookmark https://www.accessdata.fda.gov/scripts/cder/daf/. This link will take one to the FDA search page for drugs. Typing in the drug name will open the drug page, and clicking on the label link will access the "Highlights of Prescribing Information" page for every marketed drug. The "Dosage Forms and Strengths" section will list available doses.

Additionally, the area of drug release and absorption will affect dosing because of differences in bioavailability. DR/ER-MPH is a good example. Because the drug is released in the colon, absorption is less efficient than in the upper GI tract. Bioavailability compared with the same daily dose of IR MPH dosed three times a day in adults was 73.9%.[59] The optimized dose of DR/ER MPH in subjects who had previously taken other MPH products was actually higher than would be expected based solely on bioavailability. The mean dose conversion ratios ranged from 1.8 to 4.3 for DR/ER-MPH compared with a previous dose of ER stimulant monotherapy and from 4.7 to 6.0 for previous treatment with IR stimulants.[93]

Single Isomer Versus Racemic Formulation

Another factor to consider is the use of a single isomer formulation or a racemic formulation. For MPH, the d-threo-enantiomer preferentially enters the brain. Plasma concentrations are about 10 to 40 times higher for the d-threo enantiomer than those for the L-enantiomer.[94] Dose of d-MPH should be at half that of racemic MPH. One might expect fewer side effects with just the D-isomer, but no data supports this concept.

For AMPH, both the d- and l-isomers are effective.[10] At the present time, only d-AMPH and d,l-AMPH formulations are marketed. The relative potencies of the 2 isomers have been compared in vitro. The D-isomer is about 4 times as potent at releasing dopamine, and they are equipotent at releasing norepinephrine.[10] Both isomers are effective in reducing ADHD symptoms, and adverse effects are not significantly different between them .[95]

Bioequivalence

Although many of the new ER formulations were approved based on their bioequivalence to older MPH or AMPH products, some patients may respond differently based on the technology of the product. For example, MAS-XR is composed of 50% IR and 50% ER beads. Each capsule may contain a few hundred beads. AMPH-XR ODT contains millions of microparticles with different coatings of different thickness for the ER portion. Rather than releasing all at once, the ER portion is released more continuously. This gradual release mechanism may improve tolerability for some patients.

Caution also must be used when switching from branded to generic products or from one generic to another. To be bioequivalent, the product has to have drug concentrations between 80% and 125% of the reference product.[96] Therefore, if one product is on the low end ($\sim$80%) and another is on the high end ($\sim$125%), a patient may have tolerability or efficacy issues with a switch.

LONG-TERM TREATMENT
Growth

A recent meta-analysis of studies with data from at least 6 months of MPH exposure found small but statistically significant pre-versus post-dose impact on height and weight z-scores.[97] Impact on weight was largest during the first 12 months and height was largest during the first 24 to 30 months.

Although data from a meta-analysis is not available for AMPH, a 2-year study with LDX found that there was a shift to a lower z score for height, weight and BMI.

Cardiovascular Effects

A longitudinal study of all children born in Denmark between 1990 and 1999 with a mean follow-up of 9.4 years, found that among children diagnosed with ADHD and taking prescription medication compared with nonusers, there was an increased risk of cardiovascular events including arrhythmia (23%), cerebrovascular disease (9%), hypertension (8%), ischemic heart disease (2%), heart failure (2%) and pulmonary hypertension (<1%).[98]

A retrospective analysis of 171,126 insured patients aged 6 to 21 years who did not have a cardiovascular history found 0.92 new cardiac events and 3.08 new cardiac symptoms per 1,000,000 days of stimulant use.[99] Compared to no use, the odds ratio of cardiac events was 0.69 for current stimulant use and 1.18 during past stimulant use. No significant differences were seen with MPH versus AMPH use. The authors concluded that cardiovascular events were rare and not associated with stimulant use.

SUMMARY

Multiple AMPH and MPH products have been approved to treat ADHD in the past two decades. The formulations differ in the percentage of IR and ER ingredients, technology used and dosage form. The properties determine the unique pharmacokinetics of each product. As pharmacokinetics and pharmacodynamics are tightly linked, the onset and duration vary between formulations. These distinctions allow clinicians to choose among different formulations to best suit the needs of individual patients. Although the differences may seem small, they may be extremely important to a patient with difficulties at a particular time of day or tolerability issues with one formulation and not another.

CLINICS CARE POINTS

- AMPH and MPH are the most effective medications to treat ADHD
- Many AMPH and MPH formulations are available, and ER drugs also contain an IR component
- ODTs, chewable tablets and suspensions have been developed for patients who have difficulty swallowing tablets or capsules
- Formulations have different onset and duration of effect based on their pharmacokinetics
- Side effects are common with stimulant treatment, and a switch to another formulation may improve tolerability
- Patients should be monitored closely when switching between branded and generic products or from one generic to another

DISCLOSURE

Dr A.C. Childress reports receipt of research or writing support, participation on advisory boards and service as a consultant or speaker for Adlon Therapeutics, Akili Interactive, Allergan, Arbor Pharmaceuticals, Cingulate Therapeutics, Emalex Biosciences, Ironshore Pharmaceuticals, Jazz Pharmaceuticals, KemPharm, Lumos, Neos Therapeutics, Noven, Otsuka, Purdue Pharma, Rhodes Pharmaceuticals, Servier, Shire, Sunovion, Supernus Pharmaceuticals, Takeda and Tris Pharma.

REFERENCES

1. Wolraich ML, Hagan JF Jr, Allan C, et al. Clinical practice guideline for the diagnosis, evaluation, and treatment of attention-deficit/hyperactivity disorder in children and adolescents. Pediatrics 2019;144(4):e20192528.
2. Danielson ML, Bitsko RH, Ghandour RM, et al. Prevalence of parent-reported ADHD diagnosis and associated treatment among U.S. Children and adolescents, 2016. J Clin Child Adolesc Psychol 2018;47(2):199–212.
3. American Psychiatric Association. American psychiatric association. DSM-5 Task Force. Diagnostic and statistical manual of mental disorders : DSM-5. 5th edition. xliv: American Psychiatric Association; 2013. p. 947.
4. Hechtman L, Swanson JM, Sibley MH, et al. Functional adult outcomes 16 years after childhood diagnosis of attention-deficit/hyperactivity disorder: MTA results. J Am Acad Child Adolesc Psychiatry 2016;55(11):945–952 e2.
5. Faraone SV, Asherson P, Banaschewski T, et al. Attention-deficit/hyperactivity disorder. Nat Rev Dis Primers 2015;1:15020.
6. Boland H, DiSalvo M, Fried R, et al. A literature review and meta-analysis on the effects of ADHD medications on functional outcomes. J Psychiatr Res 2020;123: 21–30.
7. Joseph A, Ayyagari R, Xie M, et al. Comparative efficacy and safety of attention-deficit/hyperactivity disorder pharmacotherapies, including guanfacine extended release: a mixed treatment comparison. Eur Child Adolesc Psychiatry 2017;26(8): 875–97.
8. Faraone SV, Buitelaar J. Comparing the efficacy of stimulants for ADHD in children and adolescents using meta-analysis. Eur Child Adolesc Psychiatry 2010; 19(4):353–64.

9. Cortese S, Adamo N, Del Giovane C, et al. Comparative efficacy and tolerability of medications for attention-deficit hyperactivity disorder in children, adolescents, and adults: a systematic review and network meta-analysis. Lancet Psychiatry 2018;5(9):727–38.

10. Heal DJ, Smith SL, Gosden J, et al. Amphetamine, past and present–a pharmacological and clinical perspective. J Psychopharmacol 2013;27(6):479–96.

11. Shellenberg TP, Stoops WW, Lile JA, et al. An update on the clinical pharmacology of methylphenidate: therapeutic efficacy, abuse potential and future considerations. Expert Rev Clin Pharmacol 2020;13(8):825–33.

12. Bradley C. The behavior of children receiving benzedrine. Am J Psychiatry 1937; 94:577–85.

13. Arnold LE, Wender PH, McCloskey K, et al. Levoamphetamine and dextroamphetamine: comparative efficacy in the hyperkinetic syndrome. Assessment by target symptoms. Arch Gen Psychiatry 1972;27(6):816–22.

14. Morton WA, Stockton GG. Methylphenidate abuse and psychiatric side effects. Prim Care Companion J Clin Psychiatry 2000;2(5):159–64.

15. Childress AC. Methylphenidate HCL for the treatment of ADHD in children and adolescents. Expert Opin Pharmacother 2016;17(8):1171–8.

16. Drugs@FDA: FDA-Approved Drugs. New drug application (NDA): 018029. Available at: https://www.accessdata.fda.gov/scripts/cder/daf/index.cfm?event=overview.process&ApplNo=018029. Accessed 29 August, 2021.

17. Pelham WE Jr, Greenslade KE, Vodde-Hamilton M, et al. Relative efficacy of long-acting stimulants on children with attention deficit-hyperactivity disorder: a comparison of standard methylphenidate, sustained-release methylphenidate, sustained-release dextroamphetamine, and pemoline. Pediatrics 1990;86(2):226–37.

18. Taylor FB, Russo J. Comparing guanfacine and dextroamphetamine for the treatment of adult attention-deficit/hyperactivity disorder. J Clin Psychopharmacol 2001;21(2):223–8.

19. James RS, Sharp WS, Bastain TM, et al. Double-blind, placebo-controlled study of single-dose amphetamine formulations in ADHD. J Am Acad Child Adolesc Psychiatry 2001;40(11):1268–76.

20. Highlights of Prescribing Information Quillivant XR (methylphenidate hydrochloride) for extended-release oral suspension, CII. Available at: https://www.accessdata.fda.gov/drugsatfda_docs/label/2021/202100s018lbl.pdf. Accessed 06 September, 2021.

21. Cotempla XR-ODT (methylphenidate extended-release orally disintegrating tablets), CII. Highlights of prescribing information. Available at: https://www.accessdata.fda.gov/drugsatfda_docs/label/2017/205489s000lbl.pdf. Accessed 30 June, 2019.

22. Clavenna A, Bonati M. Pediatric pharmacoepidemiology - safety and effectiveness of medicines for ADHD. Expert Opin Drug Saf 2017;16(12):1335–45.

23. Concerta (methylphenidate HCl) extended-release tablets, CII. Highlights of prescribing information. Available at: https://www.accessdata.fda.gov/drugsatfda_docs/label/2017/021121s038lbl.pdf. Accessed 29 August, 2021.

24. Armstrong RB, Damaraju CV, Ascher S, et al. Time course of treatment effect of OROS(R) methylphenidate in children with ADHD. J Atten Disord 2012;16(8):697–705.

25. Once daily metadate CD (methylphenidate HCl, USP) extended-release capsules CII. Available at: https://www.accessdata.fda.gov/drugsatfda_docs/label/2021/021259s032lbl.pdf. Accessed 30 August, 2021.

26. Swanson JM, Wigal SB, Wigal T, et al. A comparison of once-daily extended-release methylphenidate formulations in children with attention-deficit/hyperactivity disorder in the laboratory school (the Comacs Study). Pediatrics 2004;113(3 Pt 1):e206–16.

27. Wigal S, Swanson JM, Feifel D, et al. A double-blind, placebo-controlled trial of dexmethylphenidate hydrochloride and d,l-threo-methylphenidate hydrochloride in children with attention-deficit/hyperactivity disorder. J Am Acad Child Adolesc Psychiatry 2004;43(11):1406–14.

28. Srinivas NR, Hubbard JW, Quinn D, et al. Enantioselective pharmacokinetics and pharmacodynamics of dl-threo-methylphenidate in children with attention deficit hyperactivity disorder. Clin Pharmacol Ther 1992;52(5):561–8.

29. Keating GM, Figgitt DP. Dexmethylphenidate. Drugs 2002;62(13):1899–904 [discussion: 1905-8].

30. Highlights of Prescribing Information Ritalin LA (methylphenidate hydrochloride) extended-release capsules. Available at: https://www.accessdata.fda.gov/drugsatfda_docs/label/2021/021284s043lbl.pdf. Accessed 05 September, 2021.

31. Novartis Ritalin LA® (methylphenidate hydrochloride) extended-release capsules. Available at: https://www.accessdata.fda.gov/drugsatfda_docs/label/2013/021284s020lbl.pdf. Accessed 5 September, 2021.

32. Silva R, Muniz R, Pestreich LK, et al. Efficacy of two long-acting methylphenidate formulations in children with attention- deficit/hyperactivity disorder in a laboratory classroom setting. J Child Adolesc Psychopharmacol 2005;15(4):637–54.

33. Highlights of Prescribing Information Focalin XR (dexmethylphenidate hydrochloride) extented-release capsules, for oral use, CII. Available at: https://www.accessdata.fda.gov/drugsatfda_docs/label/2021/021802s039lbl.pdf. Accessed 06 September, 2021.

34. Silva RR, Muniz R, Pestreich L, et al. Dexmethylphenidate extended-release capsules in children with attention-deficit/hyperactivity disorder. J Am Acad Child Adolesc Psychiatry 2008;47(2):199–208.

35. Brams M, Muniz R, Childress A, et al. A randomized, double-blind, crossover study of once-daily dexmethylphenidate in children with attention-deficit hyperactivity disorder: rapid onset of effect. CNS Drugs 2008;22(8):693–704.

36. Silva RR, Brams M, McCague K, et al. Extended-release dexmethylphenidate 30 mg/d versus 20 mg/d: duration of attention, behavior, and performance benefits in children with attention-deficit/hyperactivity disorder. Clin Neuropharmacol 2013;36(4):117–21.

37. Muniz R, Brams M, Mao A, et al. Efficacy and safety of extended-release dexmethylphenidate compared with d,l-methylphenidate and placebo in the treatment of children with attention-deficit/hyperactivity disorder: a 12-hour laboratory classroom study. J Child Adolesc Psychopharmacol 2008;18(3):248–56.

38. Highlights of prescribing information Daytrana® (methylphenidate transdermal system), CII. Available at: https://www.accessdata.fda.gov/drugsatfda_docs/label/2021/021514s032lbl.pdf. Accessed 10 September, 2021.

39. McGough JJ, Wigal SB, Abikoff H, et al. A randomized, double-blind, placebo-controlled, laboratory classroom assessment of methylphenidate transdermal system in children with ADHD. J Atten Disord 2006;9(3):476–85.

40. Wilens TE, Boellner SW, Lopez FA, et al. Varying the wear time of the methylphenidate transdermal system in children with attention-deficit/hyperactivity disorder. J Am Acad Child Adolesc Psychiatry 2008;47(6):700–8.

41. Warshaw EM, Paller AS, Fowler JF, et al. Practical management of cutaneous reactions to the methylphenidate transdermal system: recommendations from a dermatology expert panel consensus meeting. Clin Ther 2008;30(2):326–37.
42. Wigal SB, Childress AC, Belden HW, et al. NWP06, an extended-release oral suspension of methylphenidate, improved attention-deficit/hyperactivity disorder symptoms compared with placebo in a laboratory classroom study. J Child Adolesc Psychopharmacol 2013;23(1):3–10.
43. Childress A, Sallee FR. The use of methylphenidate hydrochloride extended-release oral suspension for the treatment of ADHD. Expert Rev Neurother 2013;13(9):979–88.
44. Childress AC, Berry SA. The single-dose pharmacokinetics of NWP06, a novel extended-release methylphenidate oral suspension. Postgrad Med 2010; 122(5):35–41.
45. Quillivant XR® CII methylphenidate HCl. Available at: https://www.trisadhd.com/quillivant-xr/. accessed 31 August 2021.
46. Highlights of Prescribing Information Quillichew ER™ (methylphenidate hydrochloride) extended-release chewable tablets, for oral use, CII. Available at: https://www.accessdata.fda.gov/drugsatfda_docs/label/2021/207960s012lbl.pdf. Accessed 04 October, 2021.
47. Childress A, Ponce De Leon B, Owens M. QuilliChew extended-release chewable tablets for the treatment of ADHD in patients ages 6 years old and above. Expert Opin Drug Deliv 2018;15(12):1263–70.
48. Abbas R, Childress AC, Nagraj P, et al. Relative bioavailability of methylphenidate extended-release chewable tablets chewed versus swallowed whole. Clin Ther 2018;40(5):733–40.
49. Wigal SB, Childress A, Berry SA, et al. Efficacy and safety of a chewable methylphenidate extended-release tablet in children with attention-deficit/hyperactivity disorder. J Child Adolesc Psychopharmacol 2017;27(8):690–9.
50. Highlights of prescribing information Aptensio XR (methylphenidate hydrochloride extended-release) Capsules for oral use, CII. Available at: https://www.accessdata.fda.gov/drugsatfda_docs/label/2021/205831s006lbl.pdf. Accessed 19 September, 2021.
51. Adjei A, Kupper RJ, Teuscher NS, et al. Steady-state bioavailability of extended-release methylphenidate (MPH-MLR) capsule vs. immediate-release (IR) methylphenidate tablets in healthy adult volunteers. Clin Drug Investig 2014;34(11):795–805.
52. Wigal SB, Greenhill LL, Nordbrock E, et al. A randomized placebo-controlled double-blind study evaluating the time course of response to methylphenidate hydrochloride extended-release capsules in children with attention-deficit/hyperactivity disorder. J Child Adolesc Psychopharmacol 2014;24(10):562–9.
53. Childress AC, Kollins SH, Foehl HC, et al. Randomized, double-blind, placebo-controlled, flexible-dose titration study of methylphenidate hydrochloride extended-release capsules (aptensio XR) in preschool children with attention-deficit/hyperactivity disorder. J Child Adolesc Psychopharmacol 2020;30(2):58–68.
54. Highlights of Prescribing Information. Cotempla XR-ODT (methylphenidate extended-release orally disintegrating tablets), CII. Available at: https://www.accessdata.fda.gov/drugsatfda_docs/label/2021/205489s007lbl.pdf. Accessed 31 August, 2021.
55. Childress A, Stark JG, McMahen R, et al. A comparison of the pharmacokinetics of methylphenidate extended-release orally disintegrating tablets with a

reference extended-release formulation of methylphenidate in healthy adults. Clin Pharmacol Drug Dev 2018;7(2):151–9.

56. Childress AC, Kollins SH, Cutler AJ, et al. Efficacy, safety, and tolerability of an extended-release orally disintegrating methylphenidate tablet in children 6-12 Years of age with attention-deficit/hyperactivity disorder in the laboratory classroom setting. J Child Adolesc Psychopharmacol 2017;27(1):66–74.

57. Engelking D, Childress AC, McMahen R, et al. How to dose attention-deficit/hyperactivity disorder medications without a grain of salt. J Child Adolesc Psychopharmacol 2018;28(8):576–7.

58. United States Pharmacopeia: Monograph naming policy for salt drug substances. In: Drug products and compounded preparations, USP General Chapter [1121] Nomenclature 2015. Rockville (MD): United States Pharmacopeial Convention, Inc. Available at: https://www.fda.gov/media/87247/download. Accessed September 8, 2021.

59. Highlights of Prescribing Information. Jornay PM® (methylphenidate hydrochloride) extended-release capsules for oral use, CII. Available at: https://www.accessdata.fda.gov/drugsatfda_docs/label/2021/209311s008lbl.pdf. Accessed 21 September, 2021.

60. Childress AC, Cutler AJ, Marraffino A, et al. A randomized, double-blind, placebo-controlled study of HLD200, a delayed-release and extended-release methylphenidate, in children with attention-deficit/hyperactivity disorder: an evaluation of safety and efficacy throughout the day and across settings. J Child Adolesc Psychopharmacol 2019. https://doi.org/10.1089/cap.2019.0070.

61. Highlights of Prescribing Information ADHANSIA XR (methylphenidate hydrochloride) extended-release capsules, for oral use, CII. Available at: https://www.accessdata.fda.gov/drugsatfda_docs/label/2021/212038s002lbl.pdf. Accessed 12 September, 2021.

62. Childress AC, Brams MN, Cutler AJ, et al. Efficacy and Safety of Multilayer, Extended-Release Methylphenidate (PRC-063) in Children 6-12 years of age with attention-deficit/hyperactivity disorder: a laboratory classroom study. J Child Adolesc Psychopharmacol 2020;30(10):580–9.

63. Childress A, Cutler AJ, Marraffino AH, et al. Randomized, double-blind, placebo-controlled, parallel-group, adult laboratory classroom study of the efficacy and safety of PRC-063 (Extended-Release methylphenidate) for the treatment of ADHD. J Atten Disord 2021. https://doi.org/10.1177/10870547211025610.

64. Highlights of Prescribing Information Azstarys (serdexmethylphenidate and dexmethylphenidate) capsules, for oral use, CII. Available at: https://www.accessdata.fda.gov/drugsatfda_docs/label/2021/212994s000lbl.pdf. Accessed 12 September 2021.

65. FDA U.S. Food & Drug Administration. NDA 212994 NDA approval. Available at: https://www.accessdata.fda.gov/drugsatfda_docs/appletter/2021/212994Orig1s000ltr.pdf. Accessed 12 September, 2021.

66. U. S. Department Of justice drug enforcement administration 21 CFR Part 1308 [docket No. DEA-808] schedules of controlled substances: placement of serdex-methylphenidate in Schedule IV. Available at: https://www.federalregister.gov/documents/2021/05/07/2021-09738/schedules-of-controlled-substances-placement-of-serdexmethylphenidate-in-schedule-iv. Accessed 12 September, 2021.

67. Highlights of Prescribing Information Dyanavel® XR (amphetamine) extended-release oral suspension, CII. Available at: https://www.accessdata.fda.gov/drugsatfda_docs/label/2019/208147s005lbl.pdf. Accessed 12 September, 2021.

68. Highlights of Prescribing Information. Adderall XR (mixed salts of a single-entity amphetamine product) extended-release capsules, for oral use, CII. Available at: https://www.accessdata.fda.gov/drugsatfda_docs/label/2019/021303s034lbl.pdf. Accessed 12 September, 2021.

69. Biederman J, Boellner SW, Childress A, et al. Lisdexamfetamine dimesylate and mixed amphetamine salts extended-release in children with ADHD: a double-blind, placebo-controlled, crossover analog classroom study. Biol Psychiatry 2007;62(9):970–6.

70. Spencer TJ, Wilens TE, Biederman J, et al. Efficacy and safety of mixed amphetamine salts extended release (Adderall XR) in the management of attention-deficit/hyperactivity disorder in adolescent patients: a 4-week, randomized, double-blind, placebo-controlled, parallel-group study. Clin Ther 2006;28(2): 266–79.

71. Highlights of Prescribing Information Vyvanse® (lisdexamfetamine dimesylate) capsules, for oral use, CII. Available at: https://www.accessdata.fda.gov/drugsatfda_docs/label/2021/021977s046,208510s003lbl.pdf. Accessed 18 September, 2021.

72. Sharman J, Pennick M. Lisdexamfetamine prodrug activation by peptidase-mediated hydrolysis in the cytosol of red blood cells. Neuropsychiatr Dis Treat 2014;10:2275–80.

73. Wigal SB, Kollins SH, Childress AC, et al. A 13-hour laboratory school study of lisdexamfetamine dimesylate in school-aged children with attention-deficit/hyperactivity disorder. Child Adolesc Psychiatry Ment Health 2009;3(1):17.

74. Wigal T, Brams M, Gasior M, et al. Randomized, double-blind, placebo-controlled, crossover study of the efficacy and safety of lisdexamfetamine dimesylate in adults with attention-deficit/hyperactivity disorder: novel findings using a simulated adult workplace environment design. Behav Brain Funct 2010;6:34.

75. Childress A, Lloyd E, Jacobson L, et al. A randomized, placebo-controlled study of lisdexamfetamine dimesylate in 4- to 5-year-old children with attention-deficit/hyperactivity disorder. Presented at the American Academy of Child and Adolescent Psychiatry Annual Meeting 2020 October;12–24.

76. Highlights of Prescribing Information ADZENYS XR-ODT (amphetamine extended-release orally disintegrating tablets), CII. Available at: https://www.accessdata.fda.gov/drugsatfda_docs/label/2017/204326s002lbl.pdf. Accessed 04 October, 2021.

77. Stark JG, Engelking D, McMahen R, et al. A randomized crossover study to assess the pharmacokinetics of a novel amphetamine extended-release orally disintegrating tablet in healthy adults. Postgrad Med 2016;128(7):648–55.

78. Adzenys ER (amphetamine) extended-release oral suspension, CII. Highlights of Prescribing Information. Available at: https://www.accessdata.fda.gov/drugsatfda_docs/label/2017/204325s000lbl.pdf. Accessed 30 June, 2019.

79. Drugs@FDA. FDA-approved drugs new drug application (NDA): 204325 company: NEOS THERAPS INC. Available at: https://www.accessdata.fda.gov/scripts/cder/daf/index.cfm?event=overview.process&ApplNo=204325. Accessed 12 September, 2021.

80. Evekeo® (amphetamine sulfate tablets, USP) CII. 2021. Available at: https://www.evekeo.com/pdfs/evekeo-pi.pdf?v=1629102837831. Accessed 04 October 2021.

81. Childress AC, Brams M, Cutler AJ, et al. The efficacy and safety of evekeo, racemic amphetamine sulfate, for treatment of attention-deficit/hyperactivity disorder symptoms: a multicenter, dose-optimized, double-blind, randomized,

placebo-controlled crossover laboratory classroom study. J Child Adolesc Psychopharmacol 2015;25(5):402–14.

82. Drugs@FDA: FDA-approved drugs new drug application (NDA): 209905 company: ARBOR PHARMS LLC. Available at: https://www.accessdata.fda.gov/scripts/cder/daf/index.cfm?event=overview.process&ApplNo=209905. Accessed 04 October, 2021.

83. Highlights of Prescribing Information Evekeo ODT (amphetamine sulfate) orally disintegrating tablets,CII. Available at: https://www.accessdata.fda.gov/drugsatfda_docs/label/2021/209905Orig1s001lbl.pdf. Accessed 12 September, 2021.

84. Zenzedi® (dextroamphetamine sulfate, USP) CII. Available at: https://www.zenzedi.com/. Accessed 05 March, 2021.

85. Childress AC, Chow H. Amphetamine extended-release oral suspension for attention-deficit/hyperactivity disorder. Expert Rev Clin Pharmacol 2019;12(10):965–71.

86. Childress AC, Wigal SB, Brams MN, et al. Efficacy and safety of amphetamine extended-release oral suspension in children with attention-deficit/hyperactivity disorder. J Child Adolesc Psychopharmacol 2018;28(5):306–13.

87. Childress AC, Pardo A, King TR, et al. Early-onset efficacy and safety pilot study of amphetamine extended-release oral suspension (AMPH EROS) in the treatment of children with attention-deficit/hyperactivity disorder. CNS Spectr 2019;24(1):191–2.

88. Highlights of Prescribing Information. Mydayis (mixed salts of a single-entity amphetamine product) extended-release capsules, for oral use, CII. Available at: https://www.accessdata.fda.gov/drugsatfda_docs/label/2017/022063s000lbl.pdf. Accessed 19 September, 2021.

89. Wigal S, Lopez F, Frick G, et al. A randomized, double-blind, 3-way crossover, analog classroom study of SHP465 mixed amphetamine salts extended-release in adolescents with ADHD. Postgrad Med 2019;131(3):212–24.

90. Hodgkins P, Shaw M, Coghill D, et al. Amfetamine and methylphenidate medications for attention-deficit/hyperactivity disorder: complementary treatment options. Eur Child Adolesc Psychiatry 2012;21(9):477–92.

91. Stein MA, Waldman ID, Charney E, et al. Dose effects and comparative effectiveness of extended release dexmethylphenidate and mixed amphetamine salts. J Child Adolesc Psychopharmacol 2011;21(6):581–8.

92. Gomeni R, Komolova M, Incledon B, et al. Model-based approach for establishing the predicted clinical response of a delayed-release and extended-release methylphenidate for the treatment of attention-deficit/hyperactivity disorder. J Clin Psychopharmacol 2020;40(4):350–8.

93. Childress AC, Uchida CL, Po MD, et al. A post hoc comparison of prior ADHD medication dose and optimized delayed-release and extended-release methylphenidate dose in a pivotal phase III trial. Clin Ther 2020;42(12):2332–40.

94. Dexmethylphenidate (focalin) for ADHD. Med Lett Drugs Ther 2002;44(1130):45–6.

95. Arnold LE, Huestis RD, Smeltzer DJ, et al. Levoamphetamine vs dextroamphetamine in minimal brain dysfunction. Replication, time response, and differential effect by diagnostic group and family rating. Arch Gen Psychiatry 1976;33(3):292–301.

96. Chow SC. Bioavailability and bioequivalence in drug development. Wiley Interdiscip Rev Comput Stat 2014;6(4):304–12.

97. Carucci S, Balia C, Gagliano A, et al. Long term methylphenidate exposure and growth in children and adolescents with ADHD. A systematic review and meta-analysis. Neurosci Biobehav Rev 2021;120:509–25.
98. Torres-Acosta N, O'Keefe JH, O'Keefe CL, et al. Cardiovascular effects of ADHD Therapies: JACC review Topic of the week. J Am Coll Cardiol 2020;76(7):858–66.
99. Olfson M, Huang C, Gerhard T, et al. Stimulants and cardiovascular events in youth with attention-deficit/hyperactivity disorder. J Am Acad Child Adolesc Psychiatry 2012;51(2):147–56.

The Pharmacokinetics and Pharmacogenomics of Psychostimulants

John S. Markowitz, PharmD[a,b],*, Philip W. Melchert, PharmD[a]

KEYWORDS

- Psychostimulants • Amphetamine • Methylphenidate • Pharmacokinetics
- Pharmacodynamics • Pharmacogenomics

KEY POINTS

- Both stimulants are rapidly absorbed with short half-lives leading to the development of multiple extended-release dosage forms. There is significant interindividual variability in the pharmacokinetic disposition of both medications.
- Amphetamine (AMP) undergoes a high degree of oxidative metabolism forming multiple inactive metabolites while methylphenidate (MPH) is primarily metabolized by hydrolysis forming one major inactive metabolite.
- At present, pharmacogenomic testing to guide the treatment of attention-deficit/ hyperactivity disorder (ADHD) cannot be routinely recommended.
- Although frequently used in combination with a variety of other medications there is little evidence that psychostimulants participate in pharmacokinetic drug interactions as a "victim" or "perpetrator."

INTRODUCTION

Attention-deficit/hyperactivity disorder (ADHD) is a common neurobehavioral disorder beginning in childhood and often persisting into adulthood with an estimated worldwide prevalence in children and adolescents between 3% and 10%.[1–3] Symptoms of ADHD typically begin during early childhood or adolescence, persist over time, are pervasive across situations and can lead to significant impairments. Childhood ADHD symptoms may persist into adulthood in 60% or more of cases.[4,5] A variety of guidelines and algorithms are available recommending treatment approaches to ADHD with both medical and nonmedical approaches typically advocated.

[a] Department of Pharmacotherapy and Translational Research, College of Pharmacy, University of Florida, Gainesville, FL 32610-0486, USA; [b] Center for Pharmacogenomics and Precision Medicine, College of Pharmacy, University of Florida, Gainesville, FL 32610-0486, USA
* Corresponding author. Department of Pharmacotherapy and Translational Research, University of Florida, 1600 SW Archer Road, RM P4-31, Gainesville, FL 32610-0486.
E-mail address: jmarkowitz@cop.ufl.edu

Child Adolesc Psychiatric Clin N Am 31 (2022) 393–416
https://doi.org/10.1016/j.chc.2022.03.003
1056-4993/22/© 2022 Elsevier Inc. All rights reserved.

childpsych.theclinics.com

Nonpharmacological treatments include interventions such as behavioral modification and social skills training.[6,7]

With regard to neuropharmacology, converging evidence points to abnormalities of the monoamines dopamine (DA) and norepinephrine (NE) involving their synthesis, metabolism, and transport.[3,8,9] Further, the catecholaminergic systems and their associated transporters, and receptors which serve as the primary neural targets of both DA and NE can be subject to influence by any number of genetic variants which may alter these proteins and compromise overall function. Likewise, the function and expression of intra- and extracellular enzymes involved in both the biosynthesis and degradation of monoamines can be subject to the influences of genetic variation. Although DA and NE have been studied and conceptualized as two separate systems, they are increasingly appreciated to overlap in numerous ways including their biosynthetic pathway, corelease from noradrenergic neurons, innervation of similar and shared intracellular signaling pathways.[10]

Psychostimulant agents used in the treatment of ADHD are believed to optimize catecholamine signaling in the prefrontal cortex and neuropsychological and neuroimaging studies have implicated the fronto-subcortical networks of the brain as being of particular significance in the underlying dysfunction in ADHD.[11–13] Perturbations in DA and NE metabolism and turnover, as well as alterations in associated transporters and receptors, are theorized as major contributors to the pathophysiology of ADHD.

The medications with the greatest efficacy in ADHD are the psychostimulants amphetamine (AMP) and methylphenidate (MPH) which primarily target central DA and NE transporters (NET). With approximately 30 distinct psychostimulant formulations available for clinical use in the US, it is noteworthy that the primary differences between these products are the dosage forms (eg, capsules, transdermal systems, oral suspensions) and the pharmaceutical technologies they use (eg, osmotic-release systems, coated beads, etc.) to disperse drug at programmed times and doses. Otherwise, notwithstanding some differences in isomer composition (ie, racemic vs scalemic [non-50:50 ratio, eg, mixed AMP salts] mixtures vs enantiopure formulations) all of these products contain either MPH or AMP. Indeed, the only psychostimulant that was FDA approved for the treatment of ADHD since MPH (Ritalin) approval in 1955 which represented a novel chemical entity was the drug pemoline (Cylert) approved in 1975. Pemoline was later associated with hepatotoxicity and subsequently withdrawn from the market in 2005. Thus, almost half a century has passed since the last psychostimulant was approved for use for ADHD in the US.

AMP and MPH have been in continuous clinical use for well more than 60 years–longer than any other agents in clinical psychopharmacology. They are also some of the most effective medications available in terms of effect size and their ability to rapidly relieve core target symptoms of the disorder. Despite this extensive track record, up to 35% of patients may not respond adequately to a given psychostimulant and may discontinue treatment or otherwise switch to nonstimulant ADHD medications.[14,15] Poor treatment response and adverse effects are the most frequently cited reasons for discontinuation. Side effects and tolerability remain an issue for many patients and common adverse "class effects" associated with psychostimulants are often dose-related and include abdominal pain, decreased appetite, headache, and insomnia.[16] Other, less common yet more concerning and serious adverse drug reactions (ADRs) can include the exacerbation of tic disorders, substantial changes in blood pressure (BP), tachycardia, and dyskinetic movements and in rare instances, psychotic symptoms. An analysis of 49 clinical trials as well as postmarketing ADR data related reports linked visual hallucinations and other psychotic symptoms while taking psychostimulants, which suggested an association.[17] It was noted in this analysis that these serious but relatively infrequent ADRs involving psychotic symptoms and significant BP elevations are more consistent with manifestations of stimulant overdose or toxicity, and suggest that the individuals experiencing these effects may have been manifesting the clinical signs of substantially elevated stimulant blood concentrations.[17] As monitoring of psychostimulant medication levels is not clinically useful nor generally performed, the detection of abnormally elevated (or lowered) systemic concentrations or identification of genetically aberrant metabolizers has had a low likelihood of being documented in the course of clinical practice. Thus, despite the extensive clinical experience with psychostimulants, there remains an unmet need to fully understand the basis for significant inter-individual differences in drug disposition, adverse events, and therapeutic response. Moreover, initial dosing and titration of psychostimulants continue to be approached on an empirical basis.

This article will briefly review the pharmacology and pharmacodynamics of the psychostimulants, discuss candidate gene association studies relevant to pharmacodynamics and mechanism of action. Next, the fundamental pharmacokinetic characteristics of the psychostimulants will be discussed, issues with MPH and AMP will be discussed as well as pharmacogenomic studies relevant to drug dispositional issues involving these agents. Potential drug–drug interaction (DDIs) liabilities will also be discussed.

PHARMACODYNAMICS

Although AMP and MPH are two of the most thoroughly studied drugs in all of the biomedicine, their theoretic mechanism(s) of action continue to be refined. Overall, the net pharmacologic effect of each of these agents is to increase the availability of both DA and NE in the neurosynapse. The molecular structures of both MPH and AMP share a phenethylamine moiety (**Fig. 1**) which superimposes on its putative neural substrates, DA and NE, which in theory provides the basis of their requisite receptor interactions. Nevertheless, there are significant differences between how these medications exert these pharmacologic effects, which will be reviewed briefly.

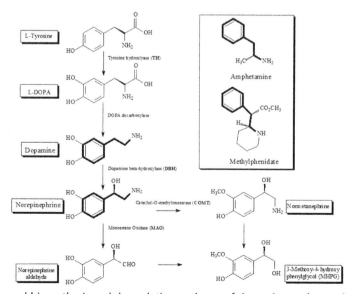

Fig. 1. General biosynthesis and degradation pathway of dopamine and norepinephrine.

Amphetamine

The preponderance of mechanistic evidence underlying the psychostimulant effects of AMP supports an AMP-induced increase in extracellular DA and NE mediated by efflux of the cytoplasmic monoamines through the DA transporter (DAT; SLC6A3) and NET (SLC6A2), respectively. AMP dramatically increases the concentrations of extraneuronal monoamines within their associated synapses through a reversal of the functional role of DAT and NET, and to a much lesser degree, serotonin (5-hydroxytryptamine [5-HT]) reuptake transporter. AMP seems to compete with endogenous monoamines for transport into the nerve terminals via DAT and NET. AMP binds to these respective transporter proteins localized on their presynaptic terminals, leading to a conformational change that moves the bound AMP to the interior of the neuron, and subsequently reverses the vesicular monoamine transporter (VMAT). This process has been described as "reverse transport" or "retro-transport," and the primary mechanism of action of AMP is that of a catecholaminergic releasing agent.[18,19] Although animal studies indicate that both d- and l-AMP release DA in the striatum and nucleus accumbens, the d-isomer seems to exhibit the greatest potency. It is known, however, that both isomers exert therapeutic effects. These intraneuronal dynamics subsequently produce a large efflux of displaced stores of monoamines into the synaptic cleft as the transporter releases the catecholamine on returning to its resting conformation.[20] There is also evidence that AMP has the additional action of inhibiting MAO and thereby inhibiting the degradation of cytosolic monoamines, potentially contributing to the molecule's therapeutic effects. In summary, recent studies suggest that AMP must be actively transported by DAT, NET as well as VMAT in tandem to induce its psychostimulant/therapeutic effects.[21]

Methylphenidate

MPH elicits its primary pharmacodynamic effects by blocking the reuptake of DA and NE into the presynaptic neuron through the inhibition of the DAT (SLC6A3) and NET (SLC6A2) thus resulting in increases in extracellular synaptic concentrations of DA and NE which may in turn bind to their respective transporters (ie, the DAT or NET) or to DA or NE receptors.[6,15] These hypothesized pharmacologic actions are supported by reductions in ligand binding observed in PET and SPECT studies. A redistribution of vesicular monoamine transporter 2 (VMAT-2) has also been reported. The pharmacologic activity of dl-MPH seems to reside almost entirely within the d-isomer.[22,23] There is some binding of d- MPH as an agonist at the 5-HT1A receptor but the significance of this observation is unclear.[24] Thus, while AMP and MPH are distinct in their pharmacologic mechanisms of action, they are primary if not unifying pharmacologic effect is to provide increased extracellular DA and NE in the neurosynapse.

Pharmacogenomic considerations related to psychostimulant pharmacodynamics

Genetics are widely believed to play a role in the etiology of ADHD and at least a partial role in treatment response to psychopharmacological agents including psychostimulants.[25] Genetic factors may likewise contribute to the potential adverse effects associated with treatments. Yet in spite of significant efforts over the last decade candidate gene studies have revealed very few variants that are consistently associated with enhanced (or diminished) responses to stimulants or to otherwise influence treatment outcomes in ADHD. As AMP and MPH both largely target the monoamine neurotransmitters DA and NE, most of the candidate gene association studies have been conducted evaluating specific variants of genes that encode for key catalytic enzymes involved in both the biosynthesis of DA and NE (which occurs intracellularly) as well as those enzymes responsible for neurotransmitter degradation (see **Fig. 1**). For example, tyrosine hydroxylase (TH), the gene encoding for the enzyme required to catalyze the conversion of the amino acid tyrosine to the DA precursor, L-3,4-dihy-droxyphenylalanine (L-DOPA), and DA β-hydroxylase (DBH) responsible for the bioconversion of DA to NE have been investigated in a number of studies.[26] Likewise, functional polymorphisms of genes encoding for prominent catalytic enzymes respon-sible for the degradation of monoamines (catechol-O-methyltransferase (COMT) and monoamine oxidase (MAO) in the extracellular space have also been targets of phar-macogenomic studies (see **Fig. 1**).[26,27] Moving beyond the processes of the biosyn-thesis and degradation of DA and NE, other "catecholaminergic gene" variants associated with transporters of monoamines, as well as both pre and postsynaptic target receptors for DA and NE have likewise been targeted for study. Some of the more well-studied of these candidate genes include the DA receptor D4 (*DRD4*) gene, DA receptor D5 (*DRD5*) gene, the DA transporter gene (*DAT1* or *SLC6A3*), the most prevalent NE receptor type in the prefrontal cortex, α-2A adrenergic receptor (*ADRA2A*), the NET gene (*NET1*; *SLC6A2*) and others.[27] To date, however, findings from these studies have not been proved consistent nor have they been reliably repli-cated and do not adequately explain variability in response to psychostimulants. Addi-tionally, it has been noted that most of these candidate gene variants fail to replicate in genome-wide association studies (GWAS).[25,27] GWAS examine the entire genome to detect common DNA variants (>1% of the population) having very specific effects; however, GWAS studies require large number of subjects to reliably map a genetic as-sociation. A limited number of GWAS studies have been conducted directed at the eti-ology of ADHD as well as its treatment.[28] An extensive discussion and analysis of ADHD GWAS studies is beyond the scope of the present review but specific and recent reviews are available.[28,29] At present, no single gene variant, gene variant com-bination, or currently available pharmacogenomics testing panel based upon mono-amine synthesis, degradation or drug pharmacodynamics can be recommended to guide the selection of stimulant or stimulant dose in the treatment of ADHD.

PHARMACOKINETICS
Amphetamine metabolism and disposition

Following the oral administration of immediate-release (IR) racemic AMP, both iso-mers are well absorbed, but bioavailability is relatively low at an estimated 25%. Dis-tribution is rapid and similar for both isomers and protein binding is approximately 15% to 40%. The steady-state volume of distribution (Vd) is estimated at 3 to 4 L/ kg. AMP is highly metabolized in the liver with two primary oxidative pathways recog-nized (**Fig. 2**). Aromatic hydroxylation occurs to the para position to form small amounts of the pharmacologically active metabolite 4-hydroxyamphetamine through a reaction reportedly catalyzed by the cytochrome P450 (CYP) 2D6 pathway.[30] 4-hydroxyamphetamine is then converted into *p*-hydroxynorephedrine by DA -β-hy-droxylase and further hydroxylation of *d*-AMP forms norephedrine (phenylpropanol-amine) in small amounts. Oxidative deamination via *N*- or α-hydroxylation is the other primary oxidative route.[31–33] Another Phase I monooxygenase, flavin-containing monooxygenase form 3 (FMO3) was reported to contribute to the *N*-oxygenation of *d*- and *l*-AMP.[34] AMP is also oxidized to inactive metabolites phenyl-acetone which is subsequently oxidized to benzoic acid, which is conjugated to glycine and excreted as hippuric acid.[31,32] AMP deamination seems to be catalyzed by CYP450 isoenzymes of the CYP2C subfamily which also proceeds in a stereoselec-tive manner.[35] Dextroamphetamine is metabolized more efficiently than *l*-AMP leading

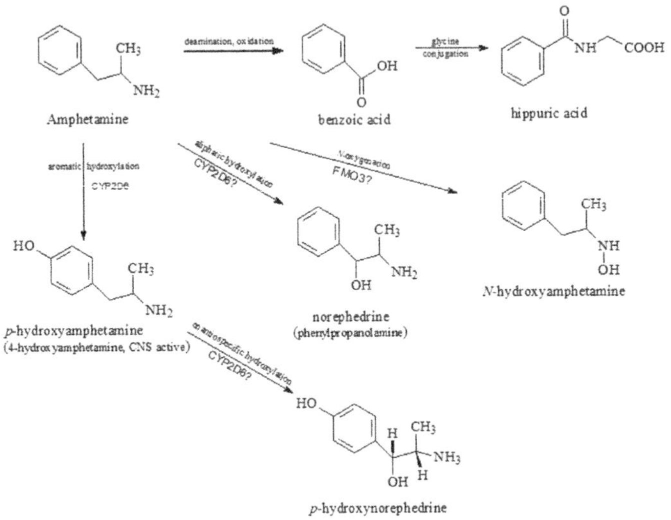

Fig. 2. Metabolism of amphetamine in humans.

to unequal amounts of isomers excreted in the urine following the administration of the racemic mixture. AMP does not seem to be a substrate or inhibitor of the P-glycoprotein (P-gp) transporter.[36]

In summary, in humans, AMP is highly metabolized by multiple enzymes to primarily inactive compounds found in relatively small amounts. The major enzymes involved in AMP's metabolism remain unclear. Anywhere from 5% to 30% of an administered dose is excreted unchanged in the urine, with the majority eliminated as benzoic acid and its corresponding glycine conjugate known as hippuric acid.

Potential sources of variability

Although there are some age-related differences in some pharmacokinetic parameters (eg, C_{max}, AUC) reported with different AMP formulations, in general, after adjustments are made for body weight and dosage there are no major differences in overall pharmacokinetics and exposure between children and adults. The influence of food and high-fat meals has been evaluated for all AMP formulations. Although there are some differences between different formulations, the following general observations can be made. With regard to IR dosage forms, little overall effects on the bioavailability or exposure to d-AMP from either an IR formulation or an initial sustained release formulation, Dexedrine Spansule, was noted.[37,38] More modern modified-release dosage forms are those which have a more specified pattern of drug release formulated to achieve a desired therapeutic objective or improved patient compliance. However, the consumption of food or a high-fat meal may significantly lengthen the time to reach T_{max} (ie, time to reach maximum plasma concentration [C_{max}]) of both the d- and l-isomers in many modified-release AMP dosage forms.[39] These delays in T_{max} vary widely among different product formulations, but may range between 2 and 4.5 hrs while not ultimately altering the overall exposure (observed area under the plasma concentration–time curve [AUC]) to most formulations.[40] To summarize, high-fat meals did not typically have significant effects on the exposure (AUC and C_{max}) to AMP formulations but tend to delay T_{max} to variable degrees. The plasma half-life ($t_{1/2}$) of IR racemic AMP is ~ 10 to 13 hrs in adults and shorter in children (~8 hrs) (**Table 1**). Studies in healthy volunteers receiving racemic AMP typically reveal a

Table 1
Comparison of enantiospecific pharmacokinetic parameters of immediate-release psychostimulants

Psychostimulant	$\sim T_{max}$ (h)	$\sim t_{1/2}$ (h)	$\sim$Vd (L/kg)	$\sim F$ (%)
dl-methylphenidate	*d*-isomer: 2	*d*-isomer: 2–3	*d*-isomer: 2.7	*d*-isomer: 23
	l-isomer: 2	*l*-isomer: 0.5–1	*l*-isomer: 1.8	*l*-isomer: 5
dl-amphetamine	*d*-isomer: 2.5	*d*-isomer: 10–11	*d*-isomer: 3–4	*d*-isomer: 25
	l-isomer: 2.5	*l*-isomer: 12–13	*l*-isomer: 3–4	*l*-isomer: 25

difference in the disposition of the AMP enantiomers with *d*-AMP having an elimination $t_{1/2}$ 1 to 2 hours shorter than *l*-AMP.[40,41] Multiple AMP dosage forms are now available, most of which permit once daily dosing (**Table 2**). Regarding the *d*-AMP prodrug lisdexamfetamine (LDX), it is a rapidly absorbed L-lysine conjugate that generally reaches its C_{max} approximately 1 hour (T_{max}) postdosing. It's elimination $t_{1/2}$ is typically less than 1 hr. Interestingly, LDX is not metabolized by human microsomes or in human hepatocytes and the primary site of hydrolytic metabolism to *d*-AMP is the red blood cell in a reaction believed to be catalyzed by unidentified peptidases.[42] The LDX capsule is not specifically formulated as an extended- or modified-release technology as the duration of activity is driven by the gradual hydrolysis releasing *d*-AMP over the day.

In general, for all AMP formulations, the AUC and the C_{max} are generally proportional to the dose. With regard to gender differences in pharmacokinetics, in general, it seems that women may have a 20%–40% higher exposure to a given dose of most of the AMP formulations than men, but these differences in overall drug exposure tend to disappear when the dose is normalized to subject weight.[40]

Amphetamine metabolism and the potential influence of genetic polymorphisms
As mentioned above, what is known about AMP metabolism is that there are multiple pathways and metabolites yet relatively few *in vitro* studies have been replicated which firmly identify major enzymes involved in its biotransformation. Although most AMP full prescribing information mentions CYP2D6 as having a role in the metabolism of AMP and CYP2D6 is mentioned in multiple FDA New Drug Applications for AMP products, no pharmaceutical company to our knowledge has submitted any original data supporting this contention to the FDA. However, as at least one report indicates that AMP serves as at least a partial substrate of the highly polymorphic enzyme/gene *CYP2D6,* the potential for genetic variability in metabolism, therapeutic response, and tolerability would seem to make it a prime candidate for pharmacogenomic testing, and indeed, this is a practice incorporated by some clinicians and commercial testing is readily available.[30,43] However, it must be borne in mind that the evidence for the involvement of CYP2D6 to date remains thin and seems to rest primarily on a single *in vitro* study.[30] Furthermore, if there is such a role *in vivo*, the degree of its involvement in the overall metabolism and clearance of AMP is unknown. We are unaware of any clinical study conducted or published demonstrating alterations in AMP disposition in individuals who are carriers of genetic variants of *CYP2D6* (eg, poor metabolizers or ultra-rapid metabolizers) versus extensive metabolizers. Likewise, there are no clinical studies assessing the influence of known CYP2D6 metabolic inhibitors (eg, paroxetine) on AMP metabolism and disposition in humans. With regard to FMO3 and its role in AMP metabolism, while a number of genetic variants have been identified that seem to influence the degree of drug oxidation by FMO3, as mentioned above, there are conflicting reports regarding the actual contribution of this oxidative enzyme

Table 2
Available amphetamine dosage forms

Composition	Proprietary Name	FDA Approval Year	Pharmaceutical Formulation/Dosage Form	Daily Dosing Frequency	T_{max} (hr)	$t_{1/2}$ (hr)	Dosage Strengths	Sprinkle/Dividing
mixed salts of d- & l-amphetamine; 3:1	Adderall®	1996	Tablet, IR	2	~7	10–12	5, 7.5, 10, 12.5, 15, 20, 30 mg	Can split/crush
D-amphetamine	Dexedrine Spansule®	1996	Capsule, SR	1–2	~8	12	5, 10, 15 mg	Can be opened/sprinkled
mixed salts of d- & l-amphetamine; 3:1	Adderall XR®	2001	Capsule, ER	Once	7–8	11–13	5, 10, 15, 20, 25, 30 mg	Can be opened/sprinkled
Lisdexamfetamine prodrug of d-amphetamine	Vyvanse®	2007	Capsule	Once	~4	~11	10, 20, 30, 40, 50, 60, 70 mg	Can be opened/sprinkled
d-amphetamine	ProCentra®	2008	Oral Solution, IR	1–2	3–4	~12	5mg/mL	N/A
dl-amphetamine	Evekeo®	2012	Tablet, IR	1–2	~2.5	10–12	5, 10 mg	Can split/crush
d-amphetamine	Zenzedi® equiv to discontinued Dexedrine® tablets	2013	Tablet, IR	1–2	~3	~12	2.5, 5, 7.5, 10, 15, 20, 30 mg	Can split/crush
mixed salts of d- & l-amphetamine ratio of 3.2:1	Dyanavel® XR	2015	Suspension, ER	Once	4	12–15	2.5 mg/mL	N/A
mixed salts of d- & l-amphetamine ratio of 3:1	Adzenys XR-ODT®	2016	Orally disintegrating tablet, ER	Once	~5	11–13	3.1, 6.3, 9.4, 12.5, 15.7, 18.8 mg	No
mixed salts of d- & l-amphetamine in the ratio of 3:1	Mydayis®	2017	Capsule, ER	Once	8	10–12	12.5, 25, 37.5, 50 mg	Can be opened/sprinkled

mixed salts of d- & l-amphetamine ratio of 3:1	Adzenys® ER	2017	Suspension, ER	Once	~5	~11	1.25 mg/mL	N/A
Lisdexamfetamine prodrug of d-amphetamine	Vyvanse®	2017	Chewable tablet	Once	~4	~11	10, 20, 30, 40, 50, 60 mg	No
dl-amphetamine	Evekeo® ODT	2019	Orally disintegrating tablet, IR	1–2	~3	10–12	5, 10, 15, 20 mg	No

Abbreviations: ER, extended release; IR, immediate release.

to AMP metabolism and disposition.[44] In summary, there have been no gene variants conclusively linked to decreased (or increased) AMP metabolism and we conclude there are insufficient data to recommend pharmacogenomic testing of any gene variant related to AMP pharmacokinetics as a means to personalize/optimize AMP pharmacotherapy.

Methylphenidate metabolism and disposition

With the exception of the enantiopure (d)-MPH products (threo-[+]-MPH, dexmethylphenidate) Focalin and Focalin XR and the recently introduced combination formulation containing the prodrug serdexmethylphenidate and d-MPH (Azstarys), all marketed MPH formulations contain a racemic (50:50) mixture of threo-RR-d- and threo-S,S-l-MPH isomers (**Table 3**). The hydrochloride salt of MPH is quite soluble in gastrointestinal fluids and it is rapidly absorbed from the small intestine to the colon. Distribution is also quite rapid and protein binding is low at 15%. The overall bioavailability of IR MPH is quite low (approximately 23% for the d-isomer vs 5% for the l-isomer) which is believed to be due to extensive and stereoselective first-pass metabolism.[45] The steady-state Vd is estimated at 2 L/kg with some differences noted between isomers (see **Table 1**). Unlike AMP, dl-MPH undergoes little oxidative metabolism and is instead subject to rapid stereoselective de-esterification (hydrolysis) to the major inactive metabolite, ritalinic acid (**Fig. 3**). Circulating concentrations of ritalinic acid greatly exceed those of the parent compound and it accounts for 60% to 80% of a dose recovered in urine. This deactivating/detoxifying process seems to be exclusively by the major hepatic esterase carboxylesterase 1 (CES1).[46]

A variety of modified-release oral dosage forms designs were introduced beginning in 2000 (see **Table 2**) and included pulsatile release and biphasic extended release, which provided intended fluctuations of plasma levels. More extensive reviews of these technologies can be found elsewhere.[45,47] The plasma half-life ($t_{1/2}$) of IR d-MPH is ~ 2 to 3 hrs (see **Table 1**). Whether an IR tablet or one of the modified-release oral dosage formulations, the C_{max} and AUC of MPH are generally proportional to the dose. CES1 mediated hydrolysis is highly stereoselective, with the catalytic efficiency of CES1 estimated to be 6- to 7-fold higher for the inactive l-isomer relative to d–MPH.[48] As a result, the plasma $t_{1/2}$ of d-MPH is markedly longer than that of l-MPH which has been reported to be ~0.5–1 hr (see **Table 1**).[22] In fact, this stereoselective metabolism is so significant, that l-MPH concentrations may fall below the analytical limits of detection within 1 to 2 hours of oral administration of racemic MPH. For example, in one enantiospecific pharmacokinetic evaluation of the OROS formulation of racemic MPH, the AUC values of l-MPH only attained only 1% of that of d-MPH.[49] In contrast to observations with racemic oral formulations is the transdermal patch formulation of racemic MPH which results in approximately equal amounts of d- and l-MPH isomers in the systemic circulation throughout the wear period.[50] This occurs presumably due to its continuous delivery through the skin which avoids the significant first-pass effect and stereoselective hepatic metabolism which influence orally administered drug. Only minor oxidative metabolism by other enzymes/pathways is known to occur including aromatic hydroxylation to form p-hydroxymethylphenidate, a metabolite with CNS activity but found in only minor amounts (~1%). A de-esterified lactam and a number of glucuronides are also formed.[51] Less than 1% of an MPH dose is excreted unchanged in the urine.

Potential sources of variability

As with AMP formulations, there are some age-related differences in some pharmacokinetic parameters (eg, C_{max}, AUC) reported with MPH. Likewise, in general, after

Table 3
Available methylphenidate dosage forms

Composition	Proprietary Name	FDA Approval Year	Pharmaceutical Formulation/ Dosage Form	Daily Dosing	T_{max} (hr)	$t_{1/2}$ (hr)	Dosage Strengths	Sprinkle/ Dividing
DL-methylphenidate	Ritalin®	1955	Tablet, IR	2–3	2	2.5–3	5, 10, 20 mg	Can split/crush
DL-methylphenidate	Methylin ER®	2000	Tablet, dissolution polymer ER, equiv to discontinued Ritalin SR®	Once	4–5	~3.5	10, 20 mg	No
DL-methylphenidate	Quillichew ER®	2015	Chewable tablet 30% IR MPH; 70% ER MPH	Once	5	5	20, 30, 40 mg	No
DL-methylphenidate	Concerta®	2000	Nondeformable tablet, osmotic release, OROS™	Once	~7	3.5	18, 27, 36, 54 mg	No
D-methylphenidate (dexmethylphenidate)	Focalin®	2001	Tablet, IR	Twice	1.5	2	2.5, 5, 10 mg	Can split/crush
DL-methylphenidate	Metadate CD®	2001	Capsule, beaded delivery 30% IR, 70% ER	Once	1.5	~7	10, 20, 30, 40, 50, 60 mg	Can be sprinkled
DL-methylphenidate	Ritalin LA®	2002	Capsule, biphasic beaded delivery, 50% IR, 50% ER	Once	2 (1st peak)	2–3	10, 20, 30, 40, 60 mg	Can be sprinkled
D-methylphenidate (dexmethylphenidate)	Focalin XR®	2005	Capsule, biphasic beaded delivery, 50% IR, 50% ER	Once	1.5 (1st peak)	3	5, 10, 15, 20, 25, 30, 35, 40 mg	Can be sprinkled

(continued on next page)

Table 3
(continued)

Composition	Proprietary Name	FDA Approval Year	Pharmaceutical Formulation/Dosage Form	Daily Dosing	T_{max} (hr)	$t_{½}$ (hr)	Dosage Strengths	Sprinkle/Dividing
dl-methylphenidate	Daytrana®	2006	Transdermal patch	Once	Depends on removal time	4–5	10, 15, 20, 30 mg	N/A
dl-methylphenidate	Quillivant XR®	2012	Suspension, reconstituted powder contains 20% IR, 80% ER	Once	4	5 (d-MPH)	10 mg/2 mL, 20 mg/4 mL, 30 mg/6 mL, 40 mg/8 mL, 50 mg/10 mL, 60 mg/12 mL	N/A
dl-methylphenidate	Aptensio XR®	2015	Capsule, outer IR layer 40% and inner CR layer 60%	Once	2	5	10, 15, 20, 30, 40, 50, 60 mg	Can be sprinkled
dl-methylphenidate	Cotempla® XR-ODT	2017	Orally disintegrating tablet, 25% IR, 75% ER MPH	Once	~5	4	8.6, 17.3, 25.9 mg	No
dl-methylphenidate	Jornay PM®	2018	Capsule, microbeads outer delayed-release layer, inner ER layer, and an IR core	Once (evening)	14	6	20, 40, 60, 80, 100 mg	Can be sprinkled

dl-methylphenidate	Adhansia XR®	2019	Capsule, multilayer release beads, 20% IR and 80% ER	Once	1.5 (1st peak)	7	25, 35, 45, 55 70, 85 mg	Can be sprinkled
d-methylphenidate & serdexmethylphenidate	Azstarys®	2021	Capsule contains IR d-MPH & prodrug of d-MPH, serdexme thylphenidate	Once	2	6: d-MPH 12: Serdex	Serdex: d-MPH ratio; 26.1 mg/5.2 mg 39.2 mg/7.8 mg 52.3 mg/10.4 mg	Can be sprinkled

Abbreviations: CR, controlled release; ER, extended release; IR, immediate release.

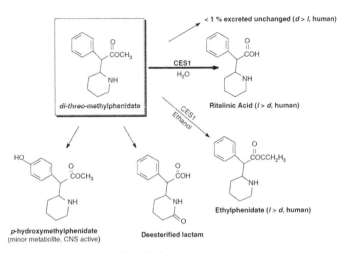

Fig. 3. Metabolism of methylphenidate in humans.

adjustments are made for body weight and dosage there are no significant differences in overall pharmacokinetics and exposure between children and adults. Regarding the fed versus fasted state, the extent of absorption of MPH from all oral dosage forms is similar when dosed in the fasting state. However, following the consumption of a high-fat meal, there is a potential for a delay in the time of peak concentrations (T_{max}), which is theorized to result from a delay in gastric emptying.[45] There are some differences between studies and formulations with some reported increased or decreased C_{max}, but in general, overall exposures as assessed by AUC are unchanged. There are several studies suggesting that there may be gender differences regarding MPH metabolism and disposition. At least two bioavailability studies which included male and female volunteers indicated that when the doses are normalized to the body weight of the subject, women have lower systemic exposure based on a mg/kg dose.[46] It has been speculated that more extensive first-pass metabolism of MPH may occur in women. The potential clinical significance of these observations is that women might require larger mg/kg doses to achieve the same MPH plasma concentration as their male counterparts. The apparent sex dimorphism in MPH bioavailability requires further study.[45]

Numerous clinical studies have demonstrated a significant *interindividual* in the metabolism and disposition in patients receiving typical doses of MPH. Interindividual variability in MPH pharmacokinetics may be particularly prominent when comparing the profiles of individual subjects after dosing with one of the long-acting formulations. This variability is well illustrated in **Fig. 4**. In this figure, "spaghetti" plots are presented depicting individual AUCs from 19 adult subjects (10 M, 9 F) participating in a healthy volunteer cross-over pharmacokinetic study comparing the two long-acting formulations Ritalin LA (*pane A*) and Concerta (*pane B*).[52] The mean values of these individual plots presented in *pane C* is quite representative of the typical profiles depicted in the two formulation's full prescribing information and promotional materials. What can be appreciated is that few of the individual subjects display a profile matching the mean profiles and some differ substantially, yet most of the prescribers assume their patients will have a profile very much mirroring the mean profiles (*pane C*) that is, that which appears in the prescribing materials. It should be noted that this type of inter-individual variability in pharmacokinetic profiles is not unique to the Ritalin LA and

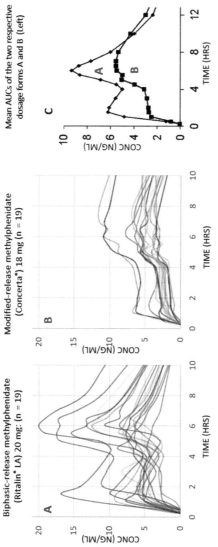

Fig. 4. Interindividual variability in long-acting methylphenidate formulations.

Concerta dosage forms, and although not routinely published it is quite typical of essentially all modified-release formulations of MPH.[53,54] With regard to *intra-subject* variability in MPH pharmacokinetics, it is generally believed to be of a smaller magnitude than that observed between subjects (ie, interindividual variability) but the issue has undergone little formal study.

In summary, MPH pharmacokinetics are generally linear and dose proportional. Absorption is rapid and oral bioavailability is low. Metabolism is almost entirely mediated by CES1, stereoselective, and forms the major inactive metabolite ritalinic acid. Clearance is rapid with little to no accumulation of the drug, even with the long-acting modified-release formulations and thus, true steady-state conditions are never really attained.

Methylphenidate metabolism and the potential influence of genetic polymorphisms

As described previously, the primary metabolic fate of MPH is to be de-esterified (hydrolyzed) into the major inactive metabolite ritalinic acid in a reaction catalyzed by CES1. There is otherwise little metabolism relevant to MPH disposition and clearance. CES1 has undergone little study relative to other drug-metabolizing enzymes such as members of the CYP450 superfamily and there is generally little clinician familiarity with the enzyme. It is, however, the most abundant drug-metabolizing enzyme (of any type) in the human liver and is responsible for an estimated 80%–95% of total hydrolytic activity in the liver. The enzyme is key in catalyzing the metabolism of an array of medications, drugs of abuse, environmental toxins, and endogenous substances.[55] Significant interindividual variability in the expression and activity of CES1 has been consistently observed and reported in the biomedical literature and this variability is likely attributable to both genetic and environmental factors, and in theory such variability could potentially result in treatment failure and/or unexpected adverse effects from a CES1 substrate medication. A single-nucleotide polymorphism (SNP) in the human *CES1* gene encoding for CES1 has been discovered which results in dysfunctional enzymatic activity, and may be one contributing factor to inter-individual variability in MPH exposure and response.[55,56] The first clinically significant *CES1* variant, the loss-of-function mutant G143E also referred to as 428G.A (rs71647871), was discovered serendipitously during the course of a healthy volunteer MPH pharmacokinetic study.[56] This variant led to gross impairments in MPH metabolism. Subsequently, this variant has been unequivocally shown *in vitro* and in clinical studies to lead to significantly impaired metabolism of MPH and other known CES1 substrates.[55–57] In a single-dose pharmacokinetic assessment, Stage and associates (2017) evaluated the influence of specific *CES1* genotypes on the pharmacokinetics of *d*-MPH in healthy subjects (n = 44).[57] G143E carriers were found to have an approximately 150% increase in MPH AUC relative to control subjects lacking the variant ($P < .0001$). It was further noted that individuals with 4 copies of *CES1* had 45% ($P = .011$) and 61% ($P = .028$) increased AUCs of *d*-MPH relative to control participants or those with fewer copies of *CES1*. Nemoda and coworkers reported the G143E variant to be associated with significantly lower MPH dosage requirements for symptom reduction in patients with ADHD.[58] In this prospective study (n = 122) children with ADHD were titrated to a dose of MPH between 10 and 30 mg in 2 doses to achieve adequate medication response. Subjects were then classified as responders or nonresponders using the ADHD Rating Scale (ADHD-RS). While there was no significant difference in response rate when comparing individuals with the variant to those without among those responding, those with the G143E variant (n = 5) required significantly lower doses (0.41 mg/kg/d vs 0.57 mg/kg/d; $P = .022$) versus those who did not carry the variant (n = 85).[58] This finding is consistent with impaired CES1 activity in G143E carriers.[59]

Thus, it seems that genetically deficient "poor metabolizers" of MPH do in fact exist and are associated with the G143E variant. The minor allele frequency (MAF) of the G143E variant is only 3% to 4% in the general population and estimated at approximately 3.7%, 4.3%, and 2%, in White, Hispanic, and African American populations, respectively, and the variant seems to be rare in Asian populations.[56]

As to whether it is clinically useful to genotype for *CES1* variants presently is open to debate. Although CES1 is recognized as the primary catalytic enzyme responsible for the metabolism of MPH, earlier nonpharmacogenomic studies evaluating plasma levels of the drug did not provide useful guidance for dosing and management of patients. There are well more than 7000 *CES1* SNPs registered in the National Center for Biotechnology Information database, the vast majority of which have not been evaluated for activity.[55] At present the field of CES1 pharmacogenomics is in its relative infancy and we would anticipate further functional variants will be discovered. At present, however, the universal genotyping for the presence of the *CES1* G143E variant (or others) cannot be recommended for all patients treated with MPH.

Drug–drug interactions

DDIs are a major source of concern in all medical disciplines and subspecialties due to their association with adverse effects, potential toxicity and increased morbidity and mortality. Additionally, DDIs resulting in ADRs and interactions are frequently a source of litigation. Because of the frequent existence of comorbid disorders in patients with ADHD which are amenable to treatment with medications and as ADHD often continues to be treated into adulthood, the concurrent use of ADHD medications with other therapeutic agents on a chronic or acute basis is often unavoidable.[60] An accumulating number of research reports, survey data, as well as analyses of health maintenance organization and prescription drug databases indicate a decade's long and continuing trend for children and adolescents diagnosed with ADHD to be concurrently treated with a psychostimulant and one or more other psychotropic medication. Among the more commonly coprescribed agents are α-2 agonists, SSRIs, second-generation antipsychotics, and anticonvulsants.[61,62]

DDIs may occur due to a number of reasons including clinician unfamiliarity with drug combinations known to be potentially problematic, the prescribing of medications by multiple clinicians–each unaware of prescribed treatments by the other, the use of over-the-counter medications or dietary supplements by the patient, and the prescribing of drug combinations which have never been assessed in a systematic fashion using modern *in vitro* screening techniques presently required by the US FDA before drug approval. This latter situation is certainly far more common for drugs that were initially approved for use many years ago such as MPH and AMP. In regard to DDIs with the psychostimulants, current full prescribing information (ie, package inserts) describe relatively few DDIs of clinical concern. In the recent past, drug prescribing materials contained a variety of cautions related to the use of stimulants with TCAs, anticonvulsants, and others. These cautions have been largely based on questionable case reports rather than formal study. Thorough reviews and assessments of most of these early stimulant DDI reports are available elsewhere.[63,64] There are in fact, relatively few published reports rigorously documenting pharmacokinetic DDIs for which the stimulants are the "victim" drugs. It should also be noted that as psychostimulant drug concentrations are seldom obtained in the clinical management of patients, this may well decrease the likelihood of discovering DDIs suspected or otherwise. Furthermore, over the extensive clinical lifetime of the psychostimulants it is only relatively recently that the respective metabolic pathways and requisite catalytic enzymes and drug transporters have been identified for MPH and AMP, and as described above for AMP and CYP2D6, there remain deficits in our understanding of the complete picture of AMP clearance.

DDIs are generally characterized as either pharmacodynamic or pharmacokinetic in nature. *Pharmacodynamic drug interactions* may be antagonistic, additive, or potentially synergistic. Since pharmacodynamic interactions are not associated with an alteration in any tissue concentration of drug they are typically suspected on the basis of diminished, exaggerated, or even toxic effects in a patient previously maintained satisfactorily on an existing medication regimen. Evidence of a pharmacodynamic interaction primarily relies on clinical observations and objective measures of drug pharmacologic effects including changes in a drug's previous effectiveness in controlling target symptoms, changes in a patient mental status or otherwise unexplained changes in one or more vital signs. *Pharmacokinetic drug interactions,* which are a focus of this article, are those that affect one or more of the ADME parameters (ie, absorption, distribution, metabolism, elimination). Relative to pharmacodynamic DDIs, pharmacokinetic interactions are more easily detected and/or confirmed through the measurement of systemic blood concentrations of the suspected agents, ideally both prior to and after a suspected perpetrator agent is added to an existing drug regimen.

Amphetamine and drug–drug interactions

As discussed previously, the metabolism of AMP is complex with no single metabolic pathway or catalytic enzyme dominating. However, both *in vitro* and available healthy volunteer studies suggest that neither *d*-AMP nor intact LDX significantly impede the activity of any of the major CYP450 enzymes. In *in vitro* models, AMP does not seem to be an inhibitor of CYP1A2, CYP2A6, CYP2B6, CYP2C8, CYP2C9, CYP2C19, CYP2D6, and CYP3A4 in human hepatic microsomal microsomes. Furthermore, in vitro assessments conducted in cultured human hepatocytes indicated that AMP was not an inducer of CYP1A2, CYP2B6, or CYP3A4/5.[65] In a healthy volunteer study using a probe drug cocktail approach, neither LDX nor *d*-AMP produced any significant effects on the substrate markers in the "Cooperstown Cocktail" (caffeine CYP1A2 substrate, dextromethorphan CYP2D6 substrate, omeprazole CYP2C19 substrate, midazolam CYP3A4 substrate), nor did these substrates seem to have any significant influence on LDX or *d*-AMP exposure.[66,67] On the other hand, one of the DDIs known to most profoundly alter the disposition of AMP is the coadministration of medications or other substance which can significantly alter urinary pH to one extreme or the other. Acidifying urine is known to greatly enhance the excretion of the parent compound while alkaline conditions have the opposite influence and significantly prolong drug half-life.[68,69] However, fortunately, there are relatively few agents which produce substantial effects on urinary pH. Citric acid and large doses of ascorbic acid can acidify urine while acetazolamide and sodium bicarbonate are examples of urinary alkalinizers. These combinations of agents seem relatively unlikely to occur, but some awareness of the potential is worthwhile. As there is some information regarding the metabolism of AMP implicating CYP2D6 it is possible that agents known to potently inhibit CYP2D6 (eg, paroxetine, quinidine) could impede the metabolism of AMP if used concurrently. In summary, there are few currently recognized pharmacokinetic interactions between AMP and CYP450 or other enzyme inhibitors.

Methylphenidate and drug–drug interactions

With respect to MPH, it is almost exclusively metabolized by the hepatic enzyme CES1 in a stereoselective manner to the major inactive metabolite, ritalinic acid. Thus, if any medications which might inhibit CES1 are coadministered with MPH on an acute or chronic basis, a decrease in MPH clearance (and potentially increased side effects or toxicity) would be anticipated for the duration of concomitant use. Although systematic DDI studies conducted in healthy human subjects are considered the gold standard for DDI confirmation, *in vitro* studies are invaluable in identifying potential DDIs. Although the exploration of CES1-mediated DDIs is in its relative infancy compared with other drug-metabolizing enzyme systems such as the CYP450, *in vitro* studies have identified several compounds from an array of therapeutic classes which can significantly inhibit CES1 activity. Such drugs are by no means contraindicated with MPH but can be regarded as suspected perpetrators because of their confirmed inhibitory effects on CES1 *in vitro*. However, we do know that *in vitro* effects are often not borne out *in vivo* for a host of reasons. For example, an *in vitro* CES1 inhibitor like montelukast which has very low dosage levels (eg, 4–5 mg/d in children) may simply be insufficient to produce significant metabolic inhibition of an abundant enzyme. We do know that neither *dl*-MPH nor ritalinic acid themselves can inhibit CES1 activity *in vitro*. On the other hand, agents which may be used concurrently with MPH which have been screened by *in vitro* methods and *not* found to significantly inhibit CES1 include; the nonstimulant ADHD medications atomoxetine, clonidine, and guanfacine, the antipsychotics clozapine, olanzapine, risperidone, paliperidone, aripiprazole, ziprasidone, quetiapine and haloperidol, the TCA imipramine, the antibiotics amoxicillin, erythromycin, and ciprofloxacin, and antihistamine diphenhydramine and decongestant phenylephrine.[70]

The concurrent use of MPH with ethanol is associated with at least two metabolic phenomena. First, consumption of ethanol (0.6 g/kg) 30 min before or after the administration of modified-release racemic MPH (Ritalin LA) as well as dexmethylphenidate (Focalin XR) resulted in significantly increased the plasma C_{max} of the second pulse of MPH by 35% ($P < .01$) and the partial $(AUC)_{4-8h}$ by 25%.[71] Secondly, in a somewhat unusual trans-esterification reaction likewise catalyzed by hepatic CES1, the methyl-group on the MPH molecule is replaced by an ethyl-group from consumed ethanol forming the metabolite ethylphenidate.[72] This too is a highly stereoselective process favoring *l*-ethylphenidate formation. Although ethylphenidate does have potent CNS activity as a psychostimulant, the amounts formed from this reaction are relatively small mitigating most of the concern over this DDI.[72] With regard to MPH participating as a potential perpetrating agent (ie, inhibiting or inducing the metabolism of coadministered agents), package insert information on potential drug interactions for some products suggests that MPH may inhibit the metabolism of a number of coadministered medications including coumarin anticoagulants, some anticonvulsants. While this may be possible, the evidence base for most of these purported interactions is quite limited. In summary, pharmacokinetic DDIs with MPH serving as the victim drug are likely to be due to combined use with medications or other substances which are CES1 inhibitors. However, essentially none of the agents identified *in vitro* as CES1 inhibitors have been evaluated for their clinical effects in this regard.

Both psychostimulants are routinely used in combination with a variety of other medications from essentially every drug class on an acute or chronic basis. There are no known pharmacokinetic interactions that represent strict contraindications, or that rise to the level of prescriber warning. Available *in vitro* data and limited clinical data suggest that neither AMP nor MPH impair the activity of any major CYP450 oxidative enzyme or drug transporter, or that other drugs which inhibit or induce these catalytic enzymes or transporter expression alter the psychostimulant's disposition. The role of CYP2D6 in AMP metabolism is not firmly established and the potential for *in vitro* CES1 inhibitors to produce clinically significant effects on the disposition of MPH has not been evaluated.

SUMMARY

The psychostimulants AMP and MPH have been in clinical use for well more than 60 years. In general, it can be stated that both stimulants are rapidly absorbed, have relatively poor bioavailability and short half-lives. The development of an array of pharmaceutical dosage forms with once daily administration has largely addressed these issues. The pharmacokinetics of both stimulants are generally linear and dose proportional although substantial interindividual variability in pharmacokinetics is in evidence. AMP is highly metabolized by several oxidative enzymes including members of the CYP450 system forming multiple metabolites with approximately 5% to 30% excreted unchanged in the urine. Although CYP2D6 is believed to play a role in AMP metabolism, the extent of that role is not well-defined. There is some evidence of stereoselectivity in metabolism when racemic AMP is administered favoring the *d*-isomer. There are as of, yet no gene variants associated with decreased (or increased) AMP metabolism. MPH is primarily metabolized by CES1 catalyzed de-esterification to the major inactive metabolite ritalinic acid. When racemic MPH is administered profound stereoselective metabolism is observed favoring the inactive *l*-isomer. Less than 1% of MPH is excreted unchanged in the urine. A loss-of-function *CES1* variant G143E (rs71647871) associated with impaired metabolism of MPH has been identified. At present, pharmacogenomic testing as an aid to guide dosing and personalize treatment cannot be recommended for either agent on a routine basis. Few significant pharmacokinetically based DDIs have been documented for either stimulant but there has been relatively little systematic clinical study of this issue with either agent.

CLINICS CARE POINTS

- When considering dosage adjustments in patients, no matter the stimulant or formulation used, pharmacokinetics are generally linear and dose proportional.
- When treating patients with amphetamine (AMP) formulations avoid the coadministration of medications or substances which can significantly alter urinary pH. For example, known urine acidifiers (ie, ascorbic acid) and known urine alkalizers (ie, sodium bicarbonate) in sufficient quantity can significantly speed or reduce AMP clearance, respectively.
- With consideration to AMP treatment, pharmacogenomic testing centered on drug-metabolizing enzymes is not recommended at present as multiple enzymes are involved in its metabolism and the significance of CYP2D6 involvement requires further clarification.
- When treating patients with methylphenidate (MPH), be cognizant of the fact individuals that a loss of function *CES1* G143E (rs71647871) variant has been documented resulting in impaired clearance. However, pharmacogenomic testing is not routinely recommended at present.
- When treating patients with MPH, be aware that coadministration with known inhibitors of CES1 can potentially impede the drug's clearance.

DISCLOSURE

The authors have nothing to disclose.

REFERENCES

1. Polanczyk GV, Salum GA, Sugaya LS, et al. Annual research review: a meta-analysis of the worldwide prevalence of mental disorders in children and adolescents. J Child Psychol Psychiatry 2015;56(3):345–65.

2. Willcutt EG. The prevalence of DSM-IV attention-deficit/hyperactivity disorder: a meta-analytic review. Neurotherapeutics 2012;9(3):490–9.

3. Warikoo N, Faraone SV. Background, clinical features and treatment of attention deficit hyperactivity disorder in children. Expert Opin Pharmacother 2013;14(14): 1885–906.

4. Faraone SV, Biederman J, Mick E. The age-dependent decline of attention deficit hyperactivity disorder: a meta-analysis of follow-up studies. Psychol Med 2006; 36(2):159–65.

5. Simon V, Czobor P, Bálint S, et al. Prevalence and correlates of adult attention-deficit hyperactivity disorder: meta-analysis. Br J Psychiatry 2009;194(3):204–11.

6. Pliszka SR. Pharmacologic treatment of attention-deficit/hyperactivity disorder: efficacy, safety and mechanisms of action. Neuropsychol Rev 2007;17(1):61–72.

7. Wolraich ML, Hagan JF, Allan C, et al. Clinical practice guideline for the diagnosis, evaluation, and treatment of attention-deficit/hyperactivity disorder in children and adolescents. Pediatrics 2019;144(4):e20192528.

8. Biederman J. Attention-deficit/hyperactivity disorder: a selective overview. Biol Psychiatry 2005;57(11):1215–20.

9. Cortese S, Faraone SV, Sergeant J. Misunderstandings of the genetics and neurobiology of ADHD: moving beyond anachronisms. Am J Med Genet B Neuropsychiatr Genet 2011;156B(5):513–6.

10. Ranjbar-Slamloo Y, Fazlali Z. Dopamine and noradrenaline in the brain; overlapping or dissociate functions? Front Mol Neurosci 2019;12:334.

11. Purper-Ouakil D, Ramoz N, Lepagnol-Bestel AM, et al. Neurobiology of attention deficit/hyperactivity disorder. Pediatr Res 2011;69(5 Pt 2):69R–76R.

12. Curatolo P, Paloscia C, D'Agati E, et al. The neurobiology of attention deficit/hyperactivity disorder. Eur J Paediatr Neurol 2009;13(4):299–304.

13. Gallo EF, Posner J. Moving towards causality in attention-deficit hyperactivity disorder: overview of neural and genetic mechanisms. Lancet Psychiatry 2016;3(6): 555–67.

14. Arnold LE. Methyiphenidate vs. amphetamine: comparative review. J Atten Disord 2000;3(4):200–11.

15. Hodgkins P, Shaw M, Coghill D, et al. Amfetamine and methylphenidate medications for attention-deficit/hyperactivity disorder: complementary treatment options. Eur Child Adolesc Psychiatry 2012;21(9):477–92.

16. Sonuga-Barke EJS, Coghill D, Wigal T, et al. Adverse reactions to methylphenidate treatment for attention-deficit/hyperactivity disorder: structure and associations with clinical characteristics and symptom control. J Child Adolesc Psychopharmacol 2009;19(6):683–90.

17. Mosholder AD, Gelperin K, Hammad TA, et al. Hallucinations and other psychotic symptoms associated with the use of attention-deficit/hyperactivity disorder drugs in children. Pediatrics 2009;123(2):611–6.

18. Glaser PEA, Thomas TC, Joyce BM, et al. Differential effects of amphetamine isomers on dopamine release in the rat striatum and nucleus accumbens core. Psychopharmacology (Berl) 2005;178(2–3):250–8.

19. Robertson SD, Matthies HJG, Galli A. A closer look at amphetamine-induced reverse transport and trafficking of the dopamine and norepinephrine transporters. Mol Neurobiol 2009;39(2):73–80.

20. Wood S, Sage JR, Shuman T, et al. Psychostimulants and cognition: a continuum of behavioral and cognitive activation. Pharmacol Rev 2014;66(1):193–221.

21. Freyberg Z, Sonders MS, Aguilar JI, et al. Mechanisms of amphetamine action illuminated through optical monitoring of dopamine synaptic vesicles in Drosophila brain. Nat Commun 2016;7:10652.
22. Markowitz JS, Patrick KS. Differential pharmacokinetics and pharmacodynamics of methylphenidate enantiomers: does chirality matter? J Clin Psychopharmacol 2008;28(3 Suppl 2):S54–61.
23. Markowitz JS, DeVane CL, Pestreich LK, et al. A comprehensive in vitro screening of d-, l-, and dl-threo-methylphenidate: an exploratory study. J Child Adolesc Psychopharmacol 2006;16(6):687–98.
24. Markowitz JS, DeVane CL, Ramamoorthy S, et al. The psychostimulant d-threo-(R,R)-methylphenidate binds as an agonist to the 5HT(1A) receptor. Pharmazie 2009;64(2):123–5.
25. Brikell I, Wimberley T, Albiñana C, et al. Genetic, clinical, and sociodemographic factors associated with stimulant treatment outcomes in ADHD. Am J Psychiatry 2021;178(9):854–64.
26. Elsayed NA, Yamamoto KM, Froehlich TE. Genetic influence on efficacy of pharmacotherapy for pediatric attention-deficit/hyperactivity disorder: overview and current status of research. CNS Drugs 2020;34(4):389–414.
27. Bruxel EM, Akutagava-Martins GC, Salatino-Oliveira A, et al. ADHD pharmacogenetics across the life cycle: new findings and perspectives. Am J Med Genet B Neuropsychiatr Genet 2014;165B(4):263–82.
28. Grimm O, Kranz TM, Reif A. Genetics of ADHD: what should the clinician know? Curr Psychiatry Rep 2020;22(4):18.
29. Faraone SV, Larsson H. Genetics of attention deficit hyperactivity disorder. Mol Psychiatry 2019;24(4):562–75.
30. Bach MV, Coutts RT, Baker GB. Involvement of CYP2D6 in the in vitro metabolism of amphetamine, two N-alkylamphetamines and their 4-methoxylated derivatives. Xenobiotica 1999;29(7):719–32.
31. Dring LG, Smith RL, Williams RT. The fate of amphetamine in man and other mammals. J Pharm Pharmacol 1966;18(6):402–4.
32. Dring LG, Smith RL, Williams RT. The metabolic fate of amphetamine in man and other species. Biochem J 1970;116(3):425–35.
33. Green CE, LeValley SE, Tyson CA. Comparison of amphetamine metabolism using isolated hepatocytes from five species including human. J Pharmacol Exp Ther 1986;237(3):931–6.
34. Cashman JR, Xiong YN, Xu L, et al. N-oxygenation of amphetamine and methamphetamine by the human flavin-containing monooxygenase (form 3): role in bioactivation and detoxication. J Pharmacol Exp Ther 1999;288(3):1251–60.
35. Shiiyama S, Soejima-Ohkuma T, Honda S, et al. Major role of the CYP2C isozymes in deamination of amphetamine and benzphetamine: evidence for the quinidine-specific inhibition of the reactions catalysed by rabbit enzyme. Xenobiotica 1997;27(4):379–87.
36. Zhu HJ, Wang JS, Donovan JL, et al. Interactions of attention-deficit/hyperactivity disorder therapeutic agents with the efflux transporter P-glycoprotein. Eur J Pharmacol 2008;578(2–3):148–58.
37. Angrist B, Corwin J, Bartlik B, et al. Early pharmacokinetics and clinical effects of oral D-amphetamine in normal subjects. Biol Psychiatry 1987;22(11):1357–68.
38. Brown GL, Ebert MH, Hunt RD. Plasma d-amphetamine absorption and elimination in hyperactive children. Psychopharmacol Bull 1978;14(3):33–5.
39. Tulloch SJ, Zhang Y, McLean A, et al. SLI381 (Adderall XR), a two-component, extended-release formulation of mixed amphetamine salts: bioavailability of three

test formulations and comparison of fasted, fed, and sprinkled administration. Pharmacotherapy 2002;22(11):1405–15.

40. Markowitz JS, Patrick KS. The clinical pharmacokinetics of amphetamines utilized in the treatment of attention-deficit/hyperactivity disorder. J Child Adolesc Psychopharmacol 2017;27(8):678–89.

41. Wan SH, Matin SB, Azarnoff DL. Kinetics, salivary excretion of amphetamine isomers, and effect of urinary pH. Clin Pharmacol Ther 1978;23(5):585–90.

42. Pennick M. Absorption of lisdexamfetamine dimesylate and its enzymatic conversion to d-amphetamine. Neuropsychiatr Dis Treat 2010;6:317–27.

43. Teh LK, Bertilsson L. Pharmacogenomics of CYP2D6: molecular genetics, interethnic differences and clinical importance. Drug Metab Pharmacokinet 2012; 27(1):55–67.

44. Yamazaki H, Shimizu M. Survey of variants of human flavin-containing monooxygenase 3 (FMO3) and their drug oxidation activities. Biochem Pharmacol 2013; 85(11):1588–93.

45. Patrick KS, González MA, Straughn AB, et al. New methylphenidate formulations for the treatment of attention-deficit/hyperactivity disorder. Expert Opin Drug Deliv 2005;2(1):121–43.

46. Markowitz JS, Straughn AB, Patrick KS. Advances in the pharmacotherapy of attention-deficit-hyperactivity disorder: focus on methylphenidate formulations. Pharmacotherapy 2003;23(10):1281–99.

47. Childress AC. Novel formulations of ADHD medications: stimulant selection and management. Focus (Am Psychiatr Publ). 2021;19(1):31–8.

48. Sun Z, Murry DJ, Sanghani SP, et al. Methylphenidate is stereoselectively hydrolyzed by human carboxylesterase CES1A1. J Pharmacol Exp Ther 2004;310(2): 469–76.

49. Modi NB, Wang B, Noveck RJ, et al. Dose-proportional and stereospecific pharmacokinetics of methylphenidate delivered using an osmotic, controlled-release oral delivery system. J Clin Pharmacol 2000;40(10):1141–9.

50. Patrick KS, Straughn AB, Perkins JS, et al. Evolution of stimulants to treat ADHD: transdermal methylphenidate. Hum Psychopharmacol 2009;24(1):1–17.

51. Faraj BA, Israili ZH, Perel JM, et al. Metabolism and disposition of methylphenidate-14C: studies in man and animals. J Pharmacol Exp Ther 1974;191(3):535–47.

52. Markowitz JS, Straughn AB, Patrick KS, et al. Pharmacokinetics of methylphenidate after oral administration of two modified-release formulations in healthy adults. Clin Pharmacokinet 2003;42(4):393–401.

53. Rochdi M, González MA, Dirksen SJH. Dose-proportional pharmacokinetics of a methylphenidate extended-release capsule. Int J Clin Pharmacol Ther 2004; 42(5):285–92.

54. Adjei A, Teuscher NS, Kupper RJ, et al. Single-dose pharmacokinetics of methylphenidate extended-release multiple layer beads administered as intact capsule or sprinkles versus methylphenidate immediate-release tablets (Ritalin®) in healthy adult volunteers. J Child Adolesc Psychopharmacol 2014;24(10): 570–8.

55. Her L, Zhu HJ. Carboxylesterase 1 and precision pharmacotherapy: pharmacogenetics and nongenetic regulators. Drug Metab Dispos 2020;48(3):230–44.

56. Zhu HJ, Patrick KS, Yuan HJ, et al. Two CES1 gene mutations lead to dysfunctional carboxylesterase 1 activity in man: clinical significance and molecular basis. Am J Hum Genet 2008;82(6):1241–8.

57. Stage C, Jürgens G, Guski LS, et al. The impact of CES1 genotypes on the pharmacokinetics of methylphenidate in healthy Danish subjects. Br J Clin Pharmacol 2017;83(7):1506–14.

58. Nemoda Z, Angyal N, Tarnok Z, et al. Carboxylesterase 1 gene polymorphism and methylphenidate response in ADHD. Neuropharmacology 2009;57(7–8): 731–3.

59. Stevens T, Sangkuhl K, Brown JT, et al. PharmGKB summary: methylphenidate pathway, pharmacokinetics/pharmacodynamics. Pharmacogenet Genomics 2019;29(6):136–54.

60. Larson K, Russ SA, Kahn RS, et al. Patterns of comorbidity, functioning, and service use for US children with ADHD, 2007. Pediatrics 2011;127(3):462–70.

61. Girand HL, Litkowiec S, Sohn M. Attention-deficit/hyperactivity disorder and psychotropic polypharmacy prescribing trends. Pediatrics 2020;146(1):e20192832.

62. Bussing R, Winterstein AG. Polypharmacy in attention deficit hyperactivity disorder treatment: current status, challenges and next steps. Curr Psychiatry Rep 2012;14(5):447–9.

63. Markowitz JS, Morrison SD, DeVane CL. Drug interactions with psychostimulants. Int Clin Psychopharmacol 1999;14(1):1–18.

64. Markowitz JS, Patrick KS. Pharmacokinetic and pharmacodynamic drug interactions in the treatment of attention-deficit hyperactivity disorder. Clin Pharmacokinet 2001;40(10):753–72.

65. 022063Orig1s000SumR.pdf. Available at: https://www.accessdata.fda.gov/drugsatfda_docs/nda/2017/022063Orig1s000SumR.pdf. Accessed March 7, 2022.

66. Krishnan S, Moncrief S. An evaluation of the cytochrome p450 inhibition potential of lisdexamfetamine in human liver microsomes. Drug Metab Dispos 2007;35(1): 180–4.

67. Ermer J, Corcoran M, Martin P. Lisdexamfetamine dimesylate effects on the pharmacokinetics of cytochrome P450 substrates in healthy adults in an open-label, randomized, crossover study. Drugs R D 2015;15(2):175–85.

68. Beckett AH, Rowland M, Turner P. Influence OF urinary PH ON excretion OF amphetamine. Lancet 1965;1(7380):303.

69. Davis JM, Kopin IJ, Lemberger L, et al. Effects of urinary pH on amphetamine metabolism. Ann N Y Acad Sci 1971;179:493–501.

70. Zhu HJ, Appel DI, Peterson YK, et al. Identification of selected therapeutic agents as inhibitors of carboxylesterase 1: potential sources of metabolic drug interactions. Toxicology 2010;270(2–3):59–65.

71. Zhu HJ, Patrick KS, Straughn AB, et al. Ethanol interactions with dexmethylphenidate and dl-methylphenidate spheroidal oral drug absorption systems in healthy volunteers. J Clin Psychopharmacol 2017;37(4):419–28.

72. Patrick KS, Straughn AB, Minhinnett RR, et al. Influence of ethanol and gender on methylphenidate pharmacokinetics and pharmacodynamics. Clin Pharmacol Ther 2007;81(3):346–53.

Nonstimulant Treatments for ADHD

Jeffrey H. Newcorn, MD[a,b],*, Beth Krone, PhD[a], Ralf W. Dittmann, MSc, MD, PhD[c]

KEYWORDS

- Nonstimulants • ADHD treatment • Psychopharmacology

KEY POINTS

- We discuss monotherapy and combined treatment of ADHD, with review of mechanism of action, pharmacokinetics, efficacy, tolerability, and safety of approved, off-label, and pipeline nonstimulants.
- Nonstimulants have an important role when response or tolerability to psychostimulants is poor, when comorbid disorders are present, or if patients prefer to use nonstimulants. There also may be advantages relative to the duration of activity.
- Four nonstimulant medications have FDA approval for ADHD–the norepinephrine reuptake inhibitors, atomoxetine and viloxazine extended release, and the α-2 long acting adrenergic agonists, clonidine extended release and guanfacine estended release.
- Characteristics of clinical response vary across drug classes, including nature of response, approach to titration, time to onset of improvement, and temporal characteristics of treatment.
- Identification of nonabusable treatments with comparable efficacy to stimulants, favorable tolerability profile and consistent effects throughout the day remains a high priority for the field.

INTRODUCTION/HISTORY/DEFINITIONS/BACKGROUND

Overview, The use of nonstimulants in ADHD has a long history; the first publication of a randomized, controlled clinical trial with imipramine was published almost 50 years ago.[1]Since then, a variety of publications have attested to the utility of nonstimulants in ADHD. Initially these medications were used "off-label" (ie, outside of FDA approval),

[a] Department of Psychiatry, Division of ADHD, Learning Disabilities, and Related Disorders, Icahn School of Medicine at Mount Sinai, 1 Gustave L Levy Place, Box 1230, New York, NY 10029, USA; [b] Department of Pediatrics, Division of ADHD, Learning Disabilities, and Related Disorders, Icahn School of Medicine at Mount Sinai, 1 Gustave L Levy Place, Box 1230, New York, NY 10029, USA; [c] Paediatric Psychopharmacology, Department of Child and Adolescent Psychiatry and Psychotherapy, Central Institute of Mental Health, Medical Faculty Mannheim, University of Heidelberg, J 5, 68159 Mannheim, Germany
* Corresponding author. Department of Psychiatry, Division of ADHD, Learning Disabilities, and Related Disorders, Icahn School of Medicine at Mount Sinai, 1 Gustave L Levy Place, Box 1230, New York, NY 10029.
E-mail address: Jeffrey.Newcorn@mssm.edu
Twitter: @beth_Krone (B.K.)

Child Adolesc Psychiatric Clin N Am 31 (2022) 417–435
https://doi.org/10.1016/j.chc.2022.03.005
1056-4993/22/© 2022 Elsevier Inc. All rights reserved.
childpsych.theclinics.com

and some continue to be used that way. However, there are now 4 nonstimulant medications that have FDA approval for ADHD—the norepinephrine (NE) reuptake inhibitors, atomoxetine (approved in 2002) and viloxazine extended release (ER; approved in 2021), and the long acting α-2 adrenergic agonists, extended release clonidine (CLON-XR; approved in 2010) and extended release guanfacine (approved in 2009).

Rationale for the development and use of nonstimulant medications in ADHD, Despite the high degree of efficacy of stimulant medications, their limitations attenuate applicability to a subgroup of individuals with ADHD—more for some individuals than others.[2] Some patients treated with stimulants do not achieve optimal symptom reduction/response, or they do not tolerate psychostimulant treatment well[3]; these are not infrequently related.[4] Time-action properties of stimulants are also problematic. Stimulants are inherently short-acting medications, and even the long-acting formulations developed during the last 20 years may not cover the entire day adequately. In addition, stimulants are controlled substances (eg, in the United States: Class II), have documented potential for abuse, and there is a substantial amount of misuse and diversion, particularly among college students and young adults.[5] Therefore, identification of nonabusable treatments for ADHD that have comparable or near comparable efficacy to stimulants, a favorable tolerability profile and consistent effects throughout the entire day is a high priority for the field.

Neurobiological basis of nonstimulant medications for ADHD, The executive control network—including the prefrontal cortex (PFC), anterior cingulate gyrus, striatum, and cerebellum—has long been implicated in the pathophysiology of ADHD.[6] The brain regions within this network are characterized by high levels of dopaminergic and/or noradrenergic neurotransmission, leading to the conceptualization of ADHD as a disorder of catecholamine function. This is attributable, in part, to an elegant series of studies illustrating that methylphenidate (MPH) binds to the dopamine (DA) transporter (see the study by Nora Volkow[7]), thereby enhancing synaptic DA. However, NE also plays an important role in the regulation of attention,[8] stimulants bind to the NE transporter and enhance synaptic NE, and NE is a potent agonist of the DA D4 receptor. Consequently, recent conceptualizations of catecholamine mechanisms in ADHD have focused on interactive properties of DA and NE neurotransmission, as well as on the modulating roles of other neurotransmitter systems. This research provides a neurobiological rationale for the use of nonstimulant agents—all of which (thus far) target NE in one way or another—in the treatment of ADHD.

Objectives, To review each of the FDA-approved nonstimulant medications in detail, provide information on medications approved for other conditions that are used off-label in ADHD and introduce several investigational medications in the ADHD pipeline. We will present information regarding mechanism of action, pharmacokinetics, efficacy, and tolerability/safety profile. In addition to reviewing the evidence-base regarding nonstimulant medications, we will offer expert opinion that may inform clinical use, including both monotherapy and combined treatment.

DISCUSSION
Nonstimulant Medications Used in ADHD

The 4 FDA-approved nonstimulant medications are described in detail below. In addition, information regarding dosing and issues related to clinical use are provided in **Table 1**.

ATOMOXETINE

Atomoxetine (ATX) was the first US Food and Drug Administration (FDA)-approved nonstimulant medication for ADHD (in 2002), and it is labeled for use in both children

Table 1
FDA-approved Nonstimulant

Drug	Class	FDA Approvals	Dose	Common Adverse Effects	Comments
ATX[a]	NRI[e]	Children <70 kg Adults >70 kg	0.5–1.4 mg/kg 40–100 mg	Sedation, nausea/vomiting, increased heart rate, and BP. Irritability. Decrease in appetite and/or growth (less than with stimulants)	Approved for once or twice daily administration. First medication specifically approved for adult ADHD. Metabolized by CYP2D6; poor metabolizers have greatly increased half-life and plasma levels. Warnings for suicidal ideation and hepatic toxicity. Best to take with food. Twice daily administration during titration may aid in reducing sedation and GI side effects. Can be administered in AM or PM/evening—effect is less robust if administered in the evening. Time to onset can be seen within weeks in excellent responders but the full effect may not be seen for up to 3 mo
VER[b]	NRI[e]	Children 6–11 Children 12–17	100–200 mg 200–400 mg	Sedation, difficulty sleeping, and decreased appetite Nausea/vomiting, irritability, and increased heart rate	Approved in children; adult data are currently under FDA review. Response (at the group level) is similar across low and higher doses but some potential for improved response with titration. Improvement often seen by 2 wk. Previously approved as an antidepressant in adults. Potential differences

(continued on next page)

Table 1
(*continued*)

Drug	Class	FDA Approvals	Dose	Common Adverse Effects	Comments
					from atomoxetine: not metabolized by CYP2D6; half-life is ~7 h; impacts several postsynaptic 5-HT receptors. Strong inhibitor of CYP1A2; may increase levels of drugs metabolized via this enzyme (eg, duloxetine, caffeine, clozapine). Also, viloxazine levels could be increased by drugs impacting CYP1A2 (eg, acetaminophen). Weak inhibitor of CYP 3A4; could increase levels of drugs metabolized via this mechanism (eg, dextromethorphan; guanfacine).
GXR[c]	α-2 agonist[f]	Children 6–17	1–4 mg (up to 7 mg in adolescents)	Sedation, decreased HR and BP, hypotension, light-headedness, dizziness, irritability, and dry mouth and/or eyes	Approved for monotherapy or combined therapy with stimulants. Sedation can be prominent when initiating therapy or raising the dose. Sequential up-titration of 1 mg/wk to minimize side effects. Discontinuation should be gradual to avoid rebound hypertension—1 mg/wk. CYP3A4 metabolized—so watch

for drug interactions. Half-life is 14–17 h; drug levels peak at ~ 6 h. Post hoc analyses support a weight-based dosing approach; target of ~.08–.10 mg/kg

| CXR[d] | α-2 agonist[f] | Children 6–17 | 0 .1–0.4 mg (bid dosing) | Sedation, decreased HR and BP, hypotension, light-headedness, dizziness, irritability, dry mouth and/or eyes | Approved for monotherapy or combined therapy with stimulants. Sedation can be prominent when initiating therapy or raising the dose. Sequential up-titration of 0.1 mg/wk to minimize side effects. Discontinuation should be gradual to avoid rebound hypertension—0.1 mg/wk. Partially metabolized via CYP2D6. Half-life is 12–16 h; drug levels peak at ~3–5 h |

[a] Atomoxetine
[b] Viloxazine extended release.
[c] Guanfacine extended release.
[d] Clonidine extended release.
[e] Norepinephrine-reuptake inhibitor.
[f] Alpha-2 adrenergic agonists.

and adults. ATX is a relatively selective NE reuptake inhibitor, which also has weak effects at the serotonin transporter, although the latter is not thought to contribute to therapeutic efficacy. ATX increases synaptic NE in multiple brain regions and DA levels in PFC.[9] However, ATX has a low potential for abuse because it does not bind to receptors associated with abuse potential and does not increase DA in the striatum or nucleus accumbens. There is also no evidence of tolerance over time.

A multitude of research has demonstrated that ATX is effective in treating core ADHD symptoms, with apparently equivalent response in inattentive and hyperactive–impulsive domains, with effect sizes that are very solid (in the moderate range overall), but somewhat lower than for stimulants.[10] Treatment is associated with a reduction in impairment across several domains of function, including child self-esteem (as reported by parents), and social and family function.[11] Review of all premarketing studies of ATX in children and adolescents[10] found that response to ATX was bimodal, with most children falling into categories of "much improved" or "nonresponders," rather than "minimally improved." This means that the effect size (ES) of 0.7 in children, which includes both responders and nonresponders, is not a very good way to portray response for this medication; it may do very well for responders, with effects near if not quite the equal of stimulants. The problem is that there is not really a good way to identify excellent responders a priori. Only onset of response by 4 weeks predicts excellent response[10]

The drug is metabolized via the cytochrome P (CYP) 2D6 system; 5% to 7% of individuals have a genetic polymorphism, which makes them poor metabolizers, and a small number of individuals are ultrarapid metabolizers. In poor metabolizers, the half-life of ATX is 19 to 21 hours (vs 4.5 hours in extensive metabolizers), and plasma medication levels are much higher for any given dose.[12] Although it is not necessary to determine CYP2D6 genotype before treatment (studies using blind titration in slow and extensive metabolizers found that end of titration doses were nearly equivalent[12]), there is some suggestion that poor metabolizers have slightly better efficacy and slightly higher adverse event (AE) rates.[12,13] ATX administration does not affect the pharmacokinetic properties of concomitant medications metabolized via CYP2D6 substrates. However, medications that alter CYP2D6 function, such as fluoxetine and paroxetine, can affect the metabolism of ATX by inducing poor metabolizer status.[14] For selected individuals, this strategy could potentially be used to extend the duration of the medication effect, and possibly enhance response.

ATX is dosed on a weight-based schedule; the target dose is 1.2 mg/kg, with a range of 1.0 to 1.4 mg/kg. The medication is effective whether administered once or twice daily. Atomoxetine maintains its effect over an extended period. Time to duration of onset of atomoxetine has been a matter of some debate. Newcorn and colleagues (2009)[10] examined predictors of response in acute trials of atomoxetine in youth, finding that early response to atomoxetine (2–4 weeks) predicted response at trial endpoint. However, De Brukyere and colleagues (2016),[11] using pooled data from short-term (10 weeks) and long-term (24 weeks) clinical trials in adults, found that although symptom reductions and global improvement scores at weeks 4 and 10 were statistically significant predictors of response at later time points, they did not fully account for improvement over time. The authors therefore recommend that the only way to determine whether a given individual will respond to atomoxetine is to treat for up to 3 months. Of course, the latter approach would be challenging for patients who are not achieving a good enough response.

The most commonly occurring AEs include sedation, nausea and vomiting, decreased appetite, weight loss, and increase in heart rate and BP (comparable to stimulants). Irritability and increased aggression can also be seen, most often in individuals with comorbid mood disorders or disruptive behavior disorders.[15] There are warnings for hepatotoxicity and suicidal ideation. In 2004, postmarketing surveillance identified 2 cases of acute hepatotoxicity (out of ~2 million exposures). Both patients had abdominal pain, jaundice, and substantially elevated liver function tests, which resolved with medication discontinuation. Recurrence of the liver function abnormalities on rechallenge in one case suggests a causal relationship.[16] Obtaining routine liver function tests before initiating ATX treatment is not recommended, owing to the very-low frequency of liver toxicity, and the fact that liver toxicity cannot be predicted from baseline laboratory indices. Atomoxetine also has a "black box" warning for suicidal ideation, due to its common mechanism of action (ie, NE reuptake inhibition) with known antidepressants, and data from premarketing clinical trials. Approximately 4 per 1000 patients treated in 12 short-term clinical trials had suicidal behavior, mainly ingestions, although intent was uncertain in almost all of these cases.[16] It should be noted that a comprehensive review did not find that ATX was more highly associated with suicidal behavior than stimulants.[15] It is nonetheless good clinical practice to obtain a careful history of mood problems and/or suicidal behavior before starting medication, to educate patients and families regarding the importance of reporting changes in mental status, and to maintain close contact with patients early in the treatment. Particular attention should be given to changes in emotional state, including sadness, tearfulness, irritability, anger, or euphoria.

Atomoxetine is not labeled for combined treatment with stimulants, and there are no controlled data that systematically evaluate this drug combination but the 2 medication classes can be used together, and ATX is sometimes used that way in practice. Potential advantages might include relatively longer duration of action, potential for lowering stimulant dose, obviating the need for an afternoon stimulant booster dose, and improving sleep (because ATX can be sedating). Potential disadvantages include sedation (if it occurs) and increased heart rate (HR) and blood pressure (BP) (because both ATX and stimulants increase HR and BP).

Alpha-2 Adrenergic Agonists

The α-2 adrenergic agonists have been used to treat ADHD for more than 3 decades, particularly in youth with comorbid tics and/or aggression. Initially, these medications were used off-label in immediate-release (IR) formulations (the only formulations available at the time) as a nonstimulant alternative in individuals with tic disorders or Tourette syndrome, based on the recognition (accepted at that time) that stimulants might precipitate or worsen tics.[17] However, the immediate release formulations have relatively short duration of action despite half-lives that are reasonably long (~12 hours for immediate release (IR) clonidine and ~16 hours for IR guanfacine). The need for multiple daily dosing as well as tolerability issues with the IR formulations (mainly sedation) led to the development of extended-release (XR) formulations. Each of the long-acting formulations is FDA-approved for both monotherapy and combined treatment with stimulants. There is also a clonidine patch (not approved for ADHD), which offers activity for approximately 5 to 7 days; however, this is rarely used. Although clinical trials indicate improvement in both inattention and hyperactive–impulsive symptoms, there seems to be a slightly better response to hyperactive/impulsive symptoms. Consequently, these medications are relegated to second line by National Institute for Healthcare Excellence and European Union (EU) regulatory.[18] Behavioral overarousal, aggression, and oppositional defiant behavior—mainly but not exclusively in association with ADHD—are frequent targets of treatment. Other frequent targets include motor or vocal tics, which may occur comorbidly or be exacerbated by stimulant treatment, and insomnia (either independent of or in association with stimulant treatment) because the α2-agonists can be fairly sedating, especially on initiating treatment. As with atomoxetine, the a2-agonists offer additional nonstimulant alternatives in cases where diversion or abuse of stimulants is suspected, or in individuals with heightened risk for substance use disorders (SUDs). Although none of the formulations of clonidine or guanfacine are FDA-approved for ADHD in adults in the United States, they may be used off-label in adults to augment ADHD treatment (mainly for overarousal, restlessness and impulsivity, or to minimize sleep disturbance) due to their well-established safety profile in the treatment of cardiovascular disease.

Initial research and the clinical use of the α2-agonists were with the IR form of clonidine, which has effects at multiple α2 subreceptors, as well as other neurotransmitter receptors. A large seminal trial of clonidine and MPH in youth with ADHD, tic disorders, or their combination indicated that the combination of MPH and clonidine was more effective than either drug alone in treating both ADHD symptoms and tics.[19] A subsequent trial, which compared the effects of immediate-release clonidine (CLON-IR), MPH, and their combination in youth with ADHD,[20] found that MPH performed better than CLON-IR but CLON-IR yielded improvement in both symptom ratings and global assessment of function. The average total daily dose of CLON-IR was roughly 0.25 mg, with administration spread over 3 daily doses, because the behavioral effects of CLON-IR last only 3 to 6 hours.

CLON-XR was developed to address limitations related to duration of effects. CLON-XR is labeled for twice daily dosing; the total daily dose ranges from 0.1 to 0.4 mg per day, with recommended dose increases limited to 0.1 mg per day weekly. In a large multisite placebo-controlled trial,[21] CLON-XR significantly improved ADHD symptoms, with the initial improvement as early as the second week of treatment with both the 0.2 mg (ie, 0.1 mg BID) and 0.4 mg (ie, 0.2 mg BID) doses. The most common AE was mild–moderate somnolence. Other AEs included changes in HR and BP (typically lower), and mild alterations of the QTc interval (corrected QT interval; with variable direction of effects, or no effects across studies). Sedation and vital sign changes tended to occur early and resolve during the course of the treatment. No significant adverse events (AEs) occurred related to changes in these parameters, and the QTc change from baseline was small. Because there is potential for rebound hypertension with clonidine, abrupt discontinuation should be avoided.

The potential utility of guanfacine for youth with ADHD has similarly been systematically evaluated, initially in youth with ADHD + tic disorders, and subsequently in youth with ADHD alone. Guanfacine is more selective for a2A-receptors than clonidine; it has a somewhat longer half-life and duration of action, and may be less sedating (although sedation is still the most common side effect). As with clonidine, initial clinical use and research were with the IR formulation but most systematic research has been with the now FDA-approved XR formulation. Guanfacine XR (GXR; doses of 1–4 mg) was found to decrease ADHD symptoms significantly in children aged 6 to 12 years, with increasing effects associated with higher weight-adjusted doses.[22,23] Adolescents aged 13 to 17 years showed less adequate response in the initial trials, due to lower weight-adjusted dosing in this group. Subsequent research using doses up to 7 mg in adolescents found the medication to be effective.[24] Adverse effects included sedation, decreased BP, and QTc changes. Sedation and BP changes generally resolved after 2 weeks and were not associated with medication discontinuation. QTc changes were minimal and did not result in adverse outcomes. Guanfacine is primarily metabolized by CYP3A4, so the dose of guanfacine may need to be increased in the presence of CYP 3A4 inducers (eg, phenobarbital, phenytoin, glucocorticoids) and reduced in the presence of CYP 3A4 inhibitors[25] (eg, erythromycin, clarithromycin, verapamil, grapefruit). Retrospective data suggest that using a weight-based approach may be helpful, with clinical improvement observed from 0.05 up to 0.12 mg/kg. This approach can be helpful in providing a target for titration. Of note, a relatively large controlled trial of guanfacine extended release conducted in adults in Japan found this medication to be effective, with an ES of ~ 0.5, comparable to what has been found for other nonstimulants in adult ADHD.[26]

Similar to other ADHD treatments, GXR was shown to maintain its therapeutic effect during the long-term.[27] Children/adolescents with ADHD who responded to GXR after 13 weeks of titration were randomized to continued treatment with active drug or placebo for 26 weeks. Treatment failure occurred in fewer of the children randomized to GXR than placebo, and time to treatment failure was significantly longer in GXR treated youth versus placebo.

In some countries (eg, United States and Australia), guanfacine XR is approved both as monotherapy and adjunctive to stimulant treatment. One large clinical trial (n = 461) in children/adolescents, showed improved core ADHD symptom control with combined guanfacine XR and stimulants over stimulants alone.[28] Another small study did not find combined guanfacine IR with D-MPH ER to perform better than D-MPH ER alone in reducing the severity of ADHD core symptoms' (n = 207) or improving working memory (n = 182).[29] Of note, discontinuation due to AEs was comparable between guanfacine IR and D-MPH (1.5% each) and was greater for combined treatment (2.9%). As expected, during acute titration, guanfacine IR decreased HR and BP, whereas D-MPH ER increased both parameters. More surprising was that combined treatment increased diastolic blood pressure but had no effects on HR or systolic blood pressure. Also of note, during the maintenance treatment, decreases in HR associated with guanfacine IR and increases in systolic blood pressure associated with D-MPH ER returned to baseline, suggesting that these effects may attenuate over time.

Similarly, a large study (n = 198) conducted in children/adolescents with CLON ER + stimulants found that the combined treatment was superior to stimulant monotherapy (ie, stimulant + placebo) in decreasing the severity of ADHD core symptoms. Another smaller trial (n = 67) of CLON IR added to stimulants in children/adolescents found no incremental benefit on ADHD core symptoms but significant effects on conduct symptoms. However, in this study, CLON was added to twice daily (i.e., bid) stimulant treatment in the combined treatment arm, whereas the stimulant monotherapy arm did not offer a third dose; perhaps, the impact of clonidine would not have been significant had a third dose of stimulant been added in the stimulant monotherapy arm. Of note, all of these trials showed good tolerability of the combination of stimulants + clonidine, with no major issues in terms of safety. This is noteworthy, because questions had initially been raised about the safety of this drug combination.

Viloxazine extended release

Viloxazine extended release (ER) is an extended release formulation of a medication previously approved in the United Kingdom and several other European countries for the treatment of depression. Viloxazine IR was never available in the United States; it was taken off the market in Europe in the early 2000s for commercial reasons but not safety concerns.[30] Viloxazine ER has documented activity at the NE transporter and several postsynaptic serotonin receptors[31]; its effects as a NE reuptake inhibitor provide a neurobiological rationale for its use in ADHD, although it is possible that serotonergic mechanisms also contribute to response. Viloxazine ER was approved by the US FDA in April, 2021, making it the first nonstimulant drug approved in over a decade (since the α-2 adrenergic agonists).

Viloxazine ER is administered once daily; the labeled dose range is 100 to 400 mg, although studies have examined doses up to 600 mg and found adequate safety in higher doses. The starting dose is 100 mg in children and 200 mg in adolescents, with target doses of 200 and 400 mg, respectively. The half-life of ~7 hours supports the once daily label. The time to peak levels is ~5 hours with a range of 3 to 9 hours after a single 200 mg dose. A high-fat meal modestly decreases levels of viloxazine and delays the time to peak by about 2 hours.

A multitude of publications have demonstrated efficacy in children and adolescents. A phase 2 study in children 6 to 12 years old tested 4 doses of viloxazine versus placebo; findings indicated comparable efficacy for each of the doses, with effect sizes ranging from 0.55 to 0.62, comparable to other nonstimulants for ADHD in children.[32] These findings were replicated in subsequent phase 3 studies, which examined the 100 and 200 mg doses in children and the 200 and 400 doses in adolescents.[33–35] Separation from placebo was seen by 2 weeks, and response seen at 2 weeks was found to predict the end of treatment outcome at 6 weeks.[36] Treatment-related AEs reported in 5% or greater of subjects included somnolence, decreased appetite, and headache; however, there was no impact on QTc.[33,34]

There are not yet sufficient data on combined treatment with stimulants to comment on whether this could yield possible augmentation of stimulant response; however, relatively small n studies examining the pharmacokinetic (pK) profiles of viloxazine XR coadministered with either MPH[37] or lisdexamfetamine[38] found relatively little alternation in the pK profiles of any of the drugs.[38] Of note, viloxazine is only partially metabolized by CYP 2D6 and drug levels are only modestly impacted by CYP 2D6 inducers. This, together with its effects at several postsynaptic serotonin receptors, and its longer half-life than ATX in CYP 2D6 extensive metabolizers, illustrate potential distinctiveness from ATX. Moreover, viloxazine ER is a beaded formulation and can be sprinkled on applesauce or pudding without altering the pK profile; this is the only nonstimulant that offers an alternative delivery option other than swallowing pills.[39] Similar to other stimulant and nonstimulant drugs for ADHD, treatment with viloxazine ER is associated with improved functional status,[35,40] with notable improvement in executive function[41] and learning and school problems.[42] In addition, because it has documented antidepressant activity, it may have a role in treating ADHD + depression and/or anxiety; however, this has not yet been studied. Note that viloxazine is a strong inhibitor of CYP 1A2 and may increase drug levels of medications metabolized via this enzyme (eg, duloxetine, caffeine, clozapine). Similarly, viloxazine levels could be increased by drugs impacting CYP 1A2, such as acetaminophen. Viloxazine is also a weak inhibitor of CYP 3A4 and could increase levels of drugs metabolized via this mechanism (eg, dextromethorphan, guanfacine).

Off-Label and Investigational Drugs

Antidepressants
Several antidepressants with noradrenergic activity have either documented or reported efficacy for ADHD—including the noradrenergic tricyclic antidepressants (TCAs; especially well-documented efficacy for desipramine[43]), the serotonin-norepinephrine reuptake inhibitors (SNRIs) (reported but not well studied),[44] bupropion[45] (fairly well studied), and even the monoamine oxidase (MAO) inhibitors (limited controlled data[46]) — although none are labeled for ADHD. Of these, bupropion is the most relevant for clinical practice.

Bupropian. Bupropion is a mixed noradrenergic–dopaminergic agent that is chemically unrelated to other known antidepressants. It is available in IR, sustained-release (SR; bid administration), and long-acting (XL; once daily administration) formulations.

Bupropion is a relatively weak inhibitor of NE and DA reuptake, and does not inhibit monoamine oxidase. Because it is metabolized by CYP2B6, there is potential for interactions with several psychotropic drugs. Multicenter studies in both children[47] and adults[48] with ADHD found that bupropion was effective, although with a lower ES than is typically seen for stimulants. Results from 5 randomized controlled studies of bupropion were evaluated in a meta-analysis (outcome: CGI-Improvement) with a pooled odds ratio of 2.42 favoring bupropion.[49] However, a recent meta-analysis examining the comparative efficacy of buproprion relative to other drugs for pediatric ADHD reported an ES of 0.32 versus placebo,[50] which is a fair bit lower than for the approved nonstimulants. Similarly, a recent Cochrane review[51] found a significant but low quality level of efficacy.

Bupropion may be particularly useful in the treatment of comorbid ADHD + mood disorders because it is an approved antidepressant in adults. In addition, similar to other nonstimulants, it may be a useful alternative to stimulants in comorbid ADHD + SUD. Bupropion has been found to reduce ADHD symptoms in trials of adolescents and adults with ADHD and comorbid SUD, often in the context of other comorbid disorders (eg, conduct disorder (CD), depression[52]). In addition, it has been shown to decrease craving and/or abuse in some of these studies. Also of note, bupropion is FDA-approved for smoking cessation treatment (under a different trade name[53]); this may be relevant to adults with ADHD, given the high association of nicotine addiction and ADHD.

The most commonly reported AEs include agitation, anxiety, decreased appetite, and insomnia. There is a slightly increased risk for drug-induced seizures at doses greater than 450 mg/d, and a black box warning regarding the risk for suicidal thoughts and behaviors. As with the stimulants, exacerbation of tic disorders has been reported.

SNRIs. Because of their partial noradrenergic mechanisms of action, the mixed SNRI medications have received limited study for ADHD. There are a variety of SNRIs, including venlafaxine, desvenlafaxine, duloxetine, milnacepran, and levomilnacepran. Note that the relative proportion of monoamine reuptake activity differs by drug.[54] Venlafaxine is the most serotonergic; desvenlafaxine and duloxetine are more balanced but strongly favoring serotonin, whereas milnacepran and levomilnacepran actually favor NE reuptake. Venlafaxine, desvenlafaxine and duloxetine exhibit very weak effects on DA reuptake, and only at higher doses. Most research to date has been with venlafaxine, including several low n controlled studies but there are also studies in children and adults with duloxetine.[55] Improvement in ADHD symptoms with venlafaxine has been seen in both parent and teacher ratings, with a generally agreeable AE profile. Open or small n controlled studies, including one comparing venlafaxine to MPH, have shown a modest degree of efficacy but are not totally convincing. Recent reviews suggested that venlafaxine may have short-term utility in treating ADHD and may be considered as an alternative agent (used off-label) in patients not tolerating or failing psychostimulants. However, it seems unlikely that doses less than 150 mg, which do not produce much effect on catecholamine neurotransmission, are likely to be effective. Moreover, given the wealth of effective medications for ADHD, it would seem the most likely use of these medications would be in patients with mood and anxiety disorders who also have ADHD symptoms.

TCAs. The TCAs have been largely replaced in clinical practice by newer antidepressants, which typically have more favorable side effect profiles. However, there is a fairly large literature supporting the efficacy of the noradrenergic TCAs, principally desipramine, in ADHD, which is important to reference. The noradrenergic TCAs basically act as SNRIs by blocking the serotonin and NE transporters, which supports their role in ADHD. In several double-blind, placebo-controlled studies, desipramine was found to be effective in the management of children with ADHD, including patients who failed to respond to psychostimulants.[56] But, there was an increased risk for elevated diastolic blood pressure and heart rate, and evidence of intraventricular conduction defects on ECG.[56] Thus, alternative noradrenergic nonstimulant options were sought, ultimately leading to the testing and approval of atomoxetine for ADHD.

Buspirone

Buspirone is an anxiolytic agent, which binds to the serotonin 5-HT1A and 5-HT2 receptors (104); it also has agonist activity at D2 autoreceptors. Because of its modest dopaminergic effects, and the role of 5-HT1A receptors in the regulation of impulse control, clinical studies have been conducted in both youth and adults with ADHD.[57] Samples were small and the effects on ADHD symptoms modest; however, this medication may have a role in the treatment of patients with ADHD and comorbid anxiety.

Glutamatergic Agents

There are limited data on the potential utility of the N-methyl-D-aspartate (NMDA) receptor antagonists amantadine[58] and memantine in youth[59] and adults[60] with ADHD. These medications have been studied in open-label studies, one comparison trial versus MPH,[61] and one augmentation trial with MPH.[62] Open studies reported positive results of treatment and acceptable tolerability. In the comparator trial, amantadine was associated with clinical improvement comparable to MPH; however, the sample was small and there was no placebo contrast. A small open-label trial in adults found improvements in both ADHD symptoms and neuropsychological test performance.[60,62] Finally, a small placebo-controlled trial using memantine adjunctive to MPH in adults with ADHD found selected improvements in executive function.[62]

Atypical Stimulants: Wakefulness and Alertness Promoting Agents

Modafinil and its R-stereoisomer, armodafinil, are novel cognitive-enhancing and wake-promoting agents, which are structurally and pharmacologically different from other agents used to treat ADHD. Modafinil and armodafinil are atypical stimulants (DEA Schedule IV in the United States) that selectively activate the cortex and modulate several different neurotransmitters, including hypocretin, histamine, NE, γ-aminobutyric acid (GABA), and glutamate. Modafinil and armodafinil are FDA approved for the treatment of narcolepsy and shift-work sleep disorder and also for adjunctive treatment of obstructive sleep apnea/hypopnea syndrome. Several years ago, a clinical development program examined the efficacy and tolerability of an investigational, extended duration formulation of modafinil.[63] Significant improvement was found for children in ratings of ADHD symptoms both at home and at school; however, adult trials with modafinil have not separated from placebo.[64] This new formulation was not approved by the FDA owing to concerns regarding possible elevated risk for Stevens–Johnson syndrome. Although further investigation is necessary to determine whether modafinil can be used safely and effectively for the treatment of ADHD, the available data[65] suggest that it may represent a viable option for some individuals who do not respond to or cannot tolerate approved stimulant and nonstimulant formulations. Of note, armodafinil has a more extended pharmacokinetic profile than modafinil and may therefore have a better effect on alertness and arousal throughout the day.

INVESTIGATIONAL COMPOUNDS

Several existing (eg, vortioxetine) and novel nonstimulant compounds (eg, dasotraline; metadoxine; fasoracetam) have been studied in clinical trials during the last several years.[66] Unfortunately, many recently studied drugs, particularly those targeting neurotransmitter systems with indirect activity on DA and NE, have failed in phase 3. Two potentially promising investigational nonstimulants for ADHD are described below.

Centanafadine. Centanafidine is a serotonin–norepinephrine–dopamine reuptake inhibitor (ratio of 14:6:1, respectively) which is currently in phase 3 trials in the United States. A recently published placebo-controlled phase 2 study in adults with ADHD evaluated the efficacy and tolerability of 400 mg (divided into 2 doses daily) centanafadine.[67] The ES versus placebo of 0.62 after 3 weeks of treatment indicates that this medication may have efficacy, which is comparable to or slightly greater than other nonstimulants (because ES of existing treatments are typically lower in adults). Observed side effects were generally mild, including decreased appetite, headaches, nausea, and diarrhea. Several cases of rash were observed in early phase trials, so ongoing research will need to document the frequency with which this may occur, and the potential clinical significance.

Mazindol XR. Mazindol is an anorexic substance, not related to amphetamines or metabolized to an amphetamine-like compound, which was approved for the treatment of obesity and also used off-label in narcolepsy. Mazindol was approved in an IR formulation as a schedule IV drug in the United States, which was withdrawn in the early 2000s for commercial reasons and not safety concerns. Mazindol binds to DA, NE, and 5-HT transporters (ie, triple reuptake inhibitor) and is also a partial agonist of orexin.[68] A small open-label pilot study of the immediate release formulation (1 mg/d) in children with ADHD reported greater than 8 hours of activity and greater than 90% improvement in ADHD symptoms after 1 week. Appetite suppression and upper abdominal pain were the most common AEs. A more extensive phase 2 study in adults with ADHD using an investigational extended release formulation[69] found robust effects on both symptom ratings (i.e., ADHD Rating Scale (ADHD-RS) scores) and functional impairment, with an ES for ADHD symptoms comparable to amphetamine. Currently, this medication is being investigated for narcolepsy but it is presumed that further study in ADHD may be undertaken.

CLINICAL USE OF NONSTIMULANTS

Because nonstimulants have a lower ES than psychostimulants (with the actual figure varying by drug and age group), most professional guidelines and treatment algorithms indicate that psychostimulants should be the first-choice medication option for youth and adults with ADHD. However, nonstimulants can have an important role if there is poor response or tolerability to psychostimulants, when certain comorbid disorders are present, or if there is patient or family preference to use a nonstimulant. Therefore, a more inclusive approach to treatment sequencing might be to simply recommend that an FDA-approved medication (stimulant or nonstimulant) be used, with the choice of which agent is selected to be directed by results of clinical trials and a variety of other clinically relevant factors. The presence of comorbid anxiety disorders or autistic spectrum disorders might represent good indications for atomoxetine. Alpha-2 agonists would potentially be a good choice for a patient with ADHD + comorbid tic disorders and/or oppositional or disruptive behavior. Bupropion or viloxazine might be reasonable drugs to recommend for someone with ADHD + comorbid depression and/or anxiety (though neither has formally been studied in these populations), due to their known antidepressant effects. All of the non-stimulants could be options for individuals with ADHD and SUD because stimulant use can be (but is not necessarily) problematic in this population. Note, however, that the above suggestions are based on clinical acumen and have received only minimal investigation.

The α-2 agonists additionally have a labeled indication for adjunctive therapy (in the United States) and can aid in mitigating increases in HR and BR or sleep disturbances that often accompany stimulant treatment. Moreover, nonstimulant medications can be used alone or in combination with stimulants to provide medication coverage throughout the day and into the evening, compensating for the restricted time-action properties of stimulants in some patients, and limiting stimulant dose. Although unstudied, the latter strategy could be useful for potentially mitigating long-term AEs of stimulants, such as growth retardation, in selected individuals.

It is important to note that while both stimulants and nonstimulants are FDA-approved for ADHD, important characteristics of clinical response often vary across the different drug classes, including the nature of response, approach to titration, expected time to onset of clinical improvement, and temporal characteristics of the treatment.

SUMMARY

There are 2 classes of FDA-approved nonstimulant medications for ADHD—the selective noradrenergic reuptake inhibitors and the α-2 adrenergic agonists. In addition, several other medication classes have been used off-label with reported efficacy and several more are being developed. Although the nonstimulant medications are, on average, not as broadly or robustly effective as the psychostimulants, they can be very helpful in treating certain patients with ADHD (and associated comorbidities)—either as monotherapy or as adjunctive agents. Controlled clinical trials comparing nonstimulant and stimulant medications that examine not only the impact on core symptoms but also a range of associated clinical and contextual variables will be essential to guide the clinical use of nonstimulants in ADHD.

There is considerable interest in developing new classes of nonstimulant medications, based on our growing knowledge regarding the multiplicity of neural circuits and neurotransmitter systems that are implicated in the pathophysiology and/or maintenance of attention, cognitive, behavioral, and emotional control—all of which are central to ADHD. It is expected that current and yet to be developed nonstimulants will have an important role in the treatment of selected subgroups of ADHD patients in the years ahead, potentially offering better opportunities to match treatments to specific clinical and neurobiological patient characteristics.

CLINICS CARE POINTS

- Currently approved nonstimulants have moderate effect sizes, although somewhat lower on average than for stimulants. More robust response is seen in a subgroup of those treated. Duration of action is typically longer than for stimulants.
- Nonstimulants can be used in monotherapy or combined treatment. Combining nonstimulants with stimulants can be an effective strategy for extending duration of coverage, improving efficacy, and limiting side effects of both medication classes.
- Atomoxetine has been shown to be effective in treating children and adults with anxiety disorders and might be a parsimonious choice for this population.

- Alpha-2 agonists improve both inattention and hyperactive–impulsive symptoms, with slightly better response to hyperactivity/impulsivity symptoms, and are often used to treat behavioral overarousal, aggression, tics, and insomnia either as comorbidity or as they emerge in treatment with stimulants.
- Norepinepherine reuptake inhibitors have cardiovascular effects more similar to stimulants than to α-2 adrenergic agonists; the α-2s may be used off-label alone or in combination with stimulants in selected adults due to their favorable cardiovascular profile.
- Among the norepinepherine reuptake inhibitors, Viloxazine extended release has documented antidepressant activity and has a longer half-life compared with ATX (except in CYP 2D6 poor metabolizers). Might this be an effective medication for depression comorbid with ADHD?
- Bupropion, an antidepressant also labeled for smoking cessation, may be particularly useful in the treatment of comorbid ADHD and depression, with evidence that it may be used successfully in context of substance use disorder.

DISCLOSURE

In the past year, Dr Newcorn is/has been an advisor and/or consultant for Adlon Therapeutics, Corium, Lumos, Medice, Myriad Neuroscience, NLS, OnDosis, Rhodes, Shire/Takeda, and Supernus. He has received research support from the National Institute on Drug Abuse, the Eunice Kennedy Shriver National Institute of Child Health and Human Development, Adlon and Shire. He also has received honoraria from for disease state presentations from Otsuka and Takeda, and served as a consultant for the US National Football League. Dr Krone has nothing to disclose. Dr Dittman has nothing to disclose.

REFERENCES

1. Rapoport JL, Quinn PO, Bradbard G, et al. Imipramine and methylphenidate treatments of hyperactive boys. A double-blind comparison. Arch Gen Psychiatry 1974;30(6):789–93.
2. Banaschewski T, Roessner V, Dittman RW, et al. Non-stimulant medications in the treatment of ADHD. Eur Child Adolesc Psychiatry 2004;13(Suppl 1):I102–16.
3. Swanson JM, Kraemer HC, Hinshaw SP, et al. Clinical relevance of the primary findings of the MTA: success rates based on severity of ADHD and ODD symptoms at the end of treatment. J Am Acad Child Adolesc Psychiatry 2001;40(2): 168–79.
4. Cortese S, Newcorn JH, Coghill D. A practical, evidence-informed approach to managing stimulant-refractory attention deficit hyperactivity disorder (ADHD). CNS Drugs 2021;35(10):1035–51.
5. Faraone SV, Rostain AL, Montano CB, et al. Systematic review: nonmedical use of prescription stimulants: risk factors, outcomes, and risk reduction strategies. J Am Acad Child Adolesc Psychiatry 2020;59(1):100–12.
6. Posner J, Polanczyk GV, Sonuga-Barke E. Attention-deficit hyperactivity disorder. Lancet 2020;395(10222):450–62.
7. Volkow ND, Wang GJ, Fowler JS, et al. Imaging the effects of methylphenidate on brain dopamine: new model on its therapeutic actions for attention-deficit/ hyperactivity disorder. Biol Psychiatry 2005;57(11):1410–5.
8. Arnsten AF, Li BM. Neurobiology of executive functions: catecholamine influences on prefrontal cortical functions. Biol Psychiatry 2005;57(11):1377–84.

9. Bymaster FP, Katner JS, Nelson DL, et al. Atomoxetine increases extracellular levels of norepinephrine and dopamine in prefrontal cortex of rat: a potential mechanism for efficacy in attention deficit/hyperactivity disorder. Neuropsychopharmacology 2002;27(5):699–711.

10. Newcorn JH, Sutton VK, Weiss MD, et al. Clinical responses to atomoxetine in attention-deficit/hyperactivity disorder: the Integrated Data Exploratory Analysis (IDEA) study. J Am Acad Child Adolesc Psychiatry 2009;48(5):511–8.

11. De Bruyckere K, Bushe C, Bartel C, et al. Relationships between functional outcomes and symptomatic improvement in atomoxetine-treated adult patients with attention-deficit/hyperactivity disorder: post hoc analysis of an integrated database. CNS Drugs 2016;30(6):541–58.

12. Michelson D, Read HA, Ruff DD, et al. CYP2D6 and clinical response to atomoxetine in children and adolescents with ADHD. J Am Acad Child Adolesc Psychiatry 2007;46(2):242–51.

13. Brown JT, Bishop JR. Atomoxetine pharmacogenetics: associations with pharmacokinetics, treatment response and tolerability. Pharmacogenomics 2015;16(13):1513–20.

14. Wernicke JF, Kratochvil CJ. Safety profile of atomoxetine in the treatment of children and adolescents with ADHD. J Clin Psychiatry 2002;63(Suppl 12):50–5.

15. Reed VA, Buitelaar JK, Anand E, et al. The safety of atomoxetine for the treatment of children and adolescents with attention-deficit/hyperactivity disorder: a comprehensive review of over a decade of research. CNS Drugs 2016;30(7):603–28.

16. Bangs ME, Tauscher-Wisniewski S, Polzer J, et al. Meta-analysis of suicide-related behavior events in patients treated with atomoxetine. J Am Acad Child Adolesc Psychiatry 2008;47(2):209–18.

17. Lowe TL, Cohen DJ, Detlor J, et al. Stimulant medications precipitate Tourette's syndrome. Jama 1982;247(8):1168–9.

18. Dalrymple RA, McKenna Maxwell L, Russell S, et al. NICE guideline review: attention deficit hyperactivity disorder: diagnosis and management (NG87). Arch Dis Child Educ Pract Ed 2020;105(5):289–93.

19. Treatment of ADHD in children with tics: a randomized controlled trial. Neurology 2002;58(4):527–36.

20. Palumbo DR, Sallee FR, Pelham WE Jr, et al. Clonidine for attention-deficit/hyperactivity disorder: I. Efficacy and tolerability outcomes. J Am Acad Child Adolesc Psychiatry 2008;47(2):180–8.

21. Jain R, Segal S, Kollins SH, et al. Clonidine extended-release tablets for pediatric patients with attention-deficit/hyperactivity disorder. J Am Acad Child Adolesc Psychiatry 2011;50(2):171–9.

22. Biederman J, Melmed RD, Patel A, et al. A randomized, double-blind, placebo-controlled study of guanfacine extended release in children and adolescents with attention-deficit/hyperactivity disorder. Pediatrics 2008;121(1):e73–84.

23. Sallee FR, McGough J, Wigal T, et al. Guanfacine extended release in children and adolescents with attention-deficit/hyperactivity disorder: a placebo-controlled trial. J Am Acad Child Adolesc Psychiatry 2009;48(2):155–65.

24. Wilens TE, Robertson B, Sikirica V, et al. A randomized, placebo-controlled trial of guanfacine extended release in adolescents with attention-deficit/hyperactivity disorder. J Am Acad Child Adolesc Psychiatry 2015;54(11):916–25.e912.

25. Schoretsanitis G, de Leon J, Eap CB, et al. Clinically significant drug-drug interactions with agents for attention-deficit/hyperactivity disorder. CNS Drugs 2019;33(12):1201–22.

26. Iwanami A, Saito K, Fujiwara M, et al. Safety and efficacy of guanfacine extended-release in adults with attention-deficit/hyperactivity disorder: an open-label, long-term, phase 3 extension study. BMC Psychiatry 2020;20(1):485.

27. Newcorn JH, Harpin V, Huss M, et al. Extended-release guanfacine hydrochloride in 6-17-year olds with ADHD: a randomised-withdrawal maintenance of efficacy study. J Child Psychol Psychiatry 2016;57(6):717–28.

28. Dittman RW, Cardo E, Nagy P, et al. Efficacy and safety of lisdexamfetaminedimesylate and atomoxetine in the treatment of attention-deficit/hyperactivity disorder: a head-to-head, randomized, double-blind, phase IIIb study. CNS Drugs 2013; 27(12):1081–92.

29. McCracken JT, McGough JJ, Loo SK, et al. Combined Stimulant and Guanfacineadministration in attention-deficit/hyperactivity disorder: a controlled, comparative study. J Am Acad Child Adolesc Psychiatry 2016;55(8):657–66.e651.

30. Findling RL, Candler SA, Nasser AF, et al. Viloxazine in the management of CNS disorders: a historical overview and current status. CNS Drugs 2021;35(6): 643–53.

31. Yu C, Garcia-Olivares J, Candler S, et al. New insights into the mechanism of action of viloxazine: serotonin and norepinephrine modulating properties. J Exp Pharmacol 2020;12:285–300.

32. Johnson JK, Liranso T, Saylor K, et al. A phase II double-blind, placebo-controlled, efficacy and safety study of SPN-812 (Extended-Release viloxazine) in children with ADHD. J Atten Disord 2020;24(2):348–58.

33. Nasser A, Hull J, Chowdhry F, et al. 113 phase 3, randomized, double-blind, placebo-controlled study (P303) assessing efficacy and safety of extended-release viloxazine in children with ADHD. CNS Spectrums 2020;25(2):273–4.

34. Nasser A, Liranso T, Adewole T, et al. A phase III, randomized, placebo-controlled trial to assess the efficacy and safety of once-daily SPN-812 (viloxazine extended-release) in the treatment of attention-deficit/hyperactivity disorder in school-age children. Clin Ther 2020;42(8):1452–66.

35. Nasser A, Hull JT, Liranso T, et al. The effect of viloxazine extended-release capsules on functional impairments associated with attention-deficit/hyperactivity disorder (ADHD) in children and adolescents in four phase 3 placebo-controlled trials. Neuropsychiatr Dis Treat 2021;17:1751–62.

36. Faraone SV, Gomeni R, Hull JT, et al. Early response to SPN-812 (viloxazine extended-release) can predict efficacy outcome in pediatric subjects with ADHD: a machine learning post-hoc analysis of four randomized clinical trials. Psychiatry Res 2021;296:113664.

37. Faison SL, Fry N, Adewole T, et al. Pharmacokinetics of coadministered viloxazine extended-release (SPN-812) and methylphenidate in healthy adults. Clin Drug Invest 2021;41(2):149–59.

38. Faison SL, Fry N, Adewole T, et al. Pharmacokinetics of coadministered viloxazine extended-release (SPN-812) and lisdexamfetamine in healthy adults. J Clin Psychopharmacol 2021;41(2):155–62.

39. Wang Z, Kosheleff AR, Adeojo LW, et al. Impact of a high-fat meal and sprinkled administration on the bioavailability and pharmacokinetics of viloxazine extended-release capsules (QelbreeTM) in Healthy Adult Subjects. Eur J Drug Metab Pharmacokinet 2021;47(1):69–79.

40. Nasser A, Kosheleff AR, Hull JT, et al. Translating attention-deficit/hyperactivity disorder rating scale-5 and weiss functional impairment rating scale-parent effectiveness scores into clinical global impressions clinical significance levels in four randomized clinical trials of SPN-812 (viloxazine extended-release) in children

and adolescents with attention-deficit/hyperactivity disorder. J Child Adolesc Psychopharmacol 2021;31(3):214–26.

41. Faraone SV, Gomeni R, Hull JT, et al. Executive function outcome of treatment with viloxazine extended-release capsules in children and adolescents with attention-deficit/hyperactivity disorder: a post-hoc analysis of four randomized clinical trials. Paediatr Drugs 2021;23(6):583–9.

42. Faraone SV, Gomeni R, Hull JT, et al. A post hoc analysis of the effect of viloxazine extended-release capsules on learning and school problems in children and adolescents with attention-deficit/hyperactivity disorder. Eur Child Adolesc Psychiatry 2021.

43. Biederman J, Baldessarini RJ, Wright V, et al. A double-blind placebo controlled study of desipramine in the treatment of ADD: III. Lack of impact of comorbidity and family history factors on clinical response. J Am Acad Child Adolesc Psychiatry 1993;32(1):199–204.

44. Wang P, Fu T, Zhang X, et al. Differentiating physicochemical properties between NDRIs and sNRIs clinically important for the treatment of ADHD. Biochim Biophys Acta Gen Subj 2017;1861(11 Pt A):2766–77.

45. Huecker MR, Smiley A, Saadabadi A. Bupropion. StatPearls. Treasure island(FL): StatPearls Publishing. Copyright © 2021. StatPearls Publishing LLC.; 2021.

46. Zametkin A, Rapoport JL, Murphy DL, et al. Treatment of hyperactive children with monoamine oxidase inhibitors. I. Clinical efficacy. Arch Gen Psychiatry 1985;42(10):962–6.

47. Conners CK, Casat CD, Gualtieri CT, et al. Bupropion hydrochloride in attention deficit disorder with hyperactivity. J Am Acad Child Adolesc Psychiatry 1996; 35(10):1314–21.

48. Wilens TE, Haight BR, Horrigan JP, et al. Bupropion XL in adults with attention-deficit/hyperactivity disorder: a randomized, placebo-controlled study. Biol Psychiatry 2005;57(7):793–801.

49. Verbeeck W, Tuinier S, Bekkering GE. Antidepressants in the treatment of adult attention-deficit hyperactivity disorder: a systematic review. Adv Ther 2009; 26(2):170–84.

50. Stuhec M, Munda B, Svab V, et al. Comparative efficacy and acceptability of atomoxetine, lisdexamfetamine, bupropion and methylphenidate in treatment of attention deficit hyperactivity disorder in children and adolescents: a meta-analysis with focus on bupropion. J Affect Disord 2015;178:149–59.

51. Verbeeck W, Bekkering GE, Van den Noortgate W, et al. Bupropion for attention deficit hyperactivity disorder (ADHD) in adults. CochraneDatabase Syst Rev 2017;10(10):Cd009504.

52. Solhkhah R, Wilens TE, Daly J, et al. Bupropion SR for the treatment of substance-abusing outpatient adolescents with attention-deficit/hyperactivity disorder and mood disorders. J Child Adolesc Psychopharmacol 2005;15(5):777–86.

53. Atripla—PIhttp://packageinserts.bms.com/pi/pi_atripla.pdf. Foster City (CA): Gilead Sciences Inc. .

54. Sansone RA, Sansone LA. Serotonin norepinephrine reuptake inhibitors: a pharmacological comparison. Innov Clin Neurosci 2014;11(3–4):37–42.

55. Boaden K, Tomlinson A, Cortese S, et al. Antidepressants in children and adolescents: meta-review of efficacy, tolerability and suicidality in acute treatment. Front Psychiatry 2020;11:717.

56. Biederman J, Baldessarini RJ, Wright V, et al. A double-blind placebo controlled study of desipramine in the treatment of ADD: I. Efficacy. J Am Acad Child Adolesc Psychiatry 1989;28(5):777–84.

57. Dittman R, Häge A, Pedraza J, et al. Non-Stimulants in the treatment of ADHD. In: Banaschewski TC D, Zuddas A, editors. Oxford textbook of attention deficit hyperactivity disorder. 1st edition. Oxford(UK): Oxford University Press; 2018. p. 393–401.
58. Hosenbocus S, Chahal R. Amantadine: a review of use in child and adolescent psychiatry. J Can Acad Child Adolesc Psychiatry 2013;22(1):55–60.
59. Findling RL, McNamara NK, Stansbrey RJ, et al. A pilot evaluation of the safety, tolerability, pharmacokinetics, and effectiveness of memantine in pediatric patients with attention-deficit/hyperactivity disorder combined type. J Child Adolesc Psychopharmacol 2007;17(1):19–33.
60. Surman CB, Hammerness PG, Petty C, et al. A pilot open label prospective study of memantine monotherapy in adults with ADHD. World J Biol Psychiatry 2013; 14(4):291–8.
61. Mohammadi MR, Kazemi MR, Zia E, et al. Amantadine versus methylphenidate in children and adolescents with attention deficit/hyperactivity disorder: a randomized, double-blind trial. Hum Psychopharmacol 2010;25(7–8):560–5.
62. Biederman J, Fried R, Tarko L, et al. Memantine in the treatment of executive function deficits in adults with ADHD. J Atten Disord 2017;21(4):343–52.
63. Swanson JM, Greenhill LL, Lopez FA, et al. Modafinil film-coated tablets in children and adolescents with attention-deficit/hyperactivity disorder: results of a randomized, double-blind, placebo-controlled, fixed-dose study followed by abrupt discontinuation. J Clin Psychiatry 2006;67(1):137–47.
64. Cortese S, Adamo N, Del Giovane C, et al. Comparative efficacy and tolerability of medications for attention-deficit hyperactivity disorder in children, adolescents, and adults: a systematic review and network meta-analysis. Lancet Psychiatry 2018;5(9):727–38.
65. Wang SM, Han C, Lee SJ, et al. Modafinil for the treatment of attention-deficit/ hyperactivity disorder: a meta-analysis. J Psychiatr Res 2017;84:292–300.
66. Nageye F, Cortese S. Beyond stimulants: a systematic review of randomised controlled trials assessing novel compounds for ADHD. Expert Rev Neurother 2019;19(7):707–17.
67. Wigal SB, Wigal T, Hobart M, et al. Safety and efficacy of centanafadine sustained-release in adults with attention-deficit hyperactivity disorder: results of phase 2 studies. Neuropsychiatr Dis Treat 2020;16:1411–26.
68. Konofal E, Zhao W, Laouénan C, et al. Pilot Phase II study of mazindol in children with attention deficit/hyperactivity disorder. Drug Des Devel Ther 2014;8: 2321–32.
69. Wigal TL, Newcorn JH, Handal N, et al. A double-blind, placebo-controlled, phase II study to determine the efficacy, safety, tolerability and pharmacokinetics of a controlled release (CR) formulation of mazindol in adults with DSM-5 attention-deficit/hyperactivity disorder (ADHD). CNS Drugs 2018;32(3):289–301.

Cardiovascular Considerations for Stimulant Class Medications

Paul Hammerness, MD[a],*, Amy Berger, BS[b], Michael C. Angelini, MA, PharmD[c], Timothy E. Wilens, MD[b]

KEYWORDS

- Cardiovascular • Stimulant • ADHD • Blood pressure • Heart rate • ECG

KEY POINTS

- Stimulant-related minor increases in blood pressure (BP) and heart rate (HR) have been well described, albeit principally reported as group-level data, in short-term treatment of healthy samples.
- Subjective complaints of a cardiovascular (CV) or cardiopulmonary nature tend to be isolated experiences and have not been associated with serious CV outcomes, noting the very low absolute risk of serious outcomes challenges detection in epidemiologic investigations.
- Recommendations regarding stimulant treatment in the presence of medical comorbidities are beginning to emerge, with future investigations needed to support sophisticated identification of risk based on structural or dynamic pathophysiology.
- Attention to stimulant-associated CV risk is an opportunity for clinicians treating pediatric attention-deficit hyperactivity disorder (ADHD) to engage in general CV risk identification and intervention, such as targeting physical inactivity, Tobacco use, and childhood obesity.

BACKGROUND

First-line treatment for attention-deficit hyperactivity disorder (ADHD) includes methylphenidate (MPH) and amphetamine (AMP)-based stimulant medications. The cardiovascular (CV) impact of stimulants has been considered for decades given inherent sympathomimetic effects.[1] CV findings on stimulants have been typically presented as clinically nonsignificant increases in resting blood pressure (BP) and heart rate (HR) in the context of short-term clinical trials, with healthy prescreened participants. Following a series of serious CV events in the setting of stimulant medications, large-scale epidemiologic studies were conducted in pediatric and adult populations. While the association between stimulants and serious CV events has not determined

[a] Psychiatry Services, Southcoast Health, 101 Page Street, New Bedford, MA, USA; [b] Child and Adolescent Psychiatry, Massachusetts General Hospital, 55 Fruit Street, Boston, MA, USA; [c] Massachusetts College of Pharmacy and Health Sciences University, Boston, MA, USA
* Corresponding author.
E-mail address: hammernessp@southcoast.org

Child Adolesc Psychiatric Clin N Am 31 (2022) 437–448
https://doi.org/10.1016/j.chc.2022.02.002
1056-4993/22/© 2022 Elsevier Inc. All rights reserved.

causality, there is no unifying mechanism to understand stimulants' impact on the CV system beyond known sympathomimetic activity. In addition, there is no understanding of mediating variables and moderating processes in the relationship between stimulants and CV outcomes, with particular uncertainty in regards to the medically complex/vulnerable patient. In this article, we will review the underlying literature on this subject as well as make clinical recommendations on screening to mitigate potentially adverse outcomes.

CURRENT EVIDENCE

Mean elevations in HR and BP on stimulants have been reported for decades. A series of studies were conducted in the 1970s–1980s, using small samples but with a targeted methodology. Readings were taken typically 1 to 2-hours postdose, principally after immediate-release MPH administration. Significant increases in HR versus placebo were described, including greater elevations in medication-naïve subjects as well as dose dependency.[2–5] With the arrival of extended duration formulations, HR and BP outcomes were reported in the context of large, placebo-controlled studies, with measurements typically ~ 8 to 10-hours postdose. Significant increases in HR (≤9 bpm) versus placebo (≤1bpm) were documented across extended-release MPH and AMP agents.[6–9]

Subsequent open extension clinical trials (6–24 months) showed persistent elevations in HR (1–5 bpm) and BP (1–5 mm Hg), consistent with a lack of tolerance to stimulants' effects on HR, and with an apparent absence of dose-dependency. Longer term, 2 to 14 year ADHD cohorts, offered nonconclusive findings given small numbers of consistent medication users, and uncertain actual exposure.[7,8,10–16] Recent naturalistic reports find unchanged BP, with significant elevations in HR,[17] and conversely, declining BP over 12 years of stimulant without significant HR change.[18] Limitations that remain in the interpretation of naturalistic reports include the nonverified medication intake and details around the collection of BP/HR.

In addition to mean HR and BP changes, some clinical reports include frequency of vital sign outliers, who are defined as exceeding a threshold (eg, ≥120/80 mm Hg) or per change from baseline (eg, increase in SBP≥20 mm Hg, HR > 25bpm), at least once on medication. Outlier rates are typically 5% to 15% in shorter and longer term treatment. When reported, outlier elevations seem sporadic, with less than 5% occurring at consecutive visits.[7,8,19–23] The clinical relevance or intervention for these outliers remains unknown.

There have been few investigations of moderators of BP/HR outcomes during therapeutic stimulant treatment. The US FDA Center for Drug Evaluation and Research conducted a novel study of stimulant formulation in healthy adults. BP and HR changes were found to be highly dependent on MPH pharmacokinetics.[24] However, in an extensive review of pediatric clinical trials (N = 5837), Hennissen (2017) found no effect of medication type or dose, along with age, gender, or comorbidity.[25]

In addition to objective BP and HR findings, subjective experiences of a possible CV or cardiopulmonary nature have been well documented in the clinical trial literature. Palpitations, tachycardia, chest pain/tightness, and dyspnea are most common, in up to ~20% of stimulant-treated subjects and can occur more frequently than on placebo. In a rare investigation of moderating/mediating variables, Hammerness[22] found elevated rates of comorbid anxiety disorders in those adolescents with consecutive CV complaints, albeit not a primary outcome with sufficient power to offer conclusions. Emergency room, naturalistic presentations document similar subjective complaints in stimulant-treated patients, yet serious events associated with complaints are rare and consistent with rates of persons not receiving stimulant medications.[12,19,23,26–29]

SERIOUS OR RARE CARDIOVASCULAR EVENTS

In the 1990s and early 2000s, serious CV events in youth prescribed stimulants raised clinical, scientific, and public health questions about the safety of ADHD treatment. The 1990s cases of sudden death involving children receiving clonidine alongside MPH[30] were not attributed to either medication or to their combination. Investigations of concomitant MPH and clonidine as well as tricyclic antidepressants subsequently shifted focus to serious CV adverse outcomes (eg, heart attack, death) associated with stimulants alone.[31] Multiple epidemiologic, registry and case control studies have been undertaken since then, with the preponderance of evidence finding no causal relationship between therapeutic stimulants and serious, life-threatening CV outcomes (ie, sudden death, myocardial infarction, and stroke). Actual rates are low, highlighting the challenge of such investigations.[32–38] When observed, rates of serious CV events on stimulants including sudden cardiac death are not different from known general population rates (1.32 per 100,000 persons in children and young adults).[39] Methodological issues limit the interpretation of positive findings,[31] yet confidence intervals for pooled estimates do not exclude a modest increase in risk.[40,41]

Taking the sum of the literature, US FDA concluded the rate of sudden death with stimulants was less than national rates and the Pediatric Advisory Committee deemed a black box warning was not indicated. Instead, FDA issued warnings about stimulants in underlying CV disease and directed the creation and implementation of Medication Guides. However, a recent evaluation of professional and consumer labels for ADHD medications registered in Australia, Canada, UK, and US finds inconsistencies in the description of stimulants' CV risk profile.[42]

Responsive to what seems to be another rare event, albeit of lower severity, a major change to US warnings occurred in 2013; "Stimulants used to treat ADHD are associated with peripheral vasculopathy, including Raynaud's phenomenon. Careful observation for digital changes is necessary during treatment."[43] Limited case report references exist in the pediatric (therapeutic) literature to support this association. For example, Yu et al (2010) described 4 boys with ADHD who developed vasculopathy following mean 6 years of stimulant exposure.[44] A recent case series (N = 16) of adults receiving treatment with AMP stimulants described generally mild vasospastic symptoms of the extremities.[45] Severe vascular manifestations were associated with a history of rheumatologic disease, found in 25% of the sample. However, is possible that peripheral vasculopathy occurs more often the literature suggests, as this adverse event is not systematically assessed for in clinical studies.

GUIDELINES AND RECOMMENDATIONS

Recommendations from American Academies of Pediatrics, Child and Adolescent Psychiatry, and American Heart Association recommend a CV focused patient and family history and physical examination for youth before the initiation of stimulant medication for ADHD.[37,46–48] The aim is to identify patients with undiagnosed underlying CV disease, for example, structural disorders (**Table 1**).

Potential cardiac origin symptoms include fainting or dizziness (exertional, emotional), chest pain (central, crushing, exertional), worsening exercise tolerance, palpitations, increased HR, extra/skipped beats, and seizures (exertional, emotional). Family member's relevant history includes sudden or unexplained death in young (<40 years), sudden death during exercise, cardiac arrhythmias, cardiomyopathy,

Table 1	
Recommendations for cardiovascular screening when using stimulant medications for ADHD	
Medical History (screening for sudden death risk)	• Personal congenital or acquired cardiac disease • Palpitations, chest pain, syncope, unexplained dizziness, fainting, shortness of breath or seizure, postexercise symptoms • Family history of premature cardiac disease (< 30 years of age), history of sudden or unexplained death including drowning or motor vehicle accident • Other medications including over the counter that affect the heart • Routine medical and family cardiac istory
Vital Signs; Routine Care	• Blood pressure/heart rate at baseline and periodically thereafter • No ECG, Holter, or exercise testing necessary in routine care
Suspicion of CV disease (eg, hypertrophic cardiomyopathy; ion channelopathies)	• Consult pediatric (or adult) specialty care, for example, cardiology, with workup as indicated by clinical history and symptoms

Recommendations derived from the American Heart Association and American Academy of Pediatrics.[32,46,63–66]

and presence of connective tissues diseases (eg, Marfan syndrome.) Any concerns before during treatment should be shared with primary care and/or specialists for the consideration of further evaluation.

Following the initiation of a stimulant, recommendations are generally to *periodically* monitor for changes in HR or BP in healthy children, with assessments recommended to occur *at every health encounter* for those at theoretic increased risk, such as in presence of complex medical conditions or concomitant medications known to increase BP.[49–55] If elevated BP is observed per appropriate protocol,[55] repeat measurements are indicated with primary/specialty care consultation, including the consideration of ambulatory BP monitoring.[56] Canadian ADHD Resource Alliance (CADDRA) Guidelines for individuals across the lifespan recommend initial BP assessment before starting medication, and then during follow-up, with closer monitoring for those with HTN or coronary heart disease. While not recommending a frequency of follow-up assessment, CADDRA recommends taking measurements while the medication is present in the system, as it may be useful to compare to findings before a dose is taken.[57]

In addition to BP monitoring, CV review during treatment can identify concerning complaints (crushing, exertional chest pain, extra/skipped beats). When present, symptoms should be communicated for shared decision making.[46,47,56,58] Thoughtful documentation of normative/baseline CV experiences before stimulant initiation, such as racing heart during exertion or with anxiety, will aid in a possible later review.

For those who do not tolerate an initial stimulant trial, such as mild subjective discomfort, without a determined contraindication to continue pharmacotherapy (eg, new/unstable CV finding), an alternate form of stimulant may be considered. Theoretically, differences in pharmacokinetics among stimulants may impact CV tolerability although this has been understudied.[24] A nonstimulant may be considered as well, given these agents offer differing CV impacts based on pharmacodynamics. While noradrenergic atomoxetine and viloxazine also result in elevations in BP/HR,[25,59,60] the converse risk (ie, hypotension, bradycardia and syncope) can occur with monotherapy or adjunctive therapy with the nonstimulant alpha-2-adrenergic agonists' clonidine and guanfacine.[61,62]

CONTROVERSIES

Although screening ECG is not recommended for healthy children/adolescents with ADHD,[37,46,56,67] previous conflicting recommendations from the American Heart Association and American Academy of Pediatrics left clinicians and families uncertain.[46,47] A follow-up joint statement clarified that ECGs were not universally mandatory,[64] yet the practice of screening ECG remained.[65]

Since early examinations, no statistically significant, clinically meaningful changes have been reported in ECG intervals in pediatric samples. A range of subjects (1%–19%) have "abnormal" ECG reports (eg, ST–T wave changes; bundle branch block) consistent with ECG variants found in similar rates in healthy individuals.[7,19,21,23,68–70] QTc prolongation during stimulant treatment when present has been modest,[71] while poor metabolizers of the nonstimulant atomoxetine have demonstrated increased QTC intervals.[69] There is no evidence that any ECG finding is associated with an increased likelihood of serious event due to stimulant medication.[37]

A retrospective study of 1470 children on ADHD medication with "abnormal" ECG in screening led to the identification of true abnormality in 0.3% of sample, at a cost to identify each case of $17,000.[72] Instead, referral is recommended if clinical CV concern (eg, palpitations, syncopal episodes) before initiation or during the course of treatment.[1,37,46,56,67]

COMPLICATIONS/CONCERNS

Concerns expressed include the uncertain impact of cumulative stimulant exposure, as well as the devolving baseline physical health of the pediatric population. At present, ADHD patients are typically prescribed an extended duration form of stimulant, year-round, with potential exposure for decades. It is not known if greater exposure over the course of the day or cumulatively over years impacts the distribution of risk.

In addition, the physical health profile of US children is concerning, with the accumulation of CV risk factors that may impact tolerability/safety of stimulant medications. While the onset of tobacco use in adolescence has a potential lifelong impact, the present-day regular/excess use of energy drinks (~30% of adolescents) especially before or during sports, may trigger palpitations and arrhythmias,[73,74] with increases of ~3 to 4 mm Hg BP documented across 15 adult studies.[75] Elevated BMI (~50% of teenagers), is particularly startling given that rates of hypertension increase with increasing adiposity; from 4% to 25%.[55] CV disease risk accumulates the earlier children develop their obesity, with detectable precursors of atherosclerosis by the time a child enters middle school.[75] All participants in health care delivery should be engaged in recognizing and monitoring individuals who are overweight or obese.[76]

In sum, data collected in past years regarding CV impact may not similarly inform risk: benefit considerations for today's patient. It is important to note these concerns reflect theoretic risk and offer areas of future investigation as well as public health engagement.

MEDICAL COMORBIDITIES

While there is no specific form of heart disease identified to be of greatest concern,[37] stimulants' CV risk may be mediated by a given patient's vulnerability. Few clinical investigations have examined specific CV populations such as a small sample of adults with ADHD and hypertension.[77–79] In a nationwide insurance database in South Korea, highest risk of arrhythmia was seen in children with Congenital Heart Disease; despite an increased relative risk, the absolute risk was low.[77] In a small sample of children (N = 28) with known long QT-syndrome, none of the children on stimulant experienced QT-related events.[80]

The Spanish Society of Pediatric Cardiology and Congenital Heart Disease recently outlined a comprehensive and individualized approach with considerations per specific cardiac condition. For example, the society recommends individualized pharmacologic treatment in those sensitive to potential tachycardia, such as in the setting of diastolic dysfunction or mitral stenosis in whom a shortening of the diastole should be avoided, or patients with systolic dysfunction in whom an increase in myocardial oxygen consumption secondary to tachycardia should be avoided.[56] Medications were not advised for a limited number of high-risk patients, including hemodynamically unstable CHD, residual hypertension, catecholaminergic polymorphic ventricular tachycardia, and frequent/complex PVCs.[56,81]

FUTURE DIRECTIONS

Critical questions remain about the mechanisms of stimulant's CV impact.[82] Abnormal sympathetic tone,[83] physiologic adaptations,[1,77] direct pathologic changes[84,85]; or peripheral vascular changes[86] are possible etiologic pathways. Finally, cardiopulmonary symptoms (eg, dyspnea) may indicate exercise-induced pulmonary arterial hypertension, diastolic dysfunction or peripheral muscle dysfunction.

Studies using dynamic assessments[77,87] and advances in methodology may be used to investigate a range of possible mechanisms. Risk may be determined to vary, according to a range of mediators (eg, age, gender, family CV history) and moderators (eg, tobacco use, stimulant dose, duration, formulation).

On the contrary, stimulant treatment of ADHD may be cardio-protective, with associated, albeit indirect, improvements in functioning and reductions in emotional reactivity.[58] As per Skinner's commentary regarding patients with long QT syndrome,[88] therapeutic stimulants may be associated with the removal of peaks in HR due to improved temper and behavioral control. In addition, stimulant treatment may lead to further indirect cardio-protection via improvements in physical health, and attention to self-care (eg, adherence to eating, sleeping, exercise regimens).[89,90]

SUMMARY

Stimulant-class medications for healthy children and adolescents with ADHD continue to be associated with mean elevations in BP ($\leq$5 mm Hg) and HR ($\leq$10 beats/min) without changes in electrocardiographic parameters. A subset (5%–15%) of children and adolescents may have a greater increase in HR or BP or may report a CV-type complaint during treatment. Serious CV events during stimulant treatment are rare and similar to groups of children not receiving stimulant medication. Despite the stability of these findings, CV may be considered dynamic, related to underlying (medical) vulnerability in a given patient, in response to alterations in prescribing, or impacted by the baseline health of the treated population. Screening includes CV-focused history before stimulant initiation, as well as monitoring of HR/BP and for novel subjective complaints in the context of treatment. Lifespan guidelines do not distinguish specific risk nor offer recommendations per age, besides that related to monitoring in the presence of increased medical comorbidities.[58]

CLINICS CARE POINTS

- Expect minor increases in HR, BP on stimulant, with outliers having greater change
- Subjective reports of a seemingly CV nature occur infrequently, without evident-associated serious CV outcomes
- Rare serious CV events occur without evident causality
- CV screening of all patients being considered for, and occurring while taking stimulant medication may identify those with underlying structural or other cardiac abnormalities—positive findings should result in collaborative care with primary and speciality care
- There remains insufficient evidence to guide risk assessment for a given patient, particularly for medically complex, although guidelines are emerging
- Opportunities exist to support public health monitoring of general CV risk factors, namely elevated BMI and BP, although stimulant attributable CV risk for such vulnerable patients is theoretic

DISCLOSURE

Dr P. Hammerness receives royalties from the following publications: *ADHD, Biographies of a Disease*, Greenwood Press, 2009; *Organize Your Mind, Organize Your Life*, Harlequin Press/Harvard University, 2012; *Straight Talk about Psychiatric Medications for Kids*, Guilford Press 2016. Dr P. Hammerness also receives royalties from Massachusetts General Hospital, owner of a copyrighted questionnaire co-developed with Dr T. E. Wilens, licensed to Ironshore Pharmaceuticals (*The Before School Functioning Questionnaire*). A. Berger has nothing to disclose. Dr M.C. Angelini has received speakers' honoraria from Alkermes, Inc. Dr T. E. Wilens is Chief, Division of Child and Adolescent Psychiatry and (Co) Director of the Center for Addiction Medicine at Massachusetts General Hospital. He receives grant support from the following sources: NIH (NIDA). Dr T. E. Wilens has published a book, Straight Talk About Psychiatric Medications for Kids (Guilford Press), and co/edited books: ADHD in Adults and Children (Cambridge University Press). Dr T. E. Wilens is co/owner of a copyrighted diagnostic questionnaire (Before School Functioning Questionnaire) and has a licensing agreement with Ironshore (BSFQ Questionnaire). He is or has been a consultant for Arbor Pharmaceuticals, 3D Therapeutics, Vallon, and Ironshore, and serves as a clinical consultant to the US National Football League (ERM Associates), US Minor/Major League Baseball; Gavin Foundation and Bay Cove Human Services.

REFERENCES

1. Hammerness PG, Perrin JM, Shelley-Abrahamson R, et al. Cardiovascular risk of stimulant treatment in pediatric attention-deficit/hyperactivity disorder: update and clinical recommendations. J Am Acad Child Adolesc Psychiatry 2011; 50(10):978–90.
2. Solanto MV, Conners CK. A dose-response and time-action analysis of autonomic and behavioral effects of methylphenidate in ADHD. Psychophysiology 1982; 19(6):658–67.
3. Kelly KL, Rapport MD, DuPaul GJ. Attention deficit disorder and methylphenidate: a multi-step analysis of dose-response effects on children's cardiovascular functioning. Int Clin Psychopharmacol 1988;3(2):167–81.

4. Tannock R, Schachar RJ, Carr RP, et al. Dose-response effects of methylphenidate on academic performance and overt behavior in hyperactive children. Pediatrics 1989;84(4):648–57.
5. Safer DJ. Relative cardiovascular safety of psychostimulants used to treat ADHD. J Child Adolesc Psychopharmacol 1992;2(4):279–90.
6. Rapport MD, Moffitt C. ADHD and methylphenidate. A review of height/weight, cardiovascular, and somatic complaint side effects. Clin Psychol Rev 2002; 22(8):1107–31.
7. Wilens TE, Spencer TJ, Biederman J. Short- and long-term cardiovascular effects of mixed amphetamine salts extended-release in adolescents with ADHD. CNS Spectrums 2005;10(S15):22–30.
8. Findling RL, Biederman J, Wilens TE, et al. Short- and long-term cardiovascular effects of mixed amphetamine salts extended release in children. J Pediatr 2005;147(3):348–54.
9. Weisler R, Adler L, Hamdani M et al. Cardiovascular outcomes in children and adults treated with lisdexamfetamine dimesylate for ADHD. Paper presented at: Annual Meeting of the American Academy of Child and Adolescent Psychiatry; Honolulu (HI); October 27-November 1, 2009.
10. McGough JJ, Biederman J, Wigal SB, et al. Long-term tolerability and effectiveness of once-daily mixed amphetamine salts (Adderall XR) in children with ADHD. J Am Acad Child Adolesc Psychiatry 2005;44(6):530–8.
11. Findling RL, Childress AC, Krishnan S, et al. Long-term effectiveness and safety of lisdexamfetamine dimesylate in school-aged children with ADHD. CNS Spectr 2008;13(7):614–20.
12. Findling RL, Wigal SB, Bukstein OG, et al. Long-term tolerability of the methylphenidate transdermal system in pediatric ADHD. Clin Ther 2009;31(8):1844–55.
13. Weisler R, Young J, Mattingly G, et al. Long-term safety and effectiveness of lisdexamfetamine dimesylate. CNS Spectr 2009;14(10):573–85.
14. Vitiello B, Elliott GR, Swanson JM, et al. Blood pressure and heart rate over 10 years in the multimodal treatment study of children with ADHD. Am J Psychiatry 2011;169(2):167–77.
15. Arcieri R, Germinario EA, Bonati M, et al. Cardiovascular measures in children and adolescents with ADHD who are new users of methylphenidate and atomoxetine. J Child Adolesc Psychopharmacol 2012;22(6):423–31.
16. Smith G. Raine ADHD study: long-term outcomes associated with stimulant medication in the treatment of ADHD in children. Perth (Western Australia): Government of Western Australia, Department of Health; 2010. Available at: http://www.health.wa.gov.au/publications/documents/MICADHD_Raine_ADHD_Study_report_022010.pdf. Accessed September 27, 2021.
17. St Amour MD, O'Leary DD, Cairney J, et al. What is the effect of ADHD stimulant medication on heart rate and blood pressure in a community sample of children? Can J Public Health 2018;109(3):395–400.
18. Conzelmann A, Müller S, Jans T, et al. Long-term cardiovascular safety of psychostimulants in children with ADHD. Int J Psychiatry Clin Pract 2019;23(2): 157–9.
19. Donner R, Michaels MA, Ambrosini PJ. Cardiovascular effects of mixed amphetamine salts extended release in the treatment of school-aged children with ADHD. Biol Psychiatry 2007;61(5):706–12.
20. Medori R, Ramos-Quiroga JA, Casas M, et al. A randomized, placebo-controlled trial of three fixed dosages of prolonged-release OROS methylphenidate in adults with ADHD. Biol Psychiatry 2008;63(10):981–9.

21. Childress AC, Spencer T, Lopez F, et al. Efficacy and safety of dexmethylphenidate extended-release capsules administered once daily to children with ADHD. J Child Adolesc Psychopharmacol 2009;19(4):351–61.
22. Hammerness P, Wilens T, Mick E, et al. Cardiovascular effects of longer-term, high-dose OROS methylphenidate in adolescents with ADHD. J Pediatr 2009; 155(1):84–9.e1.
23. Findling RL, Katic A, Rubin R, et al. A 6-month, open-label, extension study of the tolerability and effectiveness of the methylphenidate transdermal system in adolescents diagnosed with ADHD. J Child Adolesc Psychopharmacol 2010;20(5): 365–75.
24. Li L, Wang Y, Uppoor RS, et al. Exposure-response analyses of blood pressure and heart rate changes for methylphenidate in healthy adults. J Pharmacokinet Pharmacodyn 2017;44(3):245–62.
25. Hennissen L, Bakker MJ, Banaschewski T, et al. Cardiovascular effects of stimulant and non-stimulant medication for children and adolescents with ADHD. CNS Drugs 2017;31(3):199–215.
26. Cohen AL, Jhung MA, Budnitz DS. Stimulant medications and ADHD. N Engl J Med 2006;354(21):2294–5.
27. Winterstein AG, Gerhard T, Shuster J, et al. Cardiac safety of central nervous system stimulants in children and adolescents with ADHD. Pediatrics 2007;120(6): e1494–501.
28. Winterstein AG, Gerhard T, Shuster J, et al. Cardiac safety of methylphenidate versus amphetamine salts in the treatment of ADHD. Pediatrics 2009;124(1): e75–80.
29. Substance Abuse and Mental Health Services Administration, Center for Behavioral Health Statistics and Quality. (January 24, 2013). The DAWN Report: Emergency Department Visits Involving Attention Deficit/Hyperactivity Disorder Stimulant Medications. Rockville (MD).
30. Popper CW, Zimnitzky B. Child and adolescent psychopharmacology update: J Child Adolesc Psychopharmacol 1996;6(2):85–118.
31. Gould MS, Walsh BT, Munfakh JL, et al. Sudden death and use of stimulant medications in youths. Am J Psychiatry 2009;166(9):992–1001.
32. Cooper WO, Habel LA, Sox CM, et al. ADHD drugs and serious cardiovascular events in children and young adults. N Engl J Med 2011;365(20):1896–904.
33. Schelleman H, Bilker WB, Strom BL, et al. Cardiovascular events and death in children exposed and unexposed to ADHD agents. Pediatrics 2011;127(6): 1102–10.
34. Winterstein AG, Gerhard T, Kubilis P, et al. Cardiovascular safety of central nervous system stimulants in children and adolescents: population based cohort study. BMJ 2012;345:e4627.
35. Westover AN, Halm EA. Do prescription stimulants increase the risk of adverse cardiovascular events? BMC Cardiovasc Disord 2012;12:41.
36. Winterstein AG. Cardiovascular safety of stimulants in children. Curr Psychiatry Rep 2013;15(8):379.
37. Berger S. ADHD medications in children with heart disease. Curr Opin Pediatr 2016;28(5):607–12.
38. Zito JM, Burcu M. Stimulants and pediatric cardiovascular risk. J Child Adolesc Psychopharmacol 2017;27(6):538–45.
39. El-Assaad I, Al-Kindi SG, Aziz PF. Trends of out-of-hospital sudden cardiac death among children and young adults. Pediatrics 2017;140(6):e20171438.

40. Liu H, Feng W, Zhang D. Association of ADHD medications with the risk of cardio-vascular diseases. Eur Child Adolesc Psychiatry 2019;28(10):1283–93.
41. Cortese S. Pharmacologic treatment of attention deficit-hyperactivity disorder. N Engl J Med 2020;383(11):1050–6.
42. Sieluk J, Palasik B, dosReis S, et al. ADHD medications and cardiovascular adverse events in children and adolescents. Pharmacoepidemiol Drug Saf 2017;26(3):274–84.
43. Label. 2013. Available at: www.fda.gov; https://www.accessdata.fda.gov/drugsatfda_docs/label/2021/021278s029lbl.pdf.
44. Yu ZJ, Parker-Kotler C, Tran K, et al. Peripheral vasculopathy associated with psychostimulant treatment in children with ADHD. Curr Psychiatry Rep 2010; 12(2):111–5. Accessed September 28, 2021.
45. Tan G, Mintz AJ, Mintz B, et al. Peripheral vascular manifestation in patients receiving an amphetamine analog: a case series. Vasc Med 2019;24(1):50–5.
46. Perrin JM, Friedman RA, Knilans TK. Black Box Working Group; Section on Cardiology and Cardiac Surgery. Cardiovascular monitoring and stimulant drugs for attention-deficit/hyperactivity disorder. Pediatrics 2008;122(2):451–3.
47. Vetter VL, Elia J, Erickson C, et al. Cardiovascular monitoring of children and adolescents with heart disease receiving medications for attention deficit/hyperactivity disorder [corrected]. Circulation 2008;117(18):2407–23 [Erratum appears in Circulation. 2009;120(7):e55-9].
48. Gutgesell HP. Screening for cardiovascular disease in the young. Congenit Heart Dis 2011;6(2):88–97.
49. National High Blood Pressure Education Program Working Group on High Blood Pressure in Children and Adolescents. Pediatrics 2004;114(2 Suppl 4th Report): 555–76.
50. Park MK, Menard SW, Schoolfield J. Oscillometric blood pressure standards for children. Pediatr Cardiol 2005;26(5):601–7.
51. Fox K, Borer JS, Camm AJ, et al. Resting heart rate in cardiovascular disease. J Am Coll Cardiol 2007;50(9):823–30.
52. Pliszka S, AACAP Work Group on Quality Issues. Practice parameter for the assessment and treatment of children and adolescents with ADHD. J Am Acad Child Adolesc Psychiatry 2007;46(7):894–921.
53. Jouven X, Empana JP, Escolano S, et al. Relation of heart rate at rest and long-term (>20 years) death rate in initially healthy middle-aged men. Am J Cardiol 2009;103(2):279–83.
54. Cooney MT, Vartiainen E, Laatikainen T, et al. Elevated resting heart rate is an independent risk factor for cardiovascular disease in healthy men and women. Am Heart J 2010;159(4):612–9.e3 [Erratum appears in Am Heart J 2010;160(1):208. Laakitainen, Tinna [corrected to Laatikainen, Tiina]].
55. Flynn JT, Kaelber DC, Baker-Smith CM, et al. Clinical practice guideline for screening and management of high blood pressure in children and adolescents. Pediatrics 2017;140(3):e20171904 [Erratum appears in Pediatrics 2017; Erratum appears in Pediatrics 2018;142(3)].
56. Pérez-Lescure Picarzo J, Centeno Malfaz F, Collell Hernández R, et al. [Recommendations of the Spanish Society of Paediatric Cardiology and Congenital Heart Disease as regards the use of drugs in attention deficit hyperactivity disorder in children and adolescents with a known heart disease, as well as in the general paediatric population: position statement by the Spanish Paediatric Association]. An Pediatr (Engl Ed) 2020;92(2):109.e1–7.

57. Canadian attention deficit hyperactivity disorder resource alliance (CADDRA): Canadian ADHD practice guidelines. 3rd edition. Toronto (ON): CADDRA; 2011.

58. Senderey E, Sousa J, Stavitsky M. Does quality of life outweigh the cardiovascular risks of stimulant medication in a child with ADHD and hypertrophic cardiomyopathy? BMJ Case Rep 2017;2017. https://doi.org/10.1136/bcr-2017-222072. bcr2017222072.

59. Nasser A, Liranso T, Adewole T, et al. A Phase III, randomized, placebo-controlled trial to assess the Efficacy and safety of once-daily SPN-812 (viloxazine extended-release) in the treatment of attention-deficit/hyperactivity disorder in school-age children. Clin Ther 2020;42(8):1452–66.

60. QELBREE. QELBREE™ (viloxazine extended-release capsules), for oral use Initial U.S. Approval: 2021. fda.gov. 2021. Available at: https://www.accessdata.fda.gov/drugsatfda_docs/label/2021/211964s000lbl.pdf. Accessed January 25, 2022.

61. KAPVAY. Prescribing information for clonidine (Kapvay®) extended-release tablets. accessdata.fda.gov. 2010. Available at: https://www.accessdata.fda.gov/drugsatfda_docs/label/2010/022331s001s002lbl.pdf. Accessed January 28, 2022.

62. INTUNIV. Prescribing Information for INTUNIV® (guanfacine) extended-release tablets. accessdata.fda.gov. 2019. Available at: https://www.accessdata.fda.gov/drugsatfda_docs/label/2019/022037s018lbl.pdf. Accessed January 28, 2022..

63. Gutgesell H, Atkins D, Barst R, et al. Cardiovascular monitoring of children and adolescents receiving psychotropic drugs: a statement for healthcare professionals from the Committee on Congenital Cardiac Defects, Council on Cardiovascular Disease in the Young. Am Heart Assoc Circ 1999;99(7):979–82.

64. O'Keefe L. ECGs for all Adhd patients? AAP-AHA RELEASE JOINT 'CLARIFICATION' On AHA recommendation. American Academy of Pediatrics. 2008. Available at: https://www.aappublications.org/content/29/6/1.1. Accessed September 28, 2021.

65. Wilens TE, Prince JB, Spencer TJ, et al. Stimulants and sudden death: what is a physician to do? Pediatrics 2006;118(3):1215–9.

66. Ekelund U, Luan J, Sherar LB, et al. Moderate to vigorous physical activity and sedentary time and cardiometabolic risk factors in children and adolescents. JAMA 2012;307(7):704–12 [Erratum appears in JAMA 2012;307(18):1915. Sardinha L [corrected to Sardinha, L B]; Anderssen, S A [corrected to Anderson, L B]].

67. Leslie LK, Rodday AM, Saunders TS, et al. Cardiac screening prior to stimulant treatment of ADHD. Pediatrics 2012;129(2):222–30.

68. Elia J, Vetter VL. Cardiovascular effects of medications for the treatment of ADHD. Paediatr Drugs 2010;12(3):165–75.

69. Fay TB, Alpert MA. Cardiovascular effects of drugs used to treat ADHD: Part 1: epidemiology, pharmacology, and impact on hemodynamics and ventricular repolarization. Cardiol Rev 2019;27(3):113–21.

70. Vetter VL, Dugan N, Guo R, et al. A pilot study of the feasibility of heart screening for sudden cardiac arrest in healthy children. Am Heart J 2011;161(5):1000–6.e3.

71. Lamberti M, Italiano D, Guerriero L, et al. Evaluation of acute cardiovascular effects of immediate-release methylphenidate in children and adolescents with ADHD. Neuropsychiatr Dis Treat 2015;11:1169–74.

72. Mahle WT, Hebson C, Strieper MJ. Electrocardiographic screening in children with ADHD. Am J Cardiol 2009;104(9):1296–9.

73. Sanchis-Gomar F, Pareja-Galeano H, Santos-Lozano A, et al. Long-term strenuous endurance exercise and the right ventricle: is it a real matter of concern? Can J Cardiol 2015;31(10):1304.e1.
74. Grasser EK, Miles-Chan JL, Charrière N, et al. Energy drinks and their impact on the cardiovascular system: potential mechanisms. Adv Nutr 2016;7(5):950–60.
75. Armstrong S, Li JS, Skinner AC. Flattening the (BMI) curve: timing of child obesity onset and cardiovascular risk. Pediatrics 2020;146(2):e20201353.
76. Institute of Medicine (US) Committee on Assuring the health of the public in the 21st Century. The future of the Public's Health in the 21st Century. Washington (DC): National Academies Press (US); 2002.
77. Hammerness P, Zusman R, Systrom D, et al. A cardiopulmonary study of lisdexamfetamine in adults with attention-deficit/hyperactivity disorder. World J Biol Psychiatry 2013;14(4):299–306.
78. Wilens TE, Zusman RM, Hammerness PG, et al. An open-label study of the tolerability of mixed amphetamine salts in adults with attention-deficit/hyperactivity disorder and treated primary essential hypertension. J Clin Psychiatry 2006;67(5):696–702.
79. Shin JY, Roughead EE, Park BJ, et al. Cardiovascular safety of methylphenidate among children and young people with attention-deficit/hyperactivity disorder (ADHD): nationwide self controlled case series study. BMJ 2016;353:i2550 [Erratum appears in BMJ 2016;353:i3123].
80. Rohatgi RK, Bos JM, Ackerman MJ. Stimulant therapy in children with attention-deficit/hyperactivity disorder and concomitant long QT syndrome: a safe combination? Heart Rhythm 2015;12(8):1807–12.
81. Wolraich ML, Hagan JF Jr, Allan C, et al. Clinical practice guideline for the diagnosis, evaluation, and treatment of ADHD in children and adolescents. Pediatrics 2019;144(4):e20192528 [Erratum appears in Pediatrics 2020;145(3)].
82. Torres-Acosta N, O'Keefe JH, O'Keefe CL, et al. Cardiovascular effects of ADHD therapies: JACC review topic of the week. J Am Coll Cardiol 2020;76(7):858–66.
83. Bellato A, Arora I, Hollis C, et al. Is autonomic nervous system function atypical in attention deficit hyperactivity disorder (ADHD)? A systematic review of the evidence. Neurosci Biobehav Rev 2020;108:182–206.
84. Toce MS, Farias M, Bruccoleri R, et al. A case report of reversible takotsubo cardiomyopathy after amphetamine/dextroamphetamine ingestion in a 15-year-old adolescent girl. J Pediatr 2017;182:385–8.e3.
85. Mosholder AD, Taylor L, Mannheim G, et al. Incidence of heart failure and cardiomyopathy following initiation of medications for attention-deficit/hyperactivity disorder. J Clin Psychopharmacol 2018;38(5):505–8.
86. Kelly AS, Rudser KD, Dengel DR, et al. Cardiac autonomic dysfunction and arterial stiffness among children and adolescents with attention deficit hyperactivity disorder treated with stimulants. J Pediatr 2014;165(4):755–9.
87. Westover AN, Nakonezny PA, Adinoff B, et al. Impact of stimulant medication use on heart rate and systolic blood pressure during submaximal exercise treadmill testing in adolescents. J Child Adolesc Psychopharmacol 2016;26(10):889–99.
88. Skinner JR, Van Hare GF. Letter to the editor–detection of long QT syndrome in the community. Heart Rhythm 2015;12(7):e67.
89. Yoon SY, Jain U, Shapiro C. Sleep in attention-deficit/hyperactivity disorder in children and adults: past, present, and future. Sleep Med Rev 2012;16(4):371–88.
90. Kaisari P, Dourish CT, Higgs S. Attention deficit hyperactivity disorder (ADHD) and disordered eating behaviour. Clin Psychol Rev 2017;53:109–21.

Pharmacotherapy of Attention-Deficit/Hyperactivity Disorder in Individuals with Autism Spectrum Disorder

Gagan Joshi, MD[a,b,c,]*, Timothy E. Wilens, MD[b,c]

KEYWORDS

• ADHD • ASD • Comorbidity • Treatment

KEY POINTS

- There is a bidirectional asymmetrical overlap of comorbidity between attention-deficit/hyperactivity disorder (ADHD) and autism spectrum disorder (ASD).
- There is under-recognition of reciprocal comorbidity between ASD and ADHD.
- There is a lack of controlled clinical trials for ADHD with mixed amphetamine salts, in adults, and in intellectually capable populations with ASD.
- The majority of ADHD treatment trials were conducted in intellectually impaired populations with autism where the response is less than typically expected.tche response is lower
- Response to ADHD treatment appears similar in higher functioning youth with autism compared with neurotypically developing youth with ADHD.

INTRODUCTION

Autism spectrum disorder (ASD) is a highly morbid neurodevelopmental disorder characterized by varying degrees of deficits in social–emotional functioning along with restricted, repetitive behaviors and interests.[1] An increasingly higher prevalence of ASD is documented in each successive epidemiologic survey conducted in the United

[a] The Alan and Lorraine Bressler Clinical and Research Program for Autism Spectrum Disorder, Massachusetts General Hospital, 55 Fruit Street, WRN 626, Boston, MA 02114, USA; [b] Clinical and Research Program in Pediatric Psychopharmacology, Massachusetts General Hospital, Boston MA, USA; [c] Department of Psychiatry, Harvard Medical School, Boston MA, USA
* Corresponding author. The Alan and Lorraine Bressler Clinical and Research Program for Autism Spectrum Disorder, Massachusetts General Hospital, 55 Fruit Street, WRN 626, Boston, MA 02114.
E-mail address: Joshi.Gagan@MGH.Harvard.edu

States since 2000, with the latest prevalence estimated to affect 1 in 44 youth in the general population.[2] Notably, the rise in prevalence is predominantly due to increased recognition of ASD in intellectually capable populations.

There is a bidirectional although asymmetrical, overlap of comorbidity between attention-deficit/hyperactivity disorder (ADHD) and ASD. Up to three-fourths of the psychiatrically referred population with ASD suffer from ADHD, and around 15% of the ADHD population suffer from ASD.[3]

ADHD is the most common psychiatric disorder recognized in youth and adults with ASD and greatly adds to their morbidity and dysfunction, particularly in those with intact intellectual capacity.[4–6] The presence of ADHD in intellectually capable individuals with ASD significantly impairs intellectual and social functioning, particularly as individuals usually cofunction alongside typically developed peers.[3,7] Untreated ADHD in intellectually capable individuals with ASD can seriously compromise educational outcomes[8,9] and predispose individuals to increased risk for disruptive behaviors, mood dysregulation, and substance use disorders.[10]

Considering ADHD is known to respond to various pharmacologic interventions in typically developing individuals, identifying and offering disorder-specific treatments for ADHD comorbid with ASD can potentially minimize morbidity and impairments in autistic individuals. Previously, *Diagnostic and Statistical Manual* (DSM) -based diagnostic restrictions precluded recognition of ADHD in the presence of ASD, resulting in the under-recognition of coexisting ADHD in ASD populations. This limited advances in research for establishing evidence-based treatment options for ADHD in autism populations. In clinical practice, ADHD agents are the most widely prescribed medication treatment in this population.[11] Thus, there remains a gulf between limited evidence-based options and the substantial utilization of pharmacotherapy for managing ADHD in ASD populations.[7] This systematic review will evaluate the extant literature on ADHD treatments in ASD with ADHD, and treatment responses in autism compared with the typically expected response.

APPROACH
Search Criteria

We conducted a systemic search of peer-reviewed literature on controlled clinical trials with sample sizes greater than 10, published through mid-2021 that examined the safety and efficacy of ADHD medications in individuals with ASD.

Data sources: The PubMed, PsychINFO, Embase, and Medline electronic databases were searched with the combination of the following MeSH terms: [ASD OR autism OR Asperger's disorder OR pervasive developmental disorder] AND [attention-deficit/hyperactivity disorder OR hyperactivity] AND [clinical trial OR controlled trial].

Data Extraction

Trials were broadly categorized based on the class of the anti-ADHD medication (stimulants, nonstimulants) and age groups of the study populations (preschoolers, youth, adults). Data collected for the design of the trial included type of controlled trial (crossover, parallel designs), duration of the trial (in weeks), status of ADHD (diagnosis, symptoms of hyperactivity-impulsivity, inattention), study medication target dose, and the study response criteria. Tolerability response was assessed by extracting data on the rates and severity of treatment-emergent adverse events (AEs), with a particular focus on the typically expected AEs and unexpected AEs.

RESULTS
Search Overview

The search yielded 2536 articles, and through the process of elimination detailed in the search overview PRISMA (**Fig. 1**), 12 controlled trials and 3 secondary analyses related to the review for the treatment of ASD were identified.

Attention-Deficit/Hyperactivity Disorder Treatment Trials in Autism Spectrum Disorder

Of the 12 relevant articles, five original trial articles and one article on secondary analysis examined the effect of methylphenidate (MPH) on ADHD. Three original trial articles and one secondary analysis article examined the effect of atomoxetine (ATX), and one original trial article and one secondary analysis study examined the effect of guanfacine (GFC) on ADHD.

Trial Protocols

Design: All five MPH trials were crossover trials with different trial doses (low and high) and their durations ranged from 3 to 6 weeks. The maximum MPH dose was 20 mg/d for the preschooler ASD population and 0.5–0.6 mg/kg/dose for trials in older children with ASD. Both ATX trials were parallel in design. The trial duration ranged from 10 to 12 weeks, and the range of ATX maximum dose per study design was 1.2 to 1.8 mg/kg/d. Finally, the single GFC trial was an 8-week parallel design with a maximum GFC extended-release formulation dose per study design of 4 mg/d.

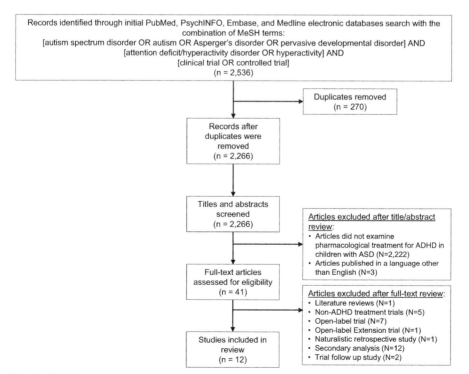

Fig. 1. PRISMA.

ADHD Status: Less than one-half of the trials (4/9) required ASD individuals to meet ADHD diagnostic criteria for participation.[12–15] All trials required hyperactivity symptom severity threshold as an eligibility criterion for participation with the exception of the Pearson and colleagues[12] and Quintana and colleagues[16] MPH trials.

ADHD Response Criteria: The primary continuous outcome measure of efficacy was identified by all the trials, except the Quintana and colleagues[16] MPH trial. In the MPH trials, the primary outcome measure assessed for hyperactivity, with the exception of the Pearson and colleagues[12] trial that assessed for both symptom domains of ADHD (ie, inattention and hyperactivity). All three ATX trials had different primary outcome measures (two parent rated and one clinician rated). Lastly, in the single GFC trial, hyperactivity was the primary outcome measure. The categorical response on the clinical global impression-improvement subscale (CGI-I) was reported by eight of nine trials. The criteria for response in four out of five trials was a combination of CGI-I$\leq$2 response and $\geq$25%-30% reduction in the informant-rated primary outcome measure. The effect size (ES) of response on the primary outcome measures was reported in five of nine trials.

Trial Participants Characteristics

All the trials were conducted in children and adolescents. The majority of the ASD participants suffered from intellectual disability (ID); conversely, the Pearson and colleagues[12] MPH trial and the Harfterkamp and colleagues[14] ATX trials were the only two trials that were conducted in predominantly intellectually intact ASD populations with intelligence quotient levels ranging from mildly impaired to majority intact. With the exception of the MPH trials by Pearson and colleagues[12] and Quintana and colleagues,[16] participants in the trials under review had high levels of irritability at baseline as documented by the mean levels of severity for irritability in the moderate range (Aberrant Behavior Checklist-irritability score $\geq$16).

Primary Efficacy Response (Attention-Deficit/Hyperactivity Disorder)

Primary Outcome Measure: The ADHD medications were significantly superior to placebo on the primary outcome measure across all the controlled trials (**Tables 1** and **2**).
CGI-I$\leq$2 Response Rate: Only one MPH trial by Pearson and colleagues[12] reported on global CGI-I$\leq$2 response rate, although the rate of placebo response and statistical significance was not provided. All nonstimulant trials reported on the CGI-I$\leq$2 response rate, and it was superior to placebo in all but one trial (ATX trial by Harfterkamp and colleagues).[14]

Secondary Efficacy Response (Autism Spectrum Disorder, Psychiatric Symptoms)

ASD Features: Autism severity response was assessed in all the trials. Whereas one trial had worsening of social withdrawal at higher MPH dosing,[17] the significant improvement in social skills was noted in other MPH trials.[12,13,18] Similarly, significant improvement in social communication and restricted-repetitive behaviors (RRBs) were observed in both ATX and GFC trials.[14,19] *Psychiatric symptoms (irritability, oppositional defiant behaviorsoppositional defiant behaviors)*: Significant improvement in irritability was reported with MPH trials.[12,13,16] In contrast, in all nonstimulant trials, no change in irritability was reported. Inconsistent improvement in oppositional defiant behaviors was noted.[12,17,19]

Table 1
Stimulants controlled trials in autism spectrum disorder

Trial — Title [Formulation] Design (Duration)	Participants — Sample Size [N]	Age [yrs] Mean (Range)	IQ Mean (Range)	Level of Irritability [ABC-IRR]	Dose Mean (Range) [mg/d]	ADHD — Primary Outcome Mean Reduction Effect Size	ADHD — Response Rate CGI-I≤2 Responder Criteria	ASD — SI [ABC-SW]	ASD — SC [ABC-IS]	ASD — RRBs [ABC-ST]	ASD — IRR [ABC-IRR]	ASD — Ψ	ASD — ODB	Tolerability — Adverse Events [N (%)] TEAE[Statistically Significant AEs] Severe AE Serious AE Dose-LAE	Tolerability — Early Terminations [N (%)] Total ET ETLE Tx-LAE	Comments
Methylphenidate																
Pre-School Children																
Ghuman et al,[18] 2009 [MPH-IR] Crossover (4-wk)	14 ASD: 12 ID: 2	4.8 ± 1 (3–6)	75 ± 18.6 (44–105)	• Irritability[5]	14.5 ± 4.6 (5–20)	Hyperactivity MPH > PBO[a]; • CPRS-R [MD = 8.9; p = SS] ↑ES: 0.97	Global- CGI-I≤2: NR; Global- CGI-I ≤2 & ≥25% ↓CPRS-R: 50% vs7%; p = NR	↓N-CBRF	↓N-CBRF	⇅ • SBS • CY-BOCS • N-CBRF	NA	NA	NA	TEAE: 7 (50) vs 0 (0); • Buccal-lingual movements[b]; Severe AEs: NR; Serious AEs: None; Dose-LAE: 9 (64)	Total ET: 3 (18) vs 0 (0); ETLE: None; Tx-LAE: 1 (6) vs 0 (0); • Dysphoria [N = 1]	• Examined Hyperactivity only • Participants with speech delay [all but 1] • Response worse than typically expected. • Exacerbation of stereotypes & emotional lability • Poorer tolerability at higher doses
School-Age Children																

(continued on next page)

Table 1
(continued)

Trial Title [Formulation] Design (Duration)	Participants Sample Size [N]	Age[yrs]/ IQ Mean (Range)	Level of Irritability [ABC-IRR]	Dose Mean (Range) [mg/d]	Efficacy [MED vs. PBO; P-value] — ADHD Primary Outcome Mean Reduction Effect Size	Response Rate CGI-I ≤2 Responder Criteria	ASD SI [ABC-SWI]	SC [ABC-IS]	RRBs [ABC-ST]	IRR [ABC-IRR]	Ψ	ODB	Tolerability — Adverse Events [N (%)] TEAE[Statistically Significant AEs] Severe AE Serious AE Dose-LAE	Early Terminations [N (%)] Total ET ETLE Tx-LAE	Comments
Pearson et al,[12] 2013 [MPH-ER/IR] Crossover (4-wk)	24	Age: 8.8 ± 1.7 (7–13) IQ: 85 ± 16.8 (46–112)	12.6 ± 10.4	AM [ER]^c LD: 0.21 MD: 0.35 HD: 0.48 Afternoon [IR]^c LD: 0.14 MD: 0.24 HD: 0.27	ADHD MPH > PBO [LD/MD/HD] • CTRS-R[NR; p = SS] ES: NR	Global-CGI-I ≤2;[d] Clinician-rated: 67% vs NR; p = NR Psychologist-rated: 79% vs NR; p = NR RC: NA	⇌ ABC	↓ ABC [MD/HD]	⇌ ABC	↓ ABC [HD]		↓ ACTeRS [MD/HD]	TEAE:[HD] • Insomnia (38%) • ↓Appetite (38%) Severe AEs: None Serious AEs: None Dose-LAE: 5 (21) • Irritability [N = 5] • ↑Stereotypy [N = 2] • ↓Sleep [N = 2]	Total ET: None ETLE: None Tx-LAE: None	• Examined ADHD • 2/3rd intellectually intact and 1/3rd with mild ID • Response as typically expected • No worsening of ASD, Mood, or Anxiety • (↑Social Skills [MPH > PBO: ACTeRS [p = SS]; SCQ [p = SS]]) High vs. Low dose • Most robust anti-ADHD response on HD • Significant improvement in irritability on HD • - More frequent AEs on HD

	N			Doses: [mg/kg/dose]	Hyperactivity	Global	↑ABC [HD]	⇌ABC [MD]	⇌ABC [MD]	⇌ABC	⇌SNAP-IV	TEAE: [LD/MD/HD]	Total ET:	
RUPP, 2005 [3]Posey et al,[24] 2007 [MPH-IR] Crossover (4-wk)	66	Age: 7.5 ± 2.2 (5–14) IQ: 62.6 ± 33 (16–135)	17 ± 10 (0–41)	LD: 0.11 ± 0.03 • 0.18 ± 0.02 MD: 0.22 ± 0.05 • 0.36 ± 0.04 HD: 0.43 ± 0.11 • 0.51 ± 0.06 (7.5–50)	MPH > PBO [LD/MD/HD] • ↑ABC-H [NR; p = 55] 1,-1ES: 0.48	CGI-I ≤2: NR CGI-I ≤2 + ≥30% ↓ PT↑ABC-H/ ≥25% ↓ P + ↑ABC-H: 49 vs 20; p = NR						• Insomnia [11%/18%/16%] • ↓Appetite [0%/24%/24%] • Emotional outburst [0%/14%/0%] • Irritability [0%/12%/0%] Severe AE: None Serious AE: None Dose-LAE: 16 (24) • HD reduced d/t AEs [N = 16]	13 (18) vs 0 (0) ETLE: None Tx-LAE: 13 (18) vs 0 (0) • Irritability [N = 6]	• Examined Hyperactivity • Majority with ID and nonverbal • Response worse than typically expected • No exacerbation of ASD features High vs. Low dose • Most robust anti-ADHD response on higher doses • Less tolerant to higher doses

(continued on next page)

Table 1
(continued)

Trial	Participants			Dose	Efficacy [MED vs. PBO; P-value]								Tolerability		Comments
					ADHD		ASD								
Title [Formulation] Design (Duration)	Sample Size [N]	Age[yrs.]/ IQ Mean (Range)	Level of Irritability [ABC-IRR]	Mean (Range) [mg/d]	Primary Outcome Mean Reduction Effect Size	Response Rate CGI-I≤2 Responder Criteria	SI [ABC-SW]	SC [ABC-IS]	RRBs [ABC-ST]	IRR [ABC-IRR]	Ψ	ODB	Adverse Events [N (%)] TEAE[Statistically Significant AEs] Severe AE Serious AE Dose-LAE	Early Terminations [N (%)] Total ET ETLE Tx-LAE	
Handen et al,[13] 2000 [MPH-IR] Crossover (3-wk)	13	Age: 7.4 ±NR (6–11) IQ: NR	15.6 ± 11	NR (NR)	Hyperactivity MPH > PBO [LD/HD] • CTRS-H[NR; p = SS] ES: NR	CGI-I ≤2: NA ≥50% ↓CTRS-H bet. MPH & PBO: 61%; p = NA	⇌ABC	↓ABC [LD/HD]	⇌ABC	⇌ABC	NA	NA	TEAE: 9 (75) vs 9 (75) • MPH vs PBO; p = NR Severe AE: 7 (58) vs 6 (50) • Irritability [N: 4 vs. 2] • Social Withdrawal [N: 3 vs. 1] Serious AE: None Dose-LAE: 2 (15) • Aggression [N = 1] • Severe staring [N = 1]	Total ET: 1 (8) vs 0 (0) ETLE: None Tx-LAE: 1 (8) vs 0 (0) • Tantrum, skin picking [N: LD = 1]	• Examined Hyperactivity only • Participants with ID [all but 1] • No worsening of ASD features (MPH ≯ PBO: CARS[NS]) • High rates of AEs on PBO High vs. Low dose • No difference in hyperactivity response between HD and LD • Sign. more AEs on HD

| Quintana et al,[16] 1995 [MPH-IR] Crossover (6-wk) | 10 | Age: 8.5 ± 1.3 (7–11) IQ: 64.3 ± 9.9 (50–84) | 11.8 ± 11.2 | NR (0.37–0.74)[e] | Hyperactivity MPH > PBO [LD/HD] • [c]ABC-H [NR; p = SS] • [c]CTRS-H [NR; p = SS] ES: NR | CGI ≤2: NA RC: NA | ⇌[ABC] | ⇌[ABC] | ⇌[ABC] | ⇌[ABC] | ↓[ABC] | NA | TEAvE: • MPH[LD] >PBO; P-value = NR • MPH[HD] >PBO; P < .05 = None Severe AE: None Serious AE: None Dose-LAE: None | Total ET: None ETLE: None Tx-LAE: None | • Examined Hyperactivity only • Majority with ID (70%) • Treatment did not worsen ASD or cause mood dysregulation • High vs. Low dose • No sign. difference in response between doses |

Abbreviations: 1, Drug versus placebo; 2, Pre versus post; 3, SNAP-IV data; 4, Optimal dose of MPH defined as the dose at which maximum improvement was recorded; ABC, aberrant behavior checklist; ABC-H, ABC-hyperactivity; ABC-IS, ABC-inappropriate speech; ABC-ST, ABC-stereotypy; ABC-SW, ABC-social withdrawal; ACTeRS, ADD-H comprehensive teacher's rating scale; ADHD, attention-deficit/hyperactive disorder; AE, adverse events; ASD, autism spectrum disorder; C, clinician-rated; CARS, childhood autism; rating Scale; CGI-I, Clinical Global Impression-Improvement subscale; CPRS-R, Children's psychiatric rating scale-revised; CY-BOCS, Children's Yale-Brown obsessive-compulsive scale; Dose-LAE, dose-limiting AE; ER, extended release; ETLE, early termination d/t lack of efficacy; HD, high dose; ID, intellectual disability; IR, immediate release; IRR, irritability; LD, low dose; MD, medium dose; MPH, methylphenidate; NA, not applicable; N-CBRF, nisonger child behavior rating form; NR, not reported; NS, statistically Not Significant; ODB, oppositional defiant behaviors; PBO, placebo; RRBs, restricted repetitive behaviors; SC, social communication; SCQ, social communication score; SI, social interaction; SNAP, swanson, Nolan, and Pelham Questionnaire; SS, statistically significant; T, teacher-rated; TEAE, treatment emergent AE; Tx-LAE, treatment-limiting AE.

[a] ASD only (Calculated from reported values).

[b] Severity significantly worse than PBO.

[c] IR mg/kg/dose.

[d] On any dose.

[e] mg/kg/d

Table 2
Nonstimulants controlled trials in autism spectrum disorder

Trial Title [Formulation] Design (Duration)	Participants Sample Size (Exposed) [N]	Participants Age[yrs]/IQ Mean (Range)	Dose Level of Irritability [ABC-IRR]	Dose Mean (Range) [mg/d]	Efficacy [MED vs. PBO: P-value] ADHD Primary Outcome Mean Reduction Effect Size	Efficacy ADHD Response Rate CGI-I ≤2 Responder Criteria	Efficacy ASD SI [ABC-SW]	Efficacy ASD SC [ABC-IS]	Efficacy ASD RRBs [ABC-ST]	Efficacy Ψ IRR [ABC-IRR]	Efficacy Ψ ODB-	Tolerability Adverse Events [N (%)] TEAE[Statistically Significant AEs] Severe AE Serious AE Dose-LAE	Tolerability Early Terminations [N (%)] Total ET ETLE Tx-LAE	Comments
Atomoxetine														
Youth														
Handen et al,[20] 2015 Parallel (10-wk)	128 (32[a]/64[b])	Age: 8.1 ± 2.1 IQ: 81.7 ± 24.3	16 ± 9.7	45 ± 22 1.4 ± 0.5[c] (1.2–1.8)[c]	ADHD ATX > PBO •[a]SNAP-IV [NR; p = SS] [z]ES: 0.80	ADHD-CGI-I ≤2: 47% vs19%; p = SS ADHD-CGI-I ≤2 & ≥30% ↓[a]SNAP: 47% vs19%; p = SS	⇌[pA]ABC	⇌ABC	⇌ABC	⇌ABC	⇌SNAP-IV	TEAE: • ↓Appetite (47%) Severe AE: None Serious AE: None Dose-LAE: None	Total ET: 11 17) vs 18 (28); p = NS ETLE: 1 (1.5) vs 4 (6) Tx-LAE: 5 (8) vs 10 (16) • Irritability [N. 4 vs. 7]	• Examined ADHD • Majority with ID [83.5%] • Efficacy less than typically expected • Tolerability as typically expected • No worsening of ASD or Mood • Less tolerated at higher doses
Harfterkamp et al,[14] 2012 [b]Harfterkamp et al,[25] 2014 Parallel (8-wk)	97 ASD: 95 ID: 2	*ATX* [N = 48] Age: 9.9 ± 2.7 (6–16) IQ: 91 ± 16 (65–132)	17.3 ± 9	NR (0.5–1.2)[d]	ADHD ATX > PBO •[c]ADHD-RS [ADHD: –8 v. –1; p = SS] ES: NR	ADHD-CGI-I ≤2: 21% vs 9%; p = NS RC: NA	⇌ABC	↓ABC	↓ABC	↓ABC	⇌CTRS-R	TEAE: 39 (81) vs 32 (65) • Nausea (29%) • ↓Appetite (27%) • Fatigue (23%) • Early waking (10%)	Total ET: 5 (10) vs 3 (6) ETLE: 1 (2) vs 0 (0) Tx-LAE: 1 (2) vs 0 (0) • Fatigue [N = 1]	• Examined ADHD • Majority without ID • Efficacy less than typically expected • Tolerability as typically expected

Study / Design	N	Age / IQ			Efficacy	Response						Adverse Events	Dropouts	Comments
							↓ABC	↓ABC	↓ABC	↓ABC	↓DSM-IV	Severe AE: None Serious AE: None Dose-LAE: None		• No worsening of stereotypes or repetitive behaviors • Decrease in fear of and resistance to change (ATX > PBO: CSBQ [p = SS]) • Most robust anti-ADHD response on higher doses
Arnold et al,[15] 2006 Crossover (12-wk)	16	Age: 9.3 ± 2.9 (5–15) IQ: NR	16 ± 9.3	44 ± 22 (20–100)	Hyperactivity ATX > PBO • ^{P}ABC-H[-5 v. 0.6; p = SS] ^{I}ES: 0.90	Global-CGI ≤2: 56% vs 25%; p = NR Global-CGI ≤2 + ≥25%↓ ABC-H: 43% vs 25%; p = NR						TEAE: 16 (100) vs NR • Upset stomach (69%) • Nausea and vomiting (67%) • Fatigue (75%) • Tachycardia (25%) Severe AE: 2 (12.5) vs 4 (25) • Agitation [N: 1 vs. 0] • Tiredness [N: 1 vs. 0] Serious AE: 1 (6) • Agitation [N = 1] Dose-LAE: None	Total D/o: 1 (6) vs 2 (13) ET/LE: 0 (0) vs 2 (13) Tx-LAE: 1 (6) vs 0 (0) • Aggression [N = 1]	• Examined Hyperactivity • Majority with ID • Titration schedule slower than typically administered • Efficacy response less than typically expected • Tolerability profile as typically expected • More pronounced effect on hyperactivity than on inattention • All participants experienced upper GI AEs

(continued on next page)

Table 2 (continued)

Trial	Participants			Dose	Efficacy [MED vs. PBO; P-value]							Tolerability		Comments
					ADHD		ASD		RRBs	Ψ		Adverse Events [N (%)]	Early Terminations [N (%)]	
Title [Formulation] Design (Duration)	Sample Size (Exposed) [N]	Age[yrs]/IQ Mean (Range)	Level of Irritability [ABC-IRR]	Mean (Range) [mg/d]	Primary Outcome Mean Reduction Effect Size	Response Rate CGI-I ≤2 Responder Criteria	SI [ABC-SW]	SC [ABC-IS]	[ABC-ST]	IRR [ABC-IRR]	ODB-	TEAE [Statistically Significant AEs] / Severe AE / Serious AE / Dose-LAE	Total ET / ETLE / Tx-LAE	
Guanfacine														
School-Age Children														
Scahill et al,[19] 2015 / Polltte et al,[26] 2018 [GFC-ER] Parallel (8-wk)	62	Age: 8.5 ± 2.3 (5–14) IQ: NR	20 ± 9.4	3 ±NR (1–4)	Hyperactivity $GFC > PBO$ • PABC-H ↓44% vs ↓13%, p = SS; ↑ES: 1.67	Global-CGI-I ≤2: 50% vs 9%; p = SS; RC: NA	⇌ABC	↓ABC	⇌ABC	⇌ABC	↓HSQ-ASD	**TEAE:** • Drowsiness (87%) • Fatigue (63%) • ↓Appetite (43%) • Dry mouth (40%) • Emotional/tearful (40%) • Irritability (37%) • Anxiety (30%) • Waking in sleep (30%) **Severe AE:** None **Serious AE:** 1 (3) • Agitation [N = 1] **Dose-LAE:** 9 (30) • Drowsiness/fatigue [NR] • Emotional (irritability) [NR]	*Total ET:* 6 (20) vs 4 (13) *ETLE:* 2 (7) vs 4 (13) *Tx-LAE:* 4 (13) • Agitation [N = 2] • Drowsiness [N = 1]	• Examined Hyperactivity • One-third without ID (34%) • Efficacy as typically expected • Tolerability worse than typically expected • Decrease in anxiety (on CASI; vs PBO p = NS) • No worsening of ASD features • Mood & anxiety related AEs

Abbreviations: 1, Drug versus placebo; 2, Pre versus post; 5, CSBQ & ABC data; 6, HSQ-ASD and CASI data; ABC, aberrant behavior checklist; ABC-H, ABC-hyperactivity; ABC-IS, ABC-inappropriate speech; ABC-ST, ABC-stereotypy; ABC-SW, ABC-social withdrawal; ADHD, attention-deficit/hyperactive disorder; ADHD-RS, ADHD-rating scale; AEs, adverse events; ASD, autism spectrum disorder; ATX, atomoxetine; bpm, beats per minute (heart rate); C, clinician-rated; CASI, child and adolescent symptom inventory; CGI-I, clinical global impression-improvement subscale; CSBQ, children's social behavior questionnaire-fear of and resistance to change; CTRS-R, Conners teacher rating scale-revised; Dose-LAE, dose-limiting AE; DSM-IV, Diagnostic and Statistical Manual Of Mental Disorders; ER, extended release; ETLE, early termination d/t lack of efficacy; GFC, guanfacine; GI AEs, gastrointestinal AEs; HSQ-ASD, home situation questionnaire-modified for ASD; ID, intellectual disability; IRR, irritability; NA, not applicable; NR, not reported; NS, statistically not significant; ODB, oppositional defiant behaviors; P, parent-rated; PBO, placebo; RRBs, restricted repetitive behaviors; SC, social communication; SI, social interaction; SNAP, swanson, Nolan, and Pelham Questionnaire; SS, statistically significant; TEAE, treatment emergent AE; Tx-LAE, treatment-limiting AE.

[a] Efficacy.
[b] Tolerability.
[c] mg/kg/d.
[d] mg/kg/d.

Tolerability Response

Typical AEs: In the MPH trials, the most common and statistically significant AEs recorded in children with ASD were insomnia, decreased appetite, emotional outbursts, and irritability.[12,17] In the preschool participants, the most common and statistically significant AE was buccal-lingual movements.[18] GI disturbances (decreased appetite, nausea and vomiting, or stomach upset) and fatigue were among the most frequently reported statistically significant AEs in the ATX trials. In the GFC trial,[19] the most common AEs included drowsiness, fatigue, decreased appetite, dry mouth, emotional/tearful, irritability, anxiety, and disturbed sleep. *Atypical AEs*: No atypical AEs were reported in any of the controlled trials under review. *Severe AEs*: No severe AEs were reported by any of the major trials under review. *Serious AEs*: Only two participants across the nine trials experienced a serious AE of agitation on ATX (N = 1) and GFC (N = 1).[15,19] *Dose-limiting AEs*: Dose-limiting AEs occurred in all but one MPH trial. Dose-limiting AEs were experienced by one-fourth of RUPP[17] trial participants, requiring dose reductions of MPH. Likewise, one-fifth of Pearson and colleagues[12] trial participants discontinued the afternoon dose of instant-release MPH due to irritability-related AEs. Two-thirds of the participants in the preschooler trial of MPH experienced dose-limiting AEs. In the GFC trial,[19] one-third of the participants experienced dose-limiting AEs including drowsiness, emotional/tearful, irritability, and/or sleep disturbance. None of the ATX trials had any dose-limiting AEs. *Treatment limiting AE*: There were few treatment-limiting AE with MPH. All three ATX trials reported treatment-limiting AEs with irritability/aggression as the most frequent reason for early termination. Agitation and fatigue-related treatment-limiting AEs were reported in the Scahill and colleagues[19] GFC trial.

DISCUSSION

Higher than expected prevalence of reciprocal comorbidity is observed between ASD and ADHD. The bidirectional comorbidity between ASD and ADHD is asymmetrically far more prevalent in intellectually capable populations with ASD than with ADHD. Clinicians should also be aware that individuals with ADHD frequently suffer from a significant burden of autistic traits that do not meet the threshold for ASD diagnosis and are associated with morbidity and dysfunction.[7]

In all the controlled trials for ADHD in youth with ASD, there was a significantly superior ADHD response to stimulant and nonstimulant treatments compared with placebo. ADHD treatments were not associated with the worsening of autism features, and oppositional behaviors. On the contrary, improvement in various domains of social functioning, irritability, and oppositional behaviors was reported with anti-ADHD treatments. A typically expected anti-ADHD agents-related treatment-emergent AE profile was observed in ASD populations with no atypical AEs.

This review assessing the empirical evidence on the response of anti-ADHD treatment in individuals with ASD makes the following salient observations. One, very limited controlled trials have been conducted to date, with nearly one-half of the trials evaluating the response of MPH in individuals with ASD. Second, the majority of controlled trials were conducted in children, a minority of them in adolescents, and none in adult populations with ASD. Third, there is no trial conducted to date on the response of amphetamine. Fourth, the majority of the trials are conducted in ASD populations with varying levels of intellectual impairments. Considering that ADHD is far more prevalent and impairing in intellectually capable populations with ASD, findings from these trials may not accurately reflect the effectiveness of these medications in intellectually intact populations with ASD. In addition, as attention is challenging to assess in lower-functioning, nonverbal ASD populations, the majority of the trials assessed ADHD response primarily on the severity of *hyperactivity*. Lastly, all ATX and GFC trials and the majority of the MPH trials included ASD participants with significant levels of irritability, which may have adversely moderated the anti-ADHD response. Among trials with high levels of irritability at participation, the majority assessed for the response of hyperactivity to anti-ADHD medications. As hyperactivity in the context of irritability could be a symptom of mood disorder and thus not responsive to treatment with anti-ADHD medications, this may have moderated the less than typically expected response of hyperactivity observed in the trials. Interestingly, although the mean severity level of irritability did not worsen with anti-ADHD treatments, treatment-emergent mood lability (irritability, emotional outbursts) was observed at a higher rate than typically expected and was the most frequent reason for dose or treatment-limiting AE,[12,13,15,17–20] thus mediating the poor response to anti-ADHD medications in this population.

Clinical implications: There are important clinical considerations based on empirical evidence (noted with reference) and clinical observation: (1) Screen for ASD in ADHD individuals with social impairments as ASD is under-recognized[7]; (2) take a nonhierarchical approach for assessing ADHD in ASD populations and refrain from attributing ADHD symptoms as sequelae or secondary features of ASD[3]; (3) confirm presence of ADHD symptoms in the absence of sensory triggers or mood lability; (4) assess for other psychopathologies frequently associated with ASD (anxiety and mood disorder)[5]; (5) manage impairing mood and anxiety symptoms before treating ADHD and treat impairing ADHD symptoms upon stabilization of mood and anxiety; (6) initiate ADHD treatment at the lowest possible dose and up titrate and small milligram increments based on tolerability to the optimal dose based on response; and (7) be clinically vigilant for treatment-emergent irritability with anti-ADHD medications in this population.[12,13,15,17–20]

Methylphenidate: Which stimulant should you choose initially? There are no ADHD trials with amphetamine and five controlled trials with MPH. Only one trial was conducted on the extended-release formulation of MPH.[12] In addition, no empirical data are available on the treatment response of MPH in ASD individuals in late adolescence and beyond. MPH response for ADHD was more robust and with lower AEs based on the severity of the study populations for autism, lability, and ID. Similar trends were seen in the improvement in social skills, irritability, and oppositional behaviors. Interestingly, MPH did not exacerbate stereotypy or oppositional behaviors in children with ASD. The differences in stimulant trial design may also have contributed to outcomes. The major differences of the ASD trial designs from the traditional stimulant trials include (1) no systematic exclusion of participants with ID or with significant anxiety and mood dysregulation; (2) lack of inattention symptom treatment outcome measure in the assessment of ADHD response; (3) primary outcome measure for ADHD response not assessed on measures that are typically applied in ADHD trials; and (4) lack of titration and shorter duration of exposure to MPH. *Clinical implications*: (1) MPH should be considered as first-line treatment for managing ADHD in ASD individuals without ID; (2) assess tolerability by offering the lowest possible dose of instant-release MPH in the morning (preferably at weekend) and continue with the MPH treatment if the single test dose is not associated with significant mood instability (irritability/agitation) and/or insomnia; (3) anticipate that the response to MPH may not be as typically expected in intellectually disabled populations; (4) use caution in up-titrating MPH to higher doses (1.25 mg/kg/d) in intellectually impaired ASD; and (5) anticipate additional improvements in irritability, oppositional behaviors and social functioning in intellectually intact individuals with ASD.

Atomoxetine: ATX was generally well tolerated by youth at a daily dose of up to 1.2 to 1.8 mg/kg, which is similar to that observed in typicals (0.5–1.8 mg/kg/d)[21] with an ES of response that was large (0.8–0.9) and comparable with the ES observed in the typicals (0.64).[21] Similar to MPH, the magnitude of response and response rate of ATX was less robust in intellectually impaired youth compared with typically developing youth (ASD: 21% vs typicals: 60%)[21] and was not superior to placebo. *Clinical implications*: (1) Based on tolerability, ATX is considered to be a first-line option for the treatment of ADHD in ASD youth with ID; (2) optimize the treatment to up to 1.8 mg/kg/d dose for optimal response; (3) splitting the dose may help improve tolerability; (4) anticipate improvement in autism-related social behaviors and autistic mannerisms in intellectually capable populations with ASD; (5) expect ASD youth to experience typically expected AEs.

Guanfacine: The only controlled trial to assess the anti-ADHD response of GFC in ASD was conducted with an extended-release formulation in children with ASD. The response in the GFC trial in ASD was similar to other traditional trials of GFC in terms of dosing, ADHD response, social behaviors, and oppositionality. However, treatment-emergent AEs occurred at higher rates in ASD compared with children with more traditional ADHD. *Clinical implications*: (1) Consider GFC as a first-line option for the treatment of ADHD in ASD individuals with co-occurring sleep disturbance and anxiety; (2) consider dosing GFC at night to minimize drowsiness and fatigue; (3) expect typical AEs, although at higher frequency in this population; (4) expect ADHD response as typically expected; (5) anticipate additional improvement in social and oppositional behaviors and autistic mannerisms.

Among the three anti-ADHD medications under review, the efficacy response of MPH and ATX was less than typically expected, whereas the response to GFC was as typically expected. The tolerability response was worse than typically expected for MPH and GFC, whereas tolerability for ATX was as typically expected. Thus, among the anti-ADHD agents, GFC had the most robust anti-ADHD response and ATX had the most favorable tolerability response. Of interest, similar response and AE rates were generally noted in intellectually capable youth with ASD compared with neurotypically developing youth.[22,23]

Evidence-Based Clinical Guidelines

As autism is under-recognized in psychiatrically referred populations in general and with ADHD in specific, and as the literature suggests that significant autistic traits and autism are highly comorbid with ADHD, it is incumbent upon treating clinicians to screen and assess for autism in individuals with ADHD. Conversely, ADHD individuals who present with impairments in social functioning that are significantly worse than expected should be assessed for autism. Other features with ADHD that should raise autism concerns are socially odd behaviors, sensory dysregulation, poor eye contact, repetitive motor mannerisms (rocking, flapping), and transitional difficulties. Also, ADHD individuals who continue to suffer from social impairments upon optimal treatment of ADHD should be assessed for ASD. More importantly, one should take a nonhierarchical approach in assessing for ADHD in ASD populations and refrain from misattributing symptoms of ADHD as associated features of ASD. As the literature suggests, the presentation of ADHD is not atypical in individuals with ASD although one should assess the role of certain autistic features like sensory dysregulation that can worsen symptom severity of ADHD. When assessing for ADHD in nonverbal and/or intellectually impaired individuals with ASD who also suffer from emotional lability/irritability it is imperative to ensure that symptoms of ADHD, in particular hyperactivity, are not present only in the context of mood dysregulation or when experiencing stress due to autism-related impairments (social, sensory, transitional distress). When ADHD in individuals with ASD is associated with high levels of mood instability/irritability, mood stabilization is essential and should precede targeted treatment for ADHD. Second-generation antipsychotics, risperidone, and aripiprazole are Food and Drug Administration approved for the treatment of irritability and agitation in autism and also improve ADHD symptoms, and the decision to treat ADHD upon stabilization of mood should be based on the persistence of functionally impairing symptoms of ADHD.

In intellectually intact ASD individuals with ADHD, treatment should target and optimize response for both hyperactive-impulsive and inattentive symptoms of ADHD and not restrict to managing only symptoms of hyperactivity-impulsivity.

In order to maximize tolerability, the anti-ADHD medication, particularly in intellectually impaired individuals with ASD, should be initiated at the lowest possible dose and, if possible, should be administered in divided dosage and follow a slower titration schedule.

In intellectually impaired ASD populations, the treatment algorithm for managing ADHD is guided by tolerability. Nonstimulants are the initial treatment of choice, and among them, GFC is the treatment of choice, particularly for those with comorbid symptoms of sleep disturbance and anxiety (autonomic arousal). Based on the evidence in this population, the extended-release formulation is preferred and, if tolerated well, then anticipate typically expected anti-ADHD response. In addition to improvement in ADHD severity, also expect improvement in autism severity (in particular RRBs), oppositional behaviors, and possibly anxiety with GFC treatment. ATX is the most well-tolerated anti-ADHD agent in this population. Based on the evidence, one should expect an anti-ADHD response to ATX treatment that is atypically more pronounced for hyperactivity than inattention in ASD populations. MPH should be considered as an alternative if treatment with both nonstimulants fail to treat ADHD, MPH should also be considered as an add-on for optimizing partial anti-ADHD response to nonstimulants. Based on the evidence that suggests a single test dose of MPH could predict treatment tolerability, if a single test dose of MPH in the morning (preferably at a weekend) is not associated with significant mood instability (irritability/agitation), then one should continue treatment with MPH. Monitor for treatment-emergent mood instability and adjust MPH dose titration accordingly. Titrate MPH to a higher daily dosage (1.25 mg/kg/d) with caution as evidence suggests that it is not well tolerated and associated with worsening of social functioning.

Based on the limited evidence on the anti-ADHD response in ASD individuals without ID, the approach for managing ADHD in this population is similar to the treatment guidelines for the typicals with few important caveats. Among the stimulants as the first line of treatment for ADHD, treatment with MPH is preferred over mixed amphetamine salts, as no empirical evidence is available on the response of mixed amphetamine salts in ASD individuals. The extended-release formulation of MPH is preferred. As suggested by the MPH extended-release trial, it may be better tolerated,[12] whereas the afternoon MPH instant-release dose was poorly tolerated. In addition to typically expected robust linear dose anti-ADHD response with MPH treatment, also expect improvement in social skills, levels of irritability, and oppositional behaviors. If MPH is not tolerated well (often due to treatment-emergent irritability), then based on tolerability, ATX could be considered as a second-line treatment. Optimize ATX dosing to up to a typically prescribed maximum daily dose (1.8 mg/kg/d). With ATX treatment expect a more pronounced response for hyperactivity than inattention and additional improvement in the levels of autism severity (social communication, RRBs, fear of and resistance to change). As evidence is lacking on the anti-ADHD response of GFC in ASD individuals without ID, clinicians should follow the clinical guidelines offered for ASD populations with ID as a proxy for GFC treatment in ASD individuals without ID.

SUMMARY

The review of the controlled anti-ADHD clinical trials in ASD offers evidence of a response that is restricted, as a majority of the trials included ASD individuals with ID, who were experiencing significant levels of mood lability (irritability) at participation, and assessed only for hyperactivity symptoms of ADHD. In addition, anti-ADHD controlled trials in intellectually capable and adult populations with ASD are lacking. Conspicuously lacking are controlled trials of amphetamine in ASD.

CLINICS CARE POINTS

- Screen for reciprocal comorbidity of ASD and ADHD as co-occurrence is highly under-recognized.
- Clinical presentation of ADHD is typical of the disorder in ASD populations.
- ADHD worsens repetitive behaviors and social impairments, and ASD related sensory hyper-reactivity worsens ADHD.
- ADHD is often comorbid with other mood and anxiety disorders in individuals with ASD.
- Treat mood instability prior to treating ADHD.
- If possible, choose extended-release formulation or split the daily dose of instant-release formulation and start anti-ADHD medication at low dose and titrate slow for improving tolerability.
- The methylphenidate response in ASD youth is worse than typically expected in the presence of ID and as typically expected in ASD youth without ID. Methylphenidate response in ASD youth without ID is also associated with improvement in social behaviors.
- In ASD youth the atomoxetine tolerability response is as typically expected though anti-ADHD response is worse than typically expected with atypically relatively more pronounced effect on hyperactivity than inattention. Additional improvement with atomoxetine treatment noted in the severity of autism in ASD youth without ID.
- The guanfacine treatment in ASD youth was associated with worse than typically expected tolerability and typically expected anti-ADHD response with additional improvement in social and oppositional behaviors.

DISCLOSURE

Gagan Joshi receives research support from Pfizer, Demarest Lloyd, Jr Foundation, and Simons Center for the Social Brain as a principal inves- tigator (PI) for investigator-initiated studies. Additionally, he receives research support from F. Hoffmann-La Roche Ltd as a site PI for multi- site trials. He received honoraria from the Governor's Council for Medical Research and Treatment of Autism in New Jersey and from the National Institute of Mental Health for grant review activities. He received speaker's honoraria from the American Academy of Child and Adolescent Psychiatry, The Israeli Society of ADHD, the Canadian Academy of Child and Adolescent Psychiatry, and the University of Jülich.

REFERENCES

1. American Psychiatric Association. Diagnostic and statistical manual of mental disorders. 5th ed. Arlington, VA: American Psychiatric Publishing; 2013.

2. Maenner MJ, Shaw KA, Bakian AV, et al. Prevalence and characteristics of autism spectrum disorder among children aged 8 years - autism and developmental disabilities monitoring network, 11 Sites, United States, 2018. MMWR Surveill Summ 2021;70(11):1–16.
3. Joshi G, Faraone SV, Wozniak J, et al. Symptom Profile of ADHD in Youth With High-Functioning Autism Spectrum Disorder: A Comparative Study in Psychiatrically Referred Populations. J Atten Disord 2017;21(10):846–55.
4. Stahlberg O, Soderstrom H, Rastam M, et al. Bipolar disorder, schizophrenia, and other psychotic disorders in adults with childhood onset AD/HD and/or autism spectrum disorders. J Neural Transm 2004;111(7):891–902.
5. Joshi G, Petty C, Wozniak J, et al. The heavy burden of psychiatric comorbidity in youth with autism spectrum disorders: a large comparative study of a psychiatrically referred population. J Autism Dev Disord 2010;40(11):1361–70.
6. Joshi G, Wozniak J, Petty C, et al. Psychiatric comorbidity and functioning in a clinically referred population of adults with autism spectrum disorders: a comparative study. J Autism Dev Disord 2013;43(6):1314–25.
7. Joshi G. Are there lessons to be learned from the prevailing patterns of psychotropic drug use in patients with autism spectrum disorder? Acta Psychiatr Scand 2017;135(1):5–7.
8. Kotte A, Joshi G, Fried R, et al. Autistic traits in children with and without ADHD. Pediatrics 2013;132(3):e612–22.
9. Joshi G, DiSalvo M, Faraone SV, et al. Predictive utility of autistic traits in youth with ADHD: a controlled 10-year longitudinal follow-up study. Eur Child Adolesc Psychiatry 2020;29(6):791–801.
10. Biederman J, Monuteaux MC, Spencer T, et al. Do stimulants protect against psychiatric disorders in youth with ADHD? A 10-year follow-up study. Pediatrics 2009;124(1):71–8.
11. Langworthy-Lam KS, Aman MG, Van Bourgondien ME. Prevalence and patterns of use of psychoactive medicines in individuals with autism in the Autism Society of North Carolina. J Child Adolesc Psychopharmacol 2002;12(4):311–21.
12. Pearson DA, Santos CW, Aman MG, et al. Effects of extended release methylphenidate treatment on ratings of attention-deficit/hyperactivity disorder (ADHD) and associated behavior in children with autism spectrum disorders and ADHD symptoms. J Child Adolesc Psychopharmacol 2013;23(5):337–51.
13. Handen BL, Johnson CR, Lubetsky M. Efficacy of methylphenidate among children with autism and symptoms of attention-deficit hyperactivity disorder. J Autism Dev Disord 2000;30(3):245–55.
14. Harfterkamp M, van de Loo-Neus G, Minderaa RB, et al. A randomized double-blind study of atomoxetine versus placebo for attention-deficit/hyperactivity disorder symptoms in children with autism spectrum disorder. J Am Acad Child Adolesc Psychiatry 2012;51(7):733–41.
15. Arnold LE, Aman MG, Cook AM, et al. Atomoxetine for hyperactivity in autism spectrum disorders: placebo-controlled crossover pilot trial. J Am Acad Child Adolesc Psychiatry 2006;45(10):1196–205.
16. Quintana H, Birmaher B, Stedge D, et al. Use of methylphenidate in the treatment of children with autistic disorder. J Autism Dev Disord 1995;25(3):283–94.
17. Research Units on Pediatric Psychopharmacology Autism Network. Randomized, controlled, crossover trial of methylphenidate in pervasive developmental disorders with hyperactivity. Arch Gen Psychiatry 2005;62(11):1266–74.
18. Ghuman JK, Aman MG, Lecavalier L, et al. Randomized, placebo-controlled, crossover study of methylphenidate for attention-deficit/hyperactivity disorder

symptoms in preschoolers with developmental disorders. J Child Adolesc Psychopharmacol 2009;19(4):329–39.

19. Scahill L, McCracken JT, King BH, et al. Extended-release guanfacine for hyperactivity in children with autism spectrum disorder. Am J Psychiatry 2015;172(12): 1197–206.

20. Handen BL, Aman MG, Arnold LE, et al. Atomoxetine, parent training, and their combination in children with autism spectrum disorder and attention-deficit/hyperactivity disorder. J Am Acad Child Adolesc Psychiatry 2015;54(11):905–15.

21. Schwartz S, Correll CU. Efficacy and safety of atomoxetine in children and adolescents with attention-deficit/hyperactivity disorder: results from a comprehensive meta-analysis and metaregression. J Am Acad Child Adolesc Psychiatry 2014;53(2):174–87.

22. Cheng JY, Chen RY, Ko JS, et al. Efficacy and safety of atomoxetine for attention-deficit/hyperactivity disorder in children and adolescents-meta-analysis and meta-regression analysis. Psychopharmacology (Berl) 2007;194(2):197–209.

23. Faraone SV, Buitelaar J. Comparing the efficacy of stimulants for ADHD in children and adolescents using meta-analysis. Eur Child Adolesc Psychiatry 2010; 19(4):353–64.

24. Posey DJ, Aman MG, McCracken JT, et al. Positive effects of methylphenidate on inattention and hyperactivity in pervasive developmental disorders: an analysis of secondary measures. Biol Psychiatry 2007;61(4):538–44.

25. Harfterkamp M, Buitelaar JK, Minderaa RB, et al. Atomoxetine in autism spectrum disorder: no effects on social functioning; some beneficial effects on stereotyped behaviors, inappropriate speech, and fear of change. J Child Adolesc Psychopharmacol 2014;24(9):481–5.

26. Politte LC, Scahill L, Figueroa J, et al. A randomized, placebo-controlled trial of extended-release guanfacine in children with autism spectrum disorder and ADHD symptoms: an analysis of secondary outcome measures. Neuropsychopharmacology 2018;43(8):1772–8.

Pharmacologic Treatment of Comorbid Attention-Deficit/ Hyperactivity Disorder and Tourette and Tic Disorders

Robert J. Jaffe, MD[a],*, Barbara J. Coffey, MD, MS[b]

KEYWORDS

- ADHD • Tics • Stimulants • α-Agonists • Tourette

KEY POINTS

- There is a bidirectional relationship between ADHD and tic disorders.
- A comprehensive medical and psychiatric evaluation is essential to treatment.
- Stimulants are the first-line pharmacotherapy to treat ADHD in patients with tic disorders.
- α-Agonists are added to simulants or used as monotherapy to treat ADHD and tics.

INTRODUCTION

Tics are defined as sudden, rapid, and recurrent, nonrhythmic motor movements or vocalizations.[1] Motor tics are movements, such as eye blinks or shoulder shrugs. Vocal, also known as phonic tics, are utterances or sounds, such as throat clearing.[2] The distinction is somewhat arbitrary, because vocalizations are produced by muscles. Both motor and phonic tics are classified as either simple or complex. Simple motor tics are brief and meaningless movements involving one muscle or muscle group, whereas complex motor tics are more purposeful and involve multiple muscle groups. Simple vocal tics, like simple motor tics, are fast and meaningless sounds. Complex vocal tics involve words or phrases, and may include obscenities (coprolalia). The Diagnostic and Statistical Manual, 5th edition, classifies motor and vocal tics based on their duration; if movements and/or sounds have been present for less than 1 year, they are classified as a provisional tic disorder. If either movements or sounds have persisted for greater than 1 year they are diagnosed as either a persistent motor or persistent vocal tic disorder.[1,2]

[a] Department of Psychiatry, Icahn School of Medicine at Mount Sinai, One Gustave L. Levy Place, Box 1230, New York, NY 10029, USA; [b] Department of Psychiatry and Behavioral Sciences, University of Miami Miller School of Medicine, 1120 Northwest Fourteenth Street, Suite 1455, Miami, FL 33136, USA
* Corresponding author. Tourette Association Center of Excellence at Mount Sinai, Department of Psychiatry, Icahn School of Medicine at Mount Sinai, One Gustave L. Levy Place, Box 1230, New York, NY 10029.
E-mail address: robert.jaffe@mountsinai.org

Child Adolesc Psychiatric Clin N Am 31 (2022) 469–477
https://doi.org/10.1016/j.chc.2022.03.004
1056-4993/22/© 2022 Elsevier Inc. All rights reserved.

Tourette disorder (TD), also referred to as Tourette syndrome, is diagnosed when an individual has multiple motor tics and one or more vocal tics, although they need not be present at the same time. The tics must have been present for at least 1 year with onset before the age of 18. The disorder is named after the French neurologist George Gilles de la Tourette, who in 1885 published a case series of nine patients with tics.[3]

Tics typically begin in early childhood with an average age of onset of 5 to 7 years. Motor tics often emerge first with a head-to-toe progression. Phonic tics typically emerge 1 to 2 years later. Tics are usually not static, and the predominant tic or tics may change at different times in the same individual. The tics wax and wane over time, and there may be long periods during which the tics are minimal or even absent. Tics usually peak before puberty around the ages of 9 to 12 and attenuate significantly by early adulthood. Intense focus, such as playing a sport or instrument, may make the tics subside or even disappear entirely at least temporarily. Conversely, tics may worsen during periods of stress and illness. Patients typically report a premonitory urge, or unpleasant sensation they feel in their body or mind, which builds up before a tic and is subsequently relieved by completing the tic. Tics are briefly suppressed with effort, which can lead to an increase in the discomfort and potential for more intense bouts.

Individuals with tic disorders, and particularly TD, often have co-occurring or comorbid psychiatric symptoms or conditions. Estimates vary, but 50% to 80% of patents with TD also meet criteria for attention-deficit/hyperactivity disorder (ADHD).[4] The relationship between TD and ADHD is bidirectional; 20% of those with ADHD may meet criteria for a tic disorder. Proposed reasons for this high overlap include a core deficit in inhibition related to frontostriatal and frontoparietal network dysfunction in cortico-striatal-thalamic-cortical tracts. Imaging studies show hyperfunctioning/overactive circuits in the basal ganglia in TD resulting in motor/cognitive/emotional disinhibition, worsened by frontal hypoactivity in ADHD. That both disorders tend to improve with time may reflect increased myelinization of prefrontal regions.[5,6]

A comprehensive diagnostic evaluation is essential in patients with tic disorders, given the high comorbidity rate not just for ADHD, but with other disorders. Twenty percent to 60% of patients with TD have obsessive-compulsive disorder, approximately 25% have a learning disorder, and 20% have an anxiety disorder. Many of these patients also have other behavioral or impulse control disorders.[4]

Diagnoses for TD and ADHD are made based on the clinical history. Structured or semistructured diagnostic interviews, such as the DISC or K-SADS, can help with reliability. The Tic Symptom Self Report is a screening questionnaire individuals and families can complete to identify tics. Clinician-scored rating scales help qualify and quantify disorder severity. The Yale-Global Tic Severity Scale (YGTSS) is considered the gold standard rating scale for tics, and assesses the following tic domains: number, frequency, intensity, complexity, and interference and tic-related impairment.[6]

It is imperative to assess the patient's self-esteem and how he or she is functioning academically, socially, and within the family. This history, along with quantitative symptom assessments, can identify which symptoms are most impairing and bothersome to the patient and family. Patients with persistent tic disorders and ADHD have more peer problems and reduced quality of life than those with either disorder alone. Indeed, much of the associated psychopathology (behavioral, emotional, neurocognitive) in TD is secondary to ADHD.[7] Given that tic disorders tend to remit independent of ADHD, and outcomes of ADHD are problematic without intervention, treatment of ADHD is usually the priority when comorbidity is present.[8]

This article next reviews current pharmacologic evidence for treatment of ADHD and tic disorders, and discusses clinical implications and treatment strategies.

RESEARCH AND CURRENT EVIDENCE IN PHARMACOTHERAPY FOR ATTENTION-DEFICIT/HYPERACTIVITY DISORDER AND TIC DISORDERS
Stimulants

In clinically referred individuals with ADHD and tic disorders, ADHD symptoms are usually more impairing than tics, and thus treatment of ADHD should be prioritized. Stimulants remain the most effective pharmacologic choice for children with ADHD, and are considered first-line. Children with ADHD and comorbid tics respond equally to stimulants as children with ADHD without tics.[9]

However, the Food and Drug Administration (FDA) lists "patients with motor tics or with a family history or diagnosis of Tourette syndrome" as a contraindication for Ritalin, and the following warning/precaution for Adderall: "Amphetamines have been reported to exacerbate motor and phonic tics and Tourette syndrome. Therefore, clinical evaluation for tics and Tourette syndrome in children and their families should precede use of stimulant medications." Cohen and colleagues[10] explain the history of case reports from the 1970s and 1980s, which led to the FDA label in 1983. These warnings have likely limited the use of an effective treatment of children with ADHD and tic disorders.[10]

There have since been several randomized controlled trials (RCTs) showing no deleterious effect of stimulants on tics. The Cohen meta-analysis examined 22 RCTs involving 2385 participants to determine the risk of new onset or worsening tics in patients with ADHD taking stimulants compared with placebo. The results showed no increase in new onset or worsening of tics in those taking stimulants. New onset or worsening of tics were reported in 5.7% of children in the stimulant group, compared with 6.5% in the placebo arm. The authors conclude that overall the risk of new onset or tic worsening associated with stimulants is similar to that of placebo. Moreover, stimulant type (methylphenidate vs amphetamine derivative), duration of action (short-acting vs long-acting), dose, and duration of treatment were not associated with a more frequent onset or worsening of tics. Crossover trials did report a greater association of new onset or worsening of tics compared with parallel-group studies, although neither group reported an association between tics and stimulant use. The study concluded that the number needed to harm from new onset or worsening tics with stimulants is 1000.[10] Thus, 1000 people would need to take a stimulant before one person would be expected to develop new or worsening tics.

α-Agonists

The α_2-agonists clonidine and guanfacine are often considered first-line pharmacologic treatment for tics.[11] Several RCTs have looked at whether they are effective at treating ADHD and comorbid tic disorders.

In 1991 Leckman and colleagues[12] reported a 26% improvement over baseline ratings in the patients treated with clonidine compared with placebo, as measured by the Tourette Syndrome Global Scale; in addition they reported a 48% reduction in the "impulsive-hyperactive" factor on the ADHD Conners Parent Questionnaire in the clonidine group compared with 6% in the placebo group.[12]

In the Treatment of ADHD and Chronic Tics (TACT) study, the Tourette Syndrome Study group reported that the combination of methylphenidate and clonidine conferred the greatest treatment effect for ADHD (1.09) and tic symptoms (0.75) compared with either medication alone or placebo.[9,13]

In contrast, Singer and colleagues[14] in a 1995 study did not show benefit of clonidine over placebo on either tic severity on the Hopkins Scale or Tourette Syndrome Severity Scale, or on ADHD on the parent global linear analogue rating of hyperactivity.

In comparing clonidine with risperidone, Gaffney and colleagues[15] showed that clonidine reduced tic severity by 26% on the YGTSS and reduced ADHD severity by 38% on the ADHD-RS. In a different study comparing clonidine with levetiracetam, Hedderick and colleagues[16] showed a small but significant decrease in mean Total Tic Score (25.2 baseline vs 21.8), but not mean total YGTSS (48.7 vs 43.1) in the clonidine group, and no difference in ADHD-RS. The latter study was limited by only including two patients with ADHD; neither study had a placebo comparator.[16]

There have been three studies that have shown a benefit for transdermal clonidine in tic disorders, but did not include any secondary ADHD outcome measures.[17–19]

In 2001 Scahill and colleagues[20] showed a 37% decrease on the teacher-rated ADHD-RS for guanfacine compared with 8% in the placebo group. For tics, the guanfacine group had a 31% decrease in tic severity on the YGTSS versus 0% in the placebo group. In contrast, a 2017 study that examined guanfacine extended release compared with placebo failed to show a significant effect of guanfacine in tic reduction compared with placebo.[21]

A 2013 meta-analysis of available studies showed α-agonists to have a significant benefit in reduction of tics compared with placebo, with a standardized mean difference (SMD) of 0.31. This study examined the impact of a comorbid ADHD diagnosis, and found that in studies that enrolled patients with tics plus ADHD, the SMD jumped to a clinically significant 0.68 for α-agonists. In studies where ADHD was excluded the SMD was 0.15. Studies that had a greater percentage of subjects with ADHD showed a greater efficacy from α-agonists in tic reduction.[11]

Overall, studies in which α-agonists have been effective reduce tic severity by about 30%, an effect likely moderated by the presence of comorbid ADHD.

Other Agents

There are two studies that examined atomoxetine. In 2005 Allen and colleagues[22] showed a decrease of 5.5 points on the YGTSS Total Tic Score in the atomoxetine group compared with 3 points in the placebo group. This difference approached but did not reach significance with a calculated effect size of 0.3. The study measured ADHD response using the ADHD-RS and found an effect size of 0.6.[22] A 2008 study did show a significant difference in response in the atomoxetine group, with a YGTSS Total Tic Score decrease of 5.1 points compared with 2 points in the placebo, yielding an effect size of 0.4. The atomoxetine group experienced a decrease in the ADHD-RS-IV-Parent:Inventory total score of 10.4 points compared with 4.4 points in the placebo arm, with an effect size of 0.57.[23] These small but statistically significant decreases may be clinically meaningful for patients depending on baseline tic severity and specific areas of improvement.

Two RCTs evaluated the tricyclic antidepressant desipramine in patients with ADHD and tic disorders after several case reports were published. Singer and colleagues[14] in 1995 reported that patients with ADHD and TD treated with desipramine had a statistically significant decrease in the parent global linear analogue comparing the child's current tics with tics anytime in the past. In contrast, participants in the desipramine group did not show a decrease in any of the standardized tic ratings used. In this same study desipramine was also superior to clonidine and placebo in reducing hyperactivity on the parent-completed global linear analogue rating scale and the hyperactivity subscale of the CBCL.[14]

In 2002 a second study reported a 30% decrease from baseline in the YGTSS global severity scores in participants treated with desipramine compared with those on placebo. Desipramine was also effective in reducing ADHD symptoms by 42% from baseline relative to placebo on the ADHD-RS.[24]

DISCUSSION

The first step in the pharmacologic treatment of individuals with comorbid ADHD and tics is a comprehensive medical and psychiatric evaluation; information should be obtained from the primary care physician, patient, parents, the school, and any involved clinicians or other services. Neuropsychological or psychometric assessment may also be helpful in disentangling ADHD symptoms from executive function difficulties and/or specific learning disorders. A thorough, detailed and multidisciplinary evaluation qualifies and quantifies problematic symptoms in the patient. This facilitates identification of which symptoms are the most problematic or distressing to prioritize for intervention.

Psychostimulants are the recommended first-line pharmacologic treatment of ADHD symptoms in patients with comorbid tic disorders. To state again, in patients whose ADHD symptoms are most problematic, stimulants should be prescribed first.

The Cohen meta-analysis makes clear that stimulants were associated with neither new onset nor worsening of tics in patients with ADHD and tic disorders. Some individuals may be particularly sensitive to the effects of stimulants and experience a transient tic increase after starting a stimulant or increasing the dose. FDA warning labels remain on many stimulants, and it is essential to discuss with the family the possibility of tic onset or increase. Attention to family history of tic disorders and/or obsessive-compulsive disorder is essential, because this may identify individuals at higher risk for the development of tics, independent of exposure to stimulants. Additionally, tics typically onset at around the same age as ADHD is recognized or diagnosed, and their onset may be entirely coincidental. Furthermore, tic fluctuations with waxing and waning are characteristic of the natural history, and it is possible that a waxing period is simultaneously occurring at the time of medication initiation. Conversely, an incidental waning period may be confused with clinical improvement on the stimulant. It is helpful to understand each individual patient's typical pattern of tic fluctuations in advance of starting treatment. Discussion of these possibilities with families before starting medication is strongly recommended.

Methylphenidate is recommended as the initial stimulant choice in this population. In the only head-to-head study of methylphenidate versus dextroamphetamine, increases in tic severity were sustained for those on high doses of dextroamphetamine.[25] For individuals treated with a stimulant in the past who experienced an increase in tics, rechallenge with a stimulant should be considered if the ADHD symptoms are not adequately controlled with nonstimulants. Methylphenidate is initiated at 5 mg for children and 10 mg for adolescents and titrated up gradually. Patients should be closely monitored for any worsening of tics. An immediate-release formulation may be helpful to start with low doses and then switched to a long-acting preparation once an effective and tolerable dose is reached. Long-acting stimulants may be less likely than their immediate-release counterparts to be associated with a tic increase, although there are no controlled studies examining this directly.

Although this article is focused on pharmacologic interventions for ADHD and tic disorders, it is important to acknowledge that there is an effective evidence-based therapy for tics called comprehensive behavioral intervention for tics (CBIT). A therapist trained in CBIT uses habit reversal training to help the patient identify premonitory urges or sensations, and to implement competing responses in lieu of the tics. By breaking the cycle of negative reinforcement, tic urges and tics themselves decrease. CBIT also helps identify antecedents and familial responses that may be reinforcing tics. CBIT has been shown to reduce tic severity by 50% and is often the first-line treatment in patients whose tics are causing significant impairment or distress.[4] These patients can address their ADHD symptoms with stimulants and tics through CBIT.

If the ADHD symptoms improve during stimulant titration but tics worsen, CBIT can facilitate reduction of tics. The stimulant dose is held or temporarily reduced while monitoring the tics. The stimulant is retitrated later on when the tics improve. If ADHD symptoms are not adequately improved and the tics have worsened, an α-agonist is added.

α-Agonists are an excellent alternative option in patients with ADHD and tic disorders. Patients with higher levels of impulsivity and hyperactivity would be ideal candidates. α-Agonists do seem to be markedly more effective in treatment of tics in patients with ADHD compared with those without; this suggests that ADHD is a moderating factor and renders α-agonists an especially appealing monotherapy in this patient population.

Guanfacine is often preferred over clonidine because it is less sedating and has a longer half-life, although there are times where sedation is a desired benefit. In choosing short- versus long-acting guanfacine, extended-release guanfacine failed to separate from placebo in the treatment of tics in its one RCT. It should be noted that dosing only went to 4 mg with a mean daily dose of 2.6 mg in the long-acting guanfacine trial, and higher doses in adolescents (up to 7 mg) were shown to be more effective when extended-release guanfacine was used to treat ADHD. Given the negative trial results, however, short-acting guanfacine would be recommended first.

Recommended dosing of immediate-release guanfacine is 0.5 mg to 1 mg nightly for children and adolescents, respectively. Guanfacine can be increased by 0.5 to 1 mg every 3 to 7 days, alternating morning and night, with the higher dose given at night to facilitate onset of sleep. It should be noted that Scahill and colleagues prescribed guanfacine three times a day, with the most common dosing schedule 1 mg at 8 AM, 0.5 mg at 3 PM, and 1 mg at 8 PM. Clinical realities make twice a day dosing much more convenient and practical for families and is therefore recommended.

Atomoxetine is another good option for patients who cannot tolerate stimulants, prefer monotherapy, have a contraindication, or for whom targeted pharmacotherapy with a stimulant plus an α-agonist has not been effective. Dosing follows the typical ADHD recommendations discussed elsewhere in this issue.

Although there is some evidence for efficacy of desipramine in patients with ADHD and tic disorders, its use is not recommended, given potential adverse effects, including cardiovascular, and the availability of safer and effective alternatives.

The antipsychotic medications aripiprazole, pimozide, and haloperidol all have FDA indications for treatment of tics in TD. There is also evidence to support the use of risperidone, a second-generation antipsychotic. The second-generation medications are generally preferred over first generations (typical) when antipsychotics are used. This class of medications is better studied for TD than ADHD, although a few studies have looked at comorbidity and shown some benefit.[26–28] Moreover, antipsychotics do usually show a greater benefit in tic reduction compared with α-agonists.[4]

However, we prefer starting with α-agonists, given their preferable adverse effect profile and higher rate of response in individuals with both TD and ADHD. Antipsychotics are good options in patients unresponsive to α-agonists and CBIT, or whose tic severity impacts their safety and well-being. In patients in which antipsychotics are added to stimulants for other reasons, tics and polypharmacy can be reduced.

Lastly, there are limited data on the use of nutraceuticals for tic disorders. Two studies from Spain showed benefit from magnesium and vitamin B_6, with the caveats that in one trial the supplements were administered intravenously, and the oral administration study was an open-label one.[29,30] A study looking at N-acetylcysteine showed no evidence for efficacy in reducing tics.[31] Omega-3 fatty acids did not reduce tic severity but did reduce tic impairment.[32] There is currently no evidence to support the use of cannabidiol or medical marijuana in the treatment of TD.

SUMMARY

It is essential to understand the frequent and bidirectional overlap of tic disorders and ADHD. A full comprehensive medical and psychiatric evaluation is necessary to separate tic symptoms from ADHD, and to prioritize the most problematic symptoms for intervention. Stimulants are the recommended first-line pharmacotherapy to treat ADHD symptoms in patients with tic disorders. CBIT is an effective behavioral therapy, which is generally considered the first-line treatment of persistent tic disorders. α-Agonists are added to stimulants if tics increase or used as monotherapy to target ADHD and tics. Atomoxetine is also an excellent option to treat ADHD and tics.

CLINICS CARE POINTS

- When evaluating patients with tic disorders, evaluate for comorbidities, such as ADHD, obsessive-compulsive disorder, anxiety, and learning disorders.
- Identify the most problematic symptoms the patient is having and treat those first.
- If tics worsen after starting a stimulant, the medication is held or temporarily reduced, retitrating when they improve.

DISCLOSURE

R.J. Jaffe: research support from Emalex and Teva/Nuvelution. B.J. Coffey Disclosures Past 12 Months: American Academy of Child and Adolescent Psychiatry, honoraria; Emalex, research support; Florida Children's Medical Services, grant support; Harvard Medical School/Psychiatry Academy, honoraria; NIMH, research support; Partners Healthcare, honoraria; Skyland Trail, advisory board; Teva/Nuvelution, research support; Scientific Advisory Board, Tourette Association of America, cochair; Medical Advisory Board, TAA-cdc Partnership.

REFERENCES

1. Diagnostic and statistical manual of mental disorders: DSM-5. 5th edition. American Psychiatric Association; 2013.
2. Scahill LD. Yale global tic severity scale. In: Volkmar FR, editor. Encyclopedia of autism spectrum disorders. New York, NY: Springer; 2013. https://doi.org/10.1007/978-1-4419-1698-3_1279. Available at.
3. Cavanna A, Seri S. George Gilles de la Tourette and his legacy. Arch Med Sci 2019;7(2):303–8.
4. Murphy TK, Lewin AB, Storch EA, et al. Practice parameter for the assessment and treatment of children and adolescents with tic disorders. J Am Acad Child Adolesc Psychiatry 2013;52(12):1341–59.
5. Leckman James F, et al. Neurobiological substrates of Tourette's disorder. J Child Adolesc Psychopharmacol 2010;20(4):237–47.
6. Robertson Mary M, et al. Gilles de la Tourette syndrome. Nat Rev Dis Primers 2017;3:16097.

7. Poh W, Payne JM, Gulenc A, et al. Chronic tic disorders in children with ADHD. Arch Dis Child 2018;103(9):847–52.
8. Spencer T, Biederman M, Coffey B, et al. The 4-year course of tic disorders in boys with attention-deficit/hyperactivity disorder. Arch Gen Psychiatry 1999; 56(9):842–7.
9. Bloch MH, Panza KE, Landeros-Weisenberger A, et al. Meta-analysis: treatment of attention-deficit/hyperactivity disorder in children with comorbid tic disorders. J Am Acad Child Adolesc Psychiatry 2009;48(9):884–93.
10. Cohen SC, Mulqueen JM, Ferracioli-Oda E, et al. Meta-analysis: risk of tics associated with psychostimulant use in randomized, placebo-controlled trials. J Am Acad Child Adolesc Psychiatry 2015;54(9):728–36.
11. Weisman H, Qureshi IA, Leckman JF, et al. Systematic review: pharmacological treatment of tic disorders: efficacy of antipsychotic and alpha-2 adrenergic agonist agents. Neurosci Biobehav Rev 2013;37(6):1162–71.
12. Leckman JF, Hardin MT, Riddle MA, et al. Clonidine treatment of Gilles de la Tourette's syndrome. Arch Gen Psychiatry 1991;48(4):324–8.
13. Treatment of ADHD in children with tics: a randomized controlled trial. Neurology 2002;58(4):527–36.
14. Singer HS, Brown J, Quaskey S, et al. The treatment of attention-deficit hyperactivity disorder in Tourette's syndrome: a double-blind placebo-controlled study with clonidine and desipramine. Pediatrics 1995;95(1):74–81.
15. Gaffney GR, Perry PJ, Lund BC, et al. Risperidone versus clonidine in the treatment of children and adolescents with Tourette's syndrome. J Am Acad Child Adolesc Psychiatry 2002;41(3):330–6.
16. Hedderick EF, Morris CM, Singer HS. Double-blind, crossover study of clonidine and levetiracetam in Tourette syndrome. Pediatr Neurol 2009;40(6):420–5.
17. Du YS, Li HF, Vance A, et al. Randomized double-blind multicentre placebo-controlled clinical trial of the clonidine adhesive patch for the treatment of tic disorders. Aust N Z J Psychiatry 2008;42(9):807–13.
18. Kang H, Zhang YF, Jiao FY, et al. [Efficacy of clonidine transdermal patch for treatment of Tourette's syndrome in children]. Zhongguo Dang Dai Er Ke Za Zhi 2009;11(7):537–9.
19. Jiao F, Zhang X, Zhang X, et al. Clinical observation on treatment of Tourette syndrome in Chinese children by clonidine adhesive patch. Eur J Paediatr Neurol 2016;20(1):80–4.
20. Scahill L, Chappell PB, Kim YS, et al. A placebo-controlled study of guanfacine in the treatment of children with tic disorders and attention deficit hyperactivity disorder. Am J Psychiatry 2001;158(7):1067–74.
21. Murphy TK, Fernandez TV, Coffey BJ, et al. Extended-release guanfacine does not show a large effect on tic severity in children with chronic tic disorders. J Child Adolesc Psychopharmacol 2017;27(9):762–70.
22. Allen AJ, Kurlan RM, Gilbert DL, et al. Atomoxetine treatment in children and adolescents with ADHD and comorbid tic disorders. Neurology 2005;65(12):1941–9.
23. Spencer TJ, Sallee FR, Gilbert DL, et al. Atomoxetine treatment of ADHD in children with comorbid Tourette syndrome. J Atten Disord 2008;11(4):470–81.
24. Spencer T, Biederman J, Coffey B, et al. A double-blind comparison of desipramine and placebo in children and adolescents with chronic tic disorder and comorbid attention-deficit/hyperactivity disorder. Arch Gen Psychiatry 2002;59(7):649–56.

25. Castellanos FX, Giedd JN, Elia J, et al. Controlled stimulant treatment of ADHD and comorbid Tourette's syndrome: effects of stimulant and dose. J Am Acad Child Adolesc Psychiatry 1997;36(5):589–96.

26. McCracken James T, et al. Effectiveness and tolerability of open label olanzapine in children and adolescents with Tourette syndrome. J Child Adolesc Psychopharmacol 2008;18(5):501–8.

27. Murphy Tanya K, et al. Open label aripiprazole in the treatment of youth with tic disorders. J Child Adolesc Psychopharmacol 2009;19(4):441–7.

28. Budman CL, et al. An open-label study of the treatment efficacy of olanzapine for Tourette's disorder. J Clin Psychiatry 2001;62(4):290–4.

29. Garcia-Lopez Rafael, et al. New therapeutic approach to Tourette syndrome in children based on a randomized placebo-controlled double-blind phase IV study of the effectiveness and safety of magnesium and vitamin B6. Trials 2009;10:16.

30. García-López Rafael, et al. An open study evaluating the efficacy and security of magnesium and vitamin B(6) as a treatment of Tourette syndrome in children. Med Clin (Barc) 2008;131(18):689–91.

31. Bloch Michael H, et al. N-acetylcysteine in the treatment of pediatric Tourette syndrome: randomized, double-blind, placebo-controlled add-on trial. J Child Adolesc Psychopharmacol 2016;26(4):327–34.

32. Gabbay Vilma, et al. A double-blind, placebo-controlled trial of ω-3 fatty acids in Tourette's disorder. Pediatrics 2012;129(6):e1493–500.

Updates in Pharmacologic Strategies for Emotional Dysregulation in Attention Deficit Hyperactivity Disorder

Raman Baweja, MD, MS*, James G. Waxmonsky, MD

KEYWORDS

- Attention deficit hyperactivity disorder • Emotion dysregulation • Irritability
- Aggression • Pharmacology

KEY POINTS

- Children with attention deficit hyperactivity disorder (ADHD) often exhibit various forms of emotional dysregulation (ED) including persistent irritability and aggression.
- Optimization of central nervous system (CNS) stimulants dose using structured ratings of tolerability and efficacy from parents and teachers may lead to appreciable reductions in aggression and irritability even in children previously treated with CNS stimulants.
- Supplementing optimization of ADHD medications with parent-focused psychosocial interventions is associated with the largest degrees of improvement in irritability, aggression, and other behavioral manifestations of ED.
- When aggression persists after CNS stimulants with psychosocial interventions, there is evidence that risperidone, and to a lesser degree, divalproex, molindone, and selective serotonin reuptake inhibitor augmentation may lead to further improvements.
- Future studies needs to identify the mechanisms by which existing ADHD treatments improve ED, markers of treatment response, and benefits of integrating pharmacotherapy with psychosocial interventions specifically designed to improve ED.

INTRODUCTION

Attention deficit hyperactivity disorder (ADHD) is one of the most common neurobehavioral disorders, affecting 5% to 7% of schoolchildren worldwide.[1] In the United States, up to 11% of youths have been diagnosed with ADHD and more than 5% of school students have been prescribed ADHD medication.[2] There are multiple evidence-based pharmacologic and psychosocial treatments for ADHD that are

Department of Psychiatry and Behavioral Health, Penn State College of Medicine, 500 University Drive, Hershey, PA 17033, USA
* Corresponding author.
E-mail address: rbaweja@pennstatehealth.psu.edu

Child Adolesc Psychiatric Clin N Am 31 (2022) 479–498
https://doi.org/10.1016/j.chc.2022.02.003
1056-4993/22/© 2022 Elsevier Inc. All rights reserved.

associated with large reductions in symptoms.[3] However, an appreciable number of youths continue to manifest persistent impairment into adolescence and adulthood even when treatments are consistently used.[4,5] Around half of the children with ADHD have significant challenges with emotional regulation.[6] Emotional dysregulation (ED) defined as a failure to modify an emotional state to achieve a goal,[7] impairs functioning at home, school, and in other social settings even when accounting for ADHD symptoms and other behavioral problems.[8-10] For example, youths with ADHD and elevated levels of ED have worse functioning than those with ADHD without prominent ED.[9,11] They are at increased risk for poor physical health and a range of future psychopathologies including suicidal behaviors,[9,12] whereas being more likely to present for behavioral health care, especially high-intensity services.[13]

EMOTION DYSREGULATION IN ATTENTION DEFICIT HYPERACTIVITY DISORDER

ED in children with ADHD has been categorized as relating to challenges with excessive reactivity to emotional stimuli, labeled emotional impulsivity, and challenges returning to a calm state, which has been described as deficient emotional self-regulation. ED covers the span of negative and positive emotions, whereas irritability is a subtype of ED that is characterized by increased proneness to anger, relative to peers. Behavioral outputs of irritability include excessive temper outbursts[14] that occur in up to 1/3 of youth with ADHD[15] and aggression, especially in children prone to appreciable impulsivity.[16] Aggression is one of the most common reasons for referrals to pediatric mental health clinics, emergency room, and inpatient units,[17] especially reactive or impulsive aggression defined as aggressive response in response to a frustrating event or perceived threat.[18] Irritability and aggression are moderately correlated (r .56),[19] suggesting that interventions improving one domain may not automatically lead to gains in the other.

There has been an increasing focus on the assessment of irritability, aggression, and other manifestations of ED in ADHD treatment trials during the past 2 decades. Both pharmacologic and psychosocial modalities have been examined. This review focuses on pharmacologic interventions for youth with ADHD and comorbid ED. Two decades ago, the conceptualization of bipolar disorder (BD) was expanded to include youth with chronic irritability otherwise known as the broad phenotype of BD, which was reconceptualized as severe mood dysregulation (SMD) and then disruptive mood dysregulation disorder (DMDD) in the *Diagnostic and Statistical Manual of Mental Disorders*, fifth edition (DSM-5).[20] SMD and DMDD are defined by the presence of persistent irritability and recurrent, excessive temper outbursts and they are considered hallmark features of the broad phenotype of BD. In most treatment studies of these disorders, ADHD was systematically assessed with the most participants meeting criteria for it. Therefore, results from these studies of broad phenotype BD, SMD, or DMDD may generalize to youth with ADHD and prominent ED.

METHODS

To be maximally inclusive of relevant treatment studies, we used a wide definition of ED that includes emotional impulsivity, deficient self-regulation, or any observable manifestation of either such as persistent irritable moods, temper outbursts, or aggression. Existing literature was ascertained in the English language, published between 1975 and September 2021, using searches of MEDLINE for the following categories: ADHD, DMDD, SMD, irritability, oppositional defiant disorder (ODD), aggression, children, adolescence, youth, nonstimulant, pharmacotherapy, drugs, stimulants, and medication. Any study enrolling participants with ADHD where outcome measures specifically assessed emotion dysregulation, irritability, or aggression have been included. Reporting on changes in total conduct disorder (CD) or ODD symptoms was not sufficient because these disorders include a range of problem behaviors beyond just ED. References from identified articles were also reviewed to ensure that all relevant articles were included. Treatment studies of other conditions where ADHD was not required for enrollment (eg, BD, CD) were included if ADHD was systematically assessed, the large majority of the participants had ADHD and outcome measures specifically assessed emotion dysregulation. **Table 1** provides a summary of the published treatment studies for children with ADHD and comorbid ED and related constructs.

RESULTS

Medication classes that have been examined for ED include central nervous system (CNS) stimulants, antipsychotics, mood stabilizers, selective serotonin reuptake inhibitors (SSRIs), and atomoxetine.

Central Nervous System Stimulants

In the first study to examine CNS stimulants for reducing aggression in youths with ED, immediate release (IR) methylphenidate (MPH) was associated with improvement in teacher-rated outbursts.[21] Since then, there is a rapidly expanding literature based for the use of CNS stimulants for the treatment of ED including youths with ADHD also meeting criteria for SMD or DMDD.

In a prospective study among adolescents with ADHD and associated ED, 6 months of open label treatment with MPH was associated with significant improvement in ED.[22] Similarly, another study in children with ADHD comorbid with ED, examined the impact of open label treatment of IR MPH over 1 year. Parents also received parent training after the first month of MPH treatment. Both ADHD and ED symptoms significantly improved with treatment. Improvement in ED was independent of improvement in ADHD symptoms.[23]

In the National Institute of Health funded Multimodal Treatment of ADHD (MTA), children with ADHD were randomly assigned to one of 4 arms for 14 months: a. community care (typically low-dose twice-daily IR MPH), b. study titrated medication (typically three-times-a-day IR MPH), c. behavioral modification therapy, or d. combination of the last 2.[24] In the post hoc analysis of MTA, CNS stimulants were associated with moderate reductions in levels of parent-rated irritability. For irritability, study-based medication treatment outperformed treatment without any pharmacotherapy. Multimodal treatment led to the greatest reduction [effect size (ES) ES = 0.82] in irritability during the 14 months of study-based treatment as compared with the other 3 arms. Irritability did not moderate the response to any treatment.[10] In a recent study evaluating the impact of extended release of CNS stimulants in the treatment naïve children over 30 months, emotional lability significantly decreased for participants with elevated levels at baseline ED and greater total medication exposure. Those with ED and lower rates of medication usage showed good tolerability of study medication but limited improvement.[25]

In an open-label study among youths with disruptive disorders and chronic aggression, participants were first optimized on CNS stimulants along with weekly behavior therapy (BT) sessions during 5 weeks before randomization to any adjunctive medication. Aggression improved to the degree that 44% of participants no longer met criteria for adjunctive pharmacotherapy.[26] There was a significant improvement in ADHD symptoms, but the ES for ADHD improvement was considerably smaller among

Table 1
Summary of the reviewed studies, and their relevant characteristics

Study	Sample	Design and Trial Length	Medication and Daily Dose Range	ED Results	Other Findings	Tolerability
Baweja et al. 2016[35]	ADHD with DMDD, N 38, mean age 9.4 (range 7–12), 72% male	6 wk open-label CNS stimulant trial	MPH equivalents dose range of 0.71–1.03 mg/kg/d	Significant decline in DSM-5 ODD IRR items on DBD-RS (ES = 0.58)	Significant decline is ADHD (ES 0.95), ODD (ES 0.5), and CD (ES 0.61) symptoms on DBD-RS, CDRS-R (ES 0.61), MSI sore (ES 0.55) but not for YMRS	No significant changes in mood related side effects (PSERS)
Baweja et al. 2021[25]	ADHD with and without persistent IRR, N:226, mean age 7.6 (range 5–12), treatment naïve, 73% male	Dose optimization for 12 wk then 27-mo open label follow-up	Average daily MPH dose 23.4 mg	Emotional lability on IOWA Conners significantly (P < .001) decreased only for IRR + participants with more medication use	For IRR + participants: significant improvement in ADHD and ODD (IOWA Conners) and impairment (IRS) with higher medication use	In IRR + participants: emotional side effects decreased (PSERS) with more medication use
Bladder et al. 2009[26]	ADHD and ODD/CD + chronic aggression (R-MOAS score >24), N 74, age range 6–13, 78% male	5 wk lead in with open-label CNS stimulants and BT followed by 8 wk of RCT of VPA vs placebo	MPH (mean dose ranges 30–66 mg) and MAS-XR (mean dose range 22–28.13 mg), VPA (mean level 68.11 mg/L)	Aggression remitted in 44% in lead in phase; RCT phase: significantly higher rate of aggression remission on VPA (57%) vs placebo (15%)	Larger decrease in ADHD symptom ratings on Conners' Global Index restless-inattentive subscale scores (P = .01) with VPA	Stimulant treatment associated with anxiety, nail biting, and appetite loss; VPA treatment with treatment-emergent sadness and insomnia
Blader et al. 2010[27]	ADHD with ODD or CD + significant aggression (R-MOAS score >24), N65, mean age 8.95 (range 6–13), 77% male	Open-label CNS stimulant optimization with BT, mean 63.26 d	OROS MPH (mean dose range 52.3–63 mg), MPH-BI (mean dose range 27.5–40 mg), MAS-XR (mean dose range 25.8–26.7 mg)	Response criteria for aggression met in 49% participants during lead in phase	Significant reductions on ADHD symptoms, ES for ADHD was higher in among responders (d = 2.02) than among those with refractory aggression (d = 0.97)	No worsening of mood-related symptoms on CDRS-R and YMRS with stimulant optimization
Blader et al, 2016[28]	ADHD with ODD or CD + significant aggression (R-MOAS score >24), N153, mean age 9.28 (range 6–13), 79% male	Open-label lead in with CNS stimulant optimization + BT, average duration 70.04 d	MPH products (76%, mean dose 49 mg), and MAS-XR (24%, mean dose 24 mg)	Aggression remitted/reduced below the severity threshold warranting adjunctive medication in 65% in lead in phase	Persistent mood symptoms at baseline did not affect the odds of remission of aggressive behavior	Subset with high irritability and low depression had more aggression at baseline but comparable treatment response

Study	Sample	Design	Dose	Results		Adverse events
Blader et al, 2021[29]	ADHD with ODD or CD + significant aggression (R-MOAS score >24), N175, mean age 9.47 (range 6–12), 81% male	Open-label lead in phase with CNS stimulants (mean duration 69 d) + BT, followed by 8 wk of RCT	MPH mean dose 41.6 mg, risperidone (mean dose 1.15 mg), VPA (mean level 77.75 mL/L)	Aggression remitted in 64% in lead in phase; RCT: greater reduction in aggression with risperidone (ES -1.32) and VPA (ES -0.91) on R-MOAS	Significant reduction with risperidone for aggression/internalizing symptoms (CBCL) and ADHD/ODD symptoms ConnGI-P, mood (CDRS) and impairment (CIS)	BMI z-scores increased significantly with risperidone (average gains 2.23 kg) than VPA (0.65 kg); neutropenia with risperidone, diffuse skin rash with VPA (n = 1 each)
Ceresoli-Borroni et al, 2020[31]	ADHD and persistent aggression (R-MOAS score >24), N152, mean age 9 (range 6–12), 97% male	3 wk open-label lead in with CNS stimulants and BT; RCT molindone vs placebo (~5.5 wk)	AMPH (44.1%, median dose 23.1 mg/d), MPH (52.5%, median dose 27.9 mg/d) or nonstimulants (2.5%); RCT phase: placebo or extended release molindone: low-dose (12/18 mg/d), medium-dose (24/36 mg/d) or high-dose (36/54 mg/d)	Aggression remitted in 6% during lead in; RCT: aggression improved significantly with low (Cohen's d .60) and medium doses (Cohen's d .59) molindone, but not with high doses (Cohen's d .04)	No significant changes from baseline in CGI-S and SNAP-IV inattention or hyperactivity/impulsivity subscales after the treatment with any dose group of molindone relative to placebo; but SNAP-IV ODD showed greater mean change with low and medium dose	Most common adverse events: headache (10.0%), sedation (8.9%), and increased appetite (7.8%)
Dickstein et al. 2009[38]	SMD (92% ADHD), N45, age range 7–17, 76% male	Single-blind, lead-in at inpatient setting (2 wk), followed by RCT 6 wk	Lithium 300 mg twice daily (target level of 0.8–1.2 mmol/L)	Significant clinical improvement in 45% during lead-in phase; RCT: no significant group differences on CGI-I or CGAS	No significant group differences on YMRS, CDRS, and PANSS	Lithium well tolerated with only 2 discontinuing
Fernandez De La Cruz et al, 2015[10]	ADHD, N579, age range 7–10, 80% male	Post hoc analysis of MTA 14-mo RCT phase	Medication vs behavioral vs combined treatment vs community care	Irritability declined for all groups: medication (ES 0.63), behavioral (ES = 0.42), combined (ES = 0.82), and community care (ES = 0.48)	Irritability did not moderate ADHD response	Not reported
Gamli et al, 2018[22]	ADHD (20% ODD 15% CD), N 82, age range 12–18, treatment naive, 52% male	Prepost design, open label study, 6 mo	MPH (dose not reported)	Significant improvement on DERS total score (P < .05)	Significant improvement on DERS for impulsivity score (P < .01)	Not reported

(continued on next page)

Table 1
(continued)

Study	Sample	Design and Trial Length	Medication and Daily Dose Range	ED Results	Other Findings	Tolerability
Kreiger et al, 2011[39]	SMD (71% ADHD), N21, mean age 10.38 (range 7–17), 43% male	Open label trial of risperidone, 8 wk	Mean dose 1.28 mg	Significant reduction of irritability score ($P < .001$) on ABC–irritability	SNAP-IV ADHD scores decreased significantly; significant improvement in depression (CDRS) and global functioning (CGAS) (all $P < 0.001$)	42% reported increased appetite, significant increase in prolactin and mean body weight (2.18 kg)
Kutlu et al, 2017[23]	ADHD and ODD/CD; 86% with ED, N 118, mean age 9 (range 7–14), 68% male	12-mo open label trial of MPH + BT with BT initiated after first month of MPH	MPH 24.2 mg	ED significantly improved (CBCL, $P < .05$); Improvement in ED independent of change in ADHD symptoms	Significantly improvement in ADHD symptoms with MPH ($P < .05$) on T-DSM-IV-S	Not reported
Pan et al, 2018[40]	ADHD + DMDD, N 31, mean age 10.67 (range 7–17), 84% male	Open label trial of MPH + aripiprazole, 6 wk	Aripiprazole mean dose 4.17 mg (range 2.5–5 mg)+ MPH mean dose 22.71 mg (range 10–45 mg)	Significant reduction in parent-rated irritability (Cohen's d = 1.26) on SNAP-IV	Significant reductions in parent-rated ODD symptoms (Cohen's d = 1.11) and inattention (Cohen's d = 1.40) on SNAP-IV	2 (7%) discontinued due to SAEs; most common side effects: appetite loss + emesis, mean weight change 2.67 kg
TOSCA Study Aman et al. 2014[30] Gadow et al. 2014[37]	ADHD and ODD/CD and serious aggression (≥ 3 on OAS-M) and severe disruptive behavior (90th percentile NCBRF D-total); N168, mean age 8.9 (rage 6–12), 77% male	3-wk lead-in of open-label CNS stimulants and BT; 6-wk RCT of risperidone vs placebo with BT continuing in RCT phase	MPH (predominantly OROS) mean dose range (45–46 mg) at week 9, Risperidone (mean dose 1.65 mg)	5% clinically remitted during lead in; RCT: significant improvement NCBRF D-total score (ES 0.50) and ABS reactive (ES 0.29) but not proactive subscale (ES 0.16); significant reduction of aggression (Cohen d's .14–.32 across subscales) on PCS	Significant reduction on ODD severity (Cohen's d = 0.27) with risperidone, but not ADHD (ES = 0.13), or CD (ES = 0.09)	Trouble falling asleep with CNS stimulants; elevated prolactin levels, GI upset and weight gain (1.8 kg at >9 wk) with risperidone

| Towbin et al, 2020[34] | SMD (98% DMDD), N69, age range 7–17, 67% male | 5 wk lead in open-label CNS stimulants then 8-wk RCT | MPH (0.8–1.2 mg/kg/d with range 10–80 mg); citalopram average dose 28.33 mg/d (range 5–40 mg/d) | Lead-in: IRR improved significantly (ES = 0.60); 16% no longer meet criteria for RCT phase; moderate effect on temper outbursts (ES = 0.54), no effect on mood between outbursts (ES = 0.08) on CGI-S | Significantly higher response on CGI-I with citalopram (35% vs 6% placebo; OR: 11.70); no differences in functional impairment between groups | No differences in adverse effects between groups; no participant exhibited hypomanic or manic symptoms |
| Winters et al, 2018[36] | ADHD + DMDD, N22, mean age 12 (range 9–15), 69% male | Open-label MPH-OROS, 4 wk | MPH-OROS average dose 61 mg (1.1 mg/kg) | Significant improvement in child-rated irritability (d = 0.57) on Irritability Scale (Youth Version), parent/child ratings of emotional lability (d = 0.85, ERC) and anger (d = 0.55, DES-IV) | Significant improvement ADHD symptoms (hyperactivity d = 0.89 and inattention d = 1.43) on ADHDRS-IV-Parent inventory | 18% rate of side effects: jittery, headaches and decreased appetite; average weight lost was <1 bs |

Abbreviations: ABC, aberrant behavior checklist; ABS, antisocial behavior scale; ADHD, attention-deficit/hyperactivity disorder; AMPH, amphetamine; BI, biphasic-release; BMI, body mass index; BT, behavioral therapy; CBCL, child behavior checklist; CD, conduct disorder; CDRS, childhood depression rating scale; CDRS-R, Childhood Depression Rating Score–Revised Scale; CGAS, Children's Global Assessment Scale; CGI-I, Clinical Global Impression's Improvement; CGI-S, clinical global impressions severity; CIS, Columbia impairment scale; ConnGI, P Conners Global Index Parent Version; CNS, central nervous system; DBD-RS, disruptive behavior disorders rating scale; DERS, difficulties in emotion regulation scale; DES-IV, Differential Emotions Scale-IV; DMDD, disruptive mood dysregulation disorder; DSM-5, diagnostic and statistical manual of mental disorders; 5th ed, ED, emotional dysregulation; ERC, emotion regulation checklist; ES, effect size; GI, gastrointestinal; IRR, irritability; IRS, impairment rating scale; MAS-XR, mixed amphetamine salts extended release; MPH, methylphenidate; MSI, mood severity index; MTA, Multimodal Treatment of ADHD; NCBRF D-To-tal, Nisonger Child Behavior Rating Form Disruptive Total; OAS–M, Overt Aggression Scale–M; ODD, oppositional defiant disorder; OROS, osmotic release oral system; PANSS, positive and negative syndrome scale; PCS, peer conflict scale; PSERS, pittsburgh side effect rating scale; RCT, randomized controlled trial; R-MOAS, Retrospective-Modified Overt Aggression Scale; SAEs, Serious Adverse Events; SMD, severe mood dysregulation; SNAP, swanson, Nolan; and Pelham; T-DSM-IV-S, Turgay DSM-IV–Based Child and Adolescent Behavior Disorders Screening and Rating Scale; TOSCA, treatment of severe childhood aggression; VPA, valproic acid; YMRS, young mania rating scale.

those with refractory aggression than among responders. Responders also showed a trend for lower average dosages of medication (52 vs 64 mg MPH), and BT (3.06 vs 7.28 sessions). Boys, especially those with higher ratings of baseline aggression and mood symptoms, were more likely to exhibit stimulant-refractory aggression. There was no worsening of mood symptoms with stimulant optimization. Initial insomnia and early waking were more prevalent at baseline among children who subsequently showed remission of aggression.[27]

In another open-label study by Blader and colleagues using a similar multistep design in children with ADHD and ODD/CD with significant aggressive behaviors, a comparable response with CNS stimulants optimization and BT was seen. Aggression reduced to below levels needed for randomization to next step pharmacotherapy in 65% of participants. Internalizing symptoms did not moderate response to CNS stimulants.[28] In the most recent study by this group using a similar design, nearly two-thirds of patients responded to CNS stimulant plus BT to the degree that they no longer met criteria for additional study treatments.[29]

In the Treatment of Severe Childhood Aggression (TOSCA) study, children with ADHD and severe aggression were first treated with parent-focused BT and open-label optimization of the CNS stimulants. Treatment was associated with significant reductions in aggression, ADHD symptoms, and other behavioral problems. Randomization to next step pharmacotherapy occurred only 3 weeks after these initial treatments were started, with 5% of participants sufficiently improved that they no longer met criteria for randomization to second stage treatments.[30]

In a study among children with ADHD and persistent impulsive aggression, participants were optimized on monotherapy treatment of ADHD with amphetamine (AMPH), MPH, or nonstimulants with all groups receiving BT over 3 weeks during the lead in phase of the trial. Nine (6%) participants improved during the lead-in period to the degree they were no longer eligible for the need for the next step randomization.[31]

Meta-analyses also document the efficacy of CNS stimulants for reducing aggression. For example, Connor reported an ES 0.84 for reduction in overt aggression and 0.69 for covert aggression. The average doses were 22.18 mg/d for MPH and 23.74 mg/d with AMPH and effect seen across parent, teacher, and clinician reports.[32] Another systematic review reported an ES of 0.9 with MPH for improving aggression in youths with ADHD.[33]

In a study among children with ADHD and SMD examining sequential treatment with CNS stimulants and citalopram, severity of irritability decreased with CNS stimulants, with 16% of participants no longer meeting criteria for adjunctive pharmacotherapy. CNS stimulants had a strong effect on hyperarousal symptoms (ES = 1.10), but only a moderate effect on temper outbursts, and no effect on mood between outbursts.[34]

In a prospective open-label trial of CNS stimulants in youth with ADHD and DMDD, both MPH and AMPH preparations were well tolerated by children and associated with clinically significant reductions in irritability as well as symptoms of ADHD and ODD. Most participants still exhibited significant impairment after the dose optimized.[35] In a small open-label study of long-acting MPH treatment among children with ADHD and DMDD during 4 weeks duration, there was a significant improvement in child-rated irritability as well as parent and child ratings of emotional lability, anger, and ADHD symptoms. Although 71% experienced reduced irritability, symptoms worsened in 19% with the remaining 10% experiencing no meaningful change in irritability. Baseline hyperactivity and irritability severity or comorbid diagnoses did not predict change in posttreatment irritability.[36]

Mood Stabilizers

In the randomized controlled trial (RCT) phase of the previously described TOSCA study, 154 participants who continued to manifest elevated levels of aggression after CNS stimulant optimization and a parenting intervention were randomly assigned to blinded risperidone or placebo for 6 additional weeks. There was a significant improvement on aggressive behavior with the addition of risperidone and on reactive subscale, but not on proactive subscale.[30] Risperidone was also associated with more improvement versus placebo on additional measures of ED, such as parent-reported aggression and ODD symptoms.[37] Prolactin elevation, weight gain, and GI upset occurred more with risperidone.[30]

In the RCT of children with disruptive disorder and severe aggression, 30 participants who had their aggression persisted after optimization of CNS stimulant dose and BT were assigned to divalproex or placebo during 8 weeks. Divalproex led to a greater reduction in aggression and larger decreases in ADHD symptoms. Divalproex treatment was overall well tolerated.[26]

Most recently, Blader compared the efficacy of risperidone, divalproex and placebo in an 8-week RCT of children with ADHD and severe aggression. All participants first received BT and open-label optimization of the CNS stimulant. In those proceeding to adjunctive care, there was a significant reduction in aggression with risperidone and divalproex as compared with placebo. Body mass index z-scores increased significantly more with risperidone than divalproex.[29]

In an RCT of molindone in children with ADHD and persistent impulsive aggression, participants were first optimized on ADHD monotherapy and BT during 3 weeks. Around 80% met criteria to continue to adjunctive treatment and were randomized to placebo, low-dose, medium-dose, or high-dose molindone during ~5.5-week alongside existing monotherapy. Aggression improved significantly with low and medium doses of molindone but not with high doses. The most common adverse events were headache, sedation, and increased appetite.[31]

A randomized controlled study of lithium, set at the National Institute of Mental Health, enrolled youths with SMD. Participants were first taken off all medications and standard behavioral procedures were implemented on the inpatient unit for 2 weeks. Approximately 45% of participants improved to the degree that they did not meet criteria for adjunctive pharmacotherapy. Participants who continued to meet criteria for SMD were assigned to lithium (mean level of .82 mmol/L) versus placebo for 6 additional weeks. There was no difference between groups across almost all outcomes. No subject was withdrawn from study due to adverse effects of lithium.[38]

In a small open-label trial of risperidone during 8 weeks in children with SMD, there was a significant reduction of irritability score. However, there were significant increases in prolactin levels and increased appetite with significant weight gain.[39] In another small open-label study in children with ADHD and DMDD, participants were simultaneously treated with MPH and aripiprazole during 6-week duration. The combination treatment was associated with significant improvement in irritability as well for externalizing symptoms, depression, anxiety, attention, and social problems. Reductions in parent-rated irritability, oppositional defiant symptoms, and inattention were comparable. The most common reported side effects were decreased appetite and vomiting.[40]

Selective Serotonin Reuptake Inhibitor

In an RCT of youth with ADHD and SMD, participants still meeting criteria for SMD after 5 weeks of open label treatment with CNS stimulants were assigned to receive citalopram or placebo for 8 additional weeks. There was a significantly higher proportion of response with citalopram. The difference in irritability severity between groups at week 8 did not reach significance, but a significant group-by-week interaction for the clinical global impressions severity (CGI-S) emerged during the trial. This difference was driven primarily by changes in the severity of temper outbursts. There were no differences in functional impairment between groups at the end of the trial. Citalopram was well tolerated with no differences in adverse effects between treatment groups.[34]

Others

There are no published randomized controlled trials or open label studies that have evaluated the efficacy of nonstimulants approved for the treatment of ADHD to reduce ED or aggression. A meta-analysis atomoxetine in pediatric ADHD studies found small positive effects of atomoxetine on child emotionality (ES = 0.28).[41]

DISCUSSION

Children with ADHD often exhibit various forms of ED including persistent irritability, explosive verbal outbursts, or even physical aggression. There is emerging evidence that pharmacologic treatments for ADHD reduce these different aspects of ED in children with SMD/DMDD and in those without a formal mood disorder. CNS stimulants seem to be a safe and tolerable treatment, with most youth showing improvements in behavior and mood. The actual rate of adverse emotional responses to CNS stimulants remains unclear as well as which youths are most prone to experience them. When aggression persists, there is evidence that risperidone, and to a lesser degree, divalproex augmentation may lead to further improvements. There is one controlled trial to support the capacity of SSRIs and molindone to reduce ED, one open label trial to support aripiprazole, and none for nonstimulants or other medications.

Multiple studies have shown the effectiveness of CNS stimulants for improving irritability, aggression, and other forms of ED among youths with ADHD. In samples selected for prominent levels of irritability or aggression, significant improvements in those constructs and other behavioral problems are seen to the degree that up to two-thirds of these youths do not need additional treatments beyond CNS stimulants and a relatively low-intensity BT.[29,42] Similarly, in the MTA, rates of concerning levels of impulsive aggression decreased from 54% to 25% after treatment.[43] Importantly, in these trials, youths already treated with CNS stimulants benefitted from a systematic dose optimization using structured rating scales from parents and teachers.[29,35] In the study by Blader and colleagues,[29] even some participants with prior antipsychotic use were able to sufficiently optimize with just CNS stimulants and BT. Adjusting doses, switching to alternate formulations of the same stimulant class to alter the onset or duration of coverage or switching stimulant classes can lead to more optimal control. In addition, there is clear evidence that both CNS stimulants and systematic behavioral interventions are effective for reducing symptoms of ADHD and ODD in youths with ED. For example, irritability was not found to moderate response to CNS stimulants in the MTA.[10] Similarly, Baweja and colleagues[35] observed robust improvements for ADHD symptoms with open label titration of CNS stimulants in youths meeting criteria for DMDD. Waxmonsky and colleagues[44] observed a comparable dose–response curve for both CNS stimulants and standardized behavior-modification program in children with and without prominent SMD symptoms.

Twenty years ago, severe persistent irritability was viewed as a sufficient criterion for BD, which is now no longer thought to be the case.[45] Even though treatment trials of BD from this era likely include youths who would no longer be classified as BD, these provide useful data on the tolerability and efficacy of CNS stimulants in children with ADHD and ED. In these studies, mixed AMPH salts and MPH were well tolerated with no concerns on drug interactions with other psychotropic agents.[46,47] For example, in a trial of MPH for pediatric BD, there was no significant change in Childhood Depression Rating Score–Revised or Young Mania Rating Scale scores after MPH was titrated.[47] However, these trials could not assess the tolerability of CNS stimulants in youths with ED not taking mood-stabilizing medication because CNS stimulants were optimized after the dose of the mood-stabilizing medication was titrated. In adults diagnosed with BD, there is evidence of increased risk of treatment-emergent mania with MPH when it is used without concomitant mood-stabilizing treatment.[48]

Emotional symptoms (irritability, mood lability) have been reported as adverse events with CNS stimulants. Recent meta-analyses of short-term randomized treatment trials of CNS stimulants reported that MPH reduced the risk of irritability, whereas AMPH worsened the risk of emotional lability.[49,50] In the Stuckelman meta-analysis, a longer duration of stimulant use correlated with the risk of increased irritability, but the range was only 1 to 8 weeks. There were no significant associations observed for dose, duration of action (short vs long-acting), age of participants, raters (clinicians vs parents and teachers), or trial design (crossover vs parallel-design).[50] It is important to note that there is evidence to support the efficacy of AMPH for improving aspects of ED in children with ADHD.[51] Other studies examining predictors of adverse emotional responses to CNS stimulants have also failed to observe that youths with elevated ED are more likely to have adverse emotional responses to CNS stimulants.[36] One study of youths with the inattentive presentation of ADHD reported that participants with low levels of baseline comorbid internalizing and ODD symptoms were most likely to experience increased emotional side effects. However, the clinical significance of this increase seems to have been slight in most cases.[52] Pretreatment assessment of emotional side effects using standardized measures followed by frequent reassessment of side effects throughout the period of dose optimization allows for more precise assessments of treatment effects for ED and other internalizing symptoms. Failure to collect structured, pretreatment ratings of irritability increase the risk of misclassifying treatment-related improvements as "medication-induced adverse events."

The collective data clearly support that safety of CNS stimulants in children with ED who do not manifest clear phasic irritability, resolving past fears about manic activation from stimulants in children with ADHD.[53] Given these findings and the preferential tolerability profile of CNS stimulants versus most other psychotropic medication classes used in children, it seems prudent to consider optimizing CNS stimulant dose and implementing behavioral treatments in youths with ADHD and prominent ED before moving to other psychotropics. This practice is consistent with published guidelines for treating aggression in youths.[54] Unfortunately, many children with ADHD are rapidly advanced to antipsychotics without stimulant optimization or, in some cases, even a single trial of a CNS stimulant.[55]

A challenging task is identifying which children with ADHD may sufficiently improve with just behavioral interventions and approved ADHD medications.[29,30,34] The variable rates of remission with these treatments across studies further complicate identification of markers of treatment response. The largest rates of remission were seen in studies using longer lead-in phases with both medication optimization and BT. An extended duration of the ADHD treatment phase may be particularly relevant when behavioral therapies are part of the initial treatment package.[27–29] However, most studies with higher remission rates were done by the same investigative team, and their entry criteria, assessment measures, and remission criteria differed from studies reporting lower rates. It has been suggested that the baseline severity may moderate response.[56] However, comorbid disruptive behavior disorders (ODD, CD) did not clearly moderate the change in ADHD symptoms in the MTA treatment arms,[24] and moderation effects for aggression were not examined in the MTA.[43] Severity of ADHD symptoms and intelligence quotient were found to moderate response to medication treatment in the MTA.[57] In the TOSCA study, greater ADHD severity predicted greater reduction in disruptive behavior symptoms across arms, whereas increased irritability but not reactive aggression, was associated with a faster response to risperidone.[58] Prominent ED also seems to be associated with larger reductions in problem behaviors with parent child interaction therapy.[59] Hence, ED may be a sign of preferential response to CNS stimulant and behavioral interventions. There has been only limited examination of dose effects of CNS stimulants for ED. Higher doses have not been clearly shown to lead to increased remission rates.[27]

Understanding how CNS stimulants improve ED may enhance the capacity to detect which children would show the largest improvements in ED after dose optimization. Blader and colleagues[26] examined if change in ADHD symptoms mediated improvement in aggression and did not find evidence to support that improved impulse control or attention drove the reductions in aggression. Additionally, there was no difference in externalizing symptoms severity between who responded to stimulants and whose aggression was refractory to stimulants.[27] Others have also found that CNS stimulants and behavioral therapies may lead to improved ED through other pathways beyond just change in ADHD symptoms.[23] Clearly, the pathways by which CNS stimulants reduce ED merit further exploration.

Several nonstimulant medications are approved for ADHD in children and have shown efficacy for improving ODD symptoms as well. Atomoxetine has been found to be efficacious in children with comorbid ODD, with the reduction in ODD symptoms related to ADHD response.[60] Furthermore, atomoxetine has been found to have moderate ES in reducing emotional lability in adults with ADHD.[61] Guanfacine extended-release has shown effectiveness for both ODD and ADHD symptoms as monotherapy as well as an adjunctive treatment to CNS stimulants.[62–64] Addition of guanfacine on stable dose of CNS stimulant was associated with significant reduction oppositional symptoms with effects sizes between 0.35 and 0.40 for the entire sample and between 0.40 and 0.52 for subgroup with baseline oppositional symptoms.[63] However, no studies of nonstimulants have used ED-specific outcome measures or recruited only youths with defined impairments in ED.

It is important to recognize that the initial lead-in phase in most adjunctive pharmacotherapy trials used parent-focused psychosocial intervention along with CNS stimulant optimization.[34] In TOSCA, a 9-week behavioral intervention was implemented with most sessions occurring after the start of the blinded adjunctive pharmacotherapy phase (risperidone vs placebo).[30] The placebo arm exhibited a nearly 30% decline in disruptive behaviors during the randomized phase. The estimated ES of 0.46 is above what is typically seen in placebo arms for pediatric ADHD trials, possibly due to the presence of the concurrent behavioral intervention.[65] Although this article focuses on pharmacologic treatments, there are numerous evidence-based psychosocial interventions found to be effective for aggression.[66] A recent review concluded that both modified and unmodified versions of currently available evidence-based psychosocial interventions are associated with reduced levels of ED. Treatments targeting symptoms of ADHD, disruptive disorders, and depression have the largest evidence based for improving ED.[67] In the MTA, the largest improvements in irritability were seen in the combined phase.[10] Several large-scale studies have observed that lower doses of medication and BT are as effective as high doses of one treatment.[68,69] Therefore, behavioral therapies may be particularly impactful for children at increased risk for side effects with medication. Implementation of behavioral interventions before pharmacotherapy for aggression is endorsed by practice guidelines,[54] and ADHD medication seems to reduce parental motivation for BT.[70] Ideally, behavior therapies in youths with ADHD are initiated before or with medication treatments. When initiated after medication, efforts to optimize engagement should be used.

There is evidence that both risperidone and divalproex can reduce aggression when it persists after BT and CNS stimulant optimization.[29,30] Adding these agents increased the observed effects sizes into the range of 0.91 to 1.32 compared with 0.7 to 0.9 seen during the lead-in phases where CNS stimulants are the only used medications.[29,32,33] Whether risperidone is used adjunctively,[29,30] or as monotherapy for aggression,[71] used doses are typically in the lower end of the dose range. However, tolerability is a concern with all atypical antipsychotics even at lower doses, with the greatest concerns over weight gain and metabolic changes.[29,30,71] These side effects can adversely affect the risk/benefit ratio even in treatment responders.[72] This is especially relevant for chronic usage as medication benefits seem to fade over time.[73] It is important to remember that none of these agents are approved for use in children with ADHD who do not meet criteria for autism spectrum disorder (ASD), schizophrenia, or BD. Although risperidone is the most well-studied atypical antipsychotic for treating aggression in children with ADHD, other agents including aripiprazole, olanzapine, quetiapine, lurasidone, paliperidone, molindone, and asenapine have been studied for those other conditions. Aripiprazole has the next largest pediatric database, with studies in ASD showing specific benefits for aggression and ED.[74] Molindone has been approved for schizophrenia in children aged 12 years and older and had good acute tolerability except for a higher risk of akathisia.[75]

Divalproex has shown effectiveness among children with disruptive behavior and significant aggression in short-term studies.[26,29] However, it was less effective than risperidone in youths diagnosed with BD in the Treatment of Early Age Mania (TEAM) study.[76] In these studies, divalproex was well tolerated, but in a longer trial, more than half of patients discontinued treatment during the first 6 months.[77] In a small retrospective chart review (mean duration 1.4 years) study, one of the most common reasons for treatment discontinuation was related to weight gain.[78] Furthermore, use of divalproex among postmenarcheal women is problematic related to its teratogenicity and possible anovulatory and androgenic effects.[29] Divalproex also has black-box warnings for hepatotoxicity and pancreatitis.[79]

Lithium was not effective in the treatment of SMD.[38] Several studies have examined the impact of lithium in children with CD and significant aggression, producing mixed results. ADHD was not always well classified in these studies, limiting the capacity to generalize results to youth with this disorder.[79–81] The TEAM study compared the efficacy of lithium, risperidone, and divalproex for improving symptoms of BD. ADHD was systematically assessed, and 93% of participants met criteria for it, whereas 32% were taking CNS stimulants. Although the impact of treatment on ED was not assessed, response rates for BD were comparable between lithium and divalproex, and both were less efficacious than risperidone.[76] Participants with ADHD had a greater probability of responding to risperidone versus lithium (response rate 2.1), compared with participants without ADHD (response rate 1).[82] These results combined with the negative trial in SMD, suggest that lithium may not be a preferred option for treating ED in youths with ADHD. Although metabolic effects are not an appreciable concern. lithium treatment requires careful monitoring and can be associated with declines in renal function, hypothyroidism, and hypercalcemia.[83]

One randomized trial found some evidence that SSRIs may improve aspects of ED in youths with ADHD optimized on stimulants.[34] A similarly designed trial examined the impact of fluoxetine during 8 weeks in youths with SMD first optimized on CNS stimulants.[84] Results are presently unpublished. Improvement in irritability and aggression with lisdexamfetamine was comparable to other open label studies on CNS stimulants. Addition of fluoxetine was well tolerated, but there was not a clear signal of efficacy for fluoxetine over placebo (McGough, personal communication). Whenever antidepressants are prescribed to children and adolescents, the black box warning for new or worsening adverse emotional effects including suicidal ideations should be reviewed with patients and families. Citalopram also carries a warning for QTc prolongation at doses of 40 mg or higher.

Although the literature based on the treatment of ED in youth with ADHD has appreciably expanded during the past decade, limitations still exist. We know little about the underlying mechanisms by which these agents produce reductions in ED or which youths with ADHD are most likely to experience meaningful reductions in ED with pharmacotherapy. This is particularly important for medications with the potential for appreciable treatment-related morbidity such as atypical antipsychotics. There is a surprising lack of controlled data for nonstimulant agents for ADHD for improving ED. Despite the widespread use of PRN medications in inpatient settings and emergency departments,[85] we also know problematically little about how to acutely resolve concerning agitation. Only a few behavioral interventions have been used in multimodal treatment studies of youths with ED, none of which were specifically designed to target ED or aggression.[29,30,42] There are now several emerging psychosocial treatments for ED that merit inclusion in multimodal trials.[67] A wide variety of tools have been used to assess treatment outcomes, impeding the ability to compare effects across studies. There are not well-established measures that capture multiple aspects of ED, with several measures focusing on physical aggression. However, irritability and aggression are only moderately correlated. Therefore, it is not clear that treatment effects in one domain will translate to the other.[19] Very little is known about the impact of treatment in school settings because few studies gathered teacher reports. Recent studies have recruited more diverse samples,[29,30] but most participants are still white males.

SUMMARY

Children with ADHD often exhibit various forms of ED including persistent irritability and aggression that are associated with significant impairment. CNS stimulants seem to be tolerable treatments for most of these youths. Optimization of CNS stimulants dose in combination with parent-focused behavioral interventions may lead to appreciable reductions in irritability and aggression. In youth with ADHD whose aggression persists after these interventions, there is the most support for the use of risperidone, with some evidence for divalproex, SSRIs, and molindone. Future studies should focus on identifying the mechanisms by which existing pharmacologic treatments improve ED, markers of treatment response and the benefits of integrating pharmacotherapy with psychosocial treatments designed to improve ED.

CLINICS CARE POINTS

- Central nervous system (CNS) stimulants are safe and well-tolerated treatment of children with attention deficit hyperactivity disorder (ADHD) and associated emotional dysregulation (ED) manifesting as irritability or aggression.

- Optimization of CNS stimulants dose in combination with parent-focused behavioral interventions leads to significant improvement in ED among youths with ADHD.
- In youths with ADHD whose aggression persists after CNS stimulants optimization and behavioral interventions, low doses of risperidone are the most well-supported medication option. Other options with some evidence of effect include divalproex, molindone, and selective serotonin reuptake inhibitors.
- When considering adjunctive medication treatments for ED and aggression, tolerability is an important concern and the risk/benefit ratio of treatment should be periodically reassessed as treatment continues.
- More studies are needed on the capacity of nonstimulant ADHD medications to improve ED.

DISCLOSURE

In the past 3 years, Dr J.G. Waxmonsky has received research funding from Supernus and served as a consultant for Adlon Therapeutics and Intracellular Therapies. Dr R. Baweja reports no biomedical financial interests or potential conflicts of interest.

REFERENCES

1. Thomas R, Sanders S, Doust J, et al. Prevalence of attention-deficit/hyperactivity disorder: a systematic review and meta-analysis. Pediatrics 2015;135(4): e994–1001.
2. Visser SN, Danielson ML, Bitsko RH, et al. Trends in the parent-report of health care provider-diagnosed and medicated attention-deficit/hyperactivity disorder: United States, 2003-2011. J Am Acad Child Adolesc Psychiatry 2014;53(1): 34–46.
3. Wolraich ML, Hagan JF, Allan C, et al. Clinical practice guideline for the diagnosis, evaluation, and treatment of attention-deficit/hyperactivity disorder in children and adolescents. Pediatrics 2019;144(4):e20192528.
4. Cherkasova MV, Roy A, Molina BSG, et al. Review: adult outcome as seen through controlled prospective follow-up studies of children with attention-deficit/hyperactivity disorder followed into adulthood. J Am Acad Child Adolesc Psychiatry 2021. https://doi.org/10.1016/j.jaac.2021.05.019.
5. Hechtman L, Swanson JM, Sibley MH, et al. Functional adult outcomes 16 years after childhood diagnosis of attention-deficit/hyperactivity disorder: MTA results. J Am Acad Child Adolesc Psychiatry 2016;55(11):945–52.
6. Shaw P, Stringaris A, Nigg J, et al. Emotion dysregulation in attention deficit hyperactivity disorder. Am J Psychiatry 2014;171(3):276–93.
7. Graziano PA, Garcia A. Attention-deficit hyperactivity disorder and children's emotion dysregulation: a meta-analysis. Clin Psychol Rev 2016;46:106–23.
8. Laporte PP, Matijasevich A, Munhoz TN, et al. Disruptive mood dysregulation disorder: symptomatic and syndromic thresholds and diagnostic Operationalization. J Am Acad Child Adolesc Psychiatry 2021;60(2):286–95.
9. Sorcher LK, Goldstein BL, Finsaas MC, et al. Preschool irritability predicts adolescent psychopathology and functional impairment: a 12-year prospective study. J Am Acad Child Adolesc Psychiatry 2021. https://doi.org/10.1016/j.jaac.2021. 08.016.
10. Fernandez de la Cruz L, Simonoff E, McGough JJ, et al. Treatment of children with attention-deficit/hyperactivity disorder (ADHD) and irritability: results from the

multimodal treatment study of children with ADHD (MTA). J Am Acad Child Adolesc Psychiatry 2015;54(1):62–70.

11. Lee CA, Milich R, Lorch EP, et al. Forming first impressions of children: the role of attention-deficit/hyperactivity disorder symptoms and emotion dysregulation. J Child Psychol Psychiatry 2018;59(5):556–64.

12. Orri M, Galera C, Turecki G, et al. Association of childhood irritability and depressive/anxious mood profiles with adolescent suicidal ideation and attempts. JAMA Psychiatry 2018;75(5):465–73.

13. Anastopoulos AD, Smith TF, Garrett ME, et al. Self-regulation of emotion, functional impairment, and comorbidity among childrenwith AD/HD. J Atten Disord 2011;15(7):583–92.

14. Spring L, Carlson GA. The phenomenology of outbursts. Child Adolesc Psychiatr Clin N Am 2021;30(2):307–19.

15. Mayes SD, Waxmonsky J, Calhoun SL, et al. Disruptive mood dysregulation disorder (DMDD) symptoms in children with autism, ADHD, and neurotypical development and impact of co-occurring ODD, depression, and anxiety. Res Autism Spectr Disord 2015;18:64–72.

16. Waschbusch DA. A meta-analytic examination of comorbid hyperactive-impulsive-attention problems and conduct problems. Psychol Bull 2002; 128(1):118.

17. Connor DF. Aggression and antisocial behavior in children and adolescents: research and treatment. New York: Guilford Press; 2004.

18. Connor DF, Steingard RJ, Cunningham JA, et al. Proactive and reactive aggression in referred children and adolescents. Am J Orthopsychiatry 2004;74(2): 129–36.

19. Zik J, Deveney CM, Ellingson JM, et al. Understanding irritability in relation to anger, aggression, and informant in a pediatric clinical population. J Am Acad Child Adolesc Psychiatry 2021. https://doi.org/10.1016/j.jaac.2021.08.012.

20. American Psychiatric Association. Diagnostic and statistical manual of mental disorders. Fifth Edition. Washington, DC: American Psychiatric Press.; 2013.

21. Gittelman-Klein R, Klein DF, Katz S, et al. Comparative effects of methylphenidate and thioridazine in hyperkinetic children: I. Clinical results. Arch Gen Psychiatry 1976;33(10):1217–31.

22. Gamli IS, Tahiroglu AY. Six months methylphenidate treatment improves emotion dysregulation in adolescents with attention deficit/hyperactivity disorder: a prospective study. Neuropsychiatr Dis Treat 2018;14:1329.

23. Kutlu A, Ardic UA, Ercan ES. Effect of methylphenidate on emotional dysregulation in children with attention-deficit/hyperactivity disorder+ oppositional defiant disorder/conduct disorder. J Clin Psychopharmacol 2017;37(2):220–5.

24. The MTA Cooperative Group. A 14-month randomized clinical trial of treatment strategies for attention-deficit/hyperactivity disorder. Arch Gen Psychiatry 1999; 56(12):1073–86.

25. Baweja R, Waschbusch DA, Pelham WE, et al. The impact of persistent irritability on the medication treatment of paediatric attention deficit hyperactivity disorder. Front Psychiatry 2021;12:699687.

26. Blader JC, Schooler NR, Jensen PS, et al. Adjunctive divalproex versus placebo for children with ADHD and aggression refractory to stimulant monotherapy. Am J Psychiatry 2009;166(12):1392–401.

27. Blader JC, Pliszka SR, Jensen PS, et al. Stimulant-responsive and stimulant-refractory aggressive behavior among children with ADHD. Pediatrics 2010; 126(4):e796–806.

28. Blader JC, Pliszka SR, Kafantaris V, et al. Prevalence and treatment outcomes of persistent negative mood among children with attention-deficit/hyperactivity disorder and aggressive behavior. J Child Adolesc Psychopharmacol 2016;26(2): 164–73.

29. Blader JC, Pliszka SR, Kafantaris V, et al. Stepped treatment for attention-deficit/ hyperactivity disorder and aggressive behavior: a randomized, controlled trial of adjunctive risperidone, divalproex sodium, or placebo after stimulant medication optimization. J Am Acad Child Adolesc Psychiatry 2021;60(2):236–51.

30. Aman MG, Bukstein OG, Gadow KD, et al. What does risperidone add to parent training and stimulant for severe aggression in child attention-deficit/hyperactivity disorder? J Am Acad Child Adolesc Psychiatry 2014;53(1):47–60 e1.

31. Ceresoli-Borroni G, Nasser A, Adewole T, et al. A double-blind, randomized study of extended-release molindone for impulsive aggression in ADHD. J Atten Disord 2021;25(11):1564–77.

32. Connor DF, Glatt SJ, Lopez ID, et al. Psychopharmacology and aggression. I: a meta-analysis of stimulant effects on overt/covert aggression-related behaviors in ADHD. J Am Acad Child Adolesc Psychiatry 2002;41(3):253–61.

33. Pappadopulos E, Woolston S, Chait A, et al. Pharmacotherapy of aggression in children and adolescents: efficacy and effect size. J Can Acad Child Adolesc Psychiatry 2006;15(1):27–39.

34. Towbin K, Vidal-Ribas P, Brotman MA, et al. A double-blind randomized placebo-controlled trial of citalopram adjunctive to stimulant medication in youth with chronic severe irritability. J Am Acad Child Adolesc Psychiatry 2020;59(3): 350–61.

35. Baweja R, Belin PJ, Humphrey HH, et al. The effectiveness and tolerability of central nervous system stimulants in school-age children with attention-deficit/ hyperactivity disorder and disruptive mood dysregulation disorder across home and school. J Child Adolesc Psychopharmacol 2016;26(2):154–63.

36. Winters DE, Fukui S, Leibenluft E, et al. Improvements in irritability with open-label methylphenidate treatment in youth with comorbid attention deficit/hyperactivity disorder and disruptive mood dysregulation disorder. J Child Adolesc Psychopharmacol 2018;28(5):298–305.

37. Gadow KD, Arnold LE, Molina BSG, et al. Risperidone added to parent training and stimulant medication: effects on attention-deficit/hyperactivity disorder, oppositional defiant disorder, conduct disorder, and peer aggression. J Am Acad Child Adolesc Psychiatry 2014;53(9):948–59.

38. Dickstein DP, Towbin KE, Van Der Veen JW, et al. Randomized double-blind placebo-controlled trial of lithium in youths with severe mood dysregulation. J Child Adolesc Psychopharmacol 2009;19(1):61–73.

39. Krieger FV, Pheula GF, Coelho R, et al. An open-label trial of risperidone in children and adolescents with severe mood dysregulation. J Child Adolesc Psychopharmacol 2011;21(3):237–43.

40. Pan P-Y, Fu A-T, Yeh C-B. Aripiprazole/methylphenidate combination in children and adolescents with disruptive mood dysregulation disorder and attention-deficit/hyperactivity disorder: an open-label study. J Child Adolesc Psychopharmacol 2018;28(10):682–9.

41. Schwartz S, Correll CU. Efficacy and safety of atomoxetine in children and adolescents with attention-deficit/hyperactivity disorder: results from a comprehensive meta-analysis and metaregression. J Am Acad Child Adolesc Psychiatry 2014;53(2):174–87.

42. Waxmonsky JG, Waschbusch DA, Belin P, et al. A randomized clinical trial of an integrative group therapy for children with severe mood dysregulation. J Am Acad Child Adolesc Psychiatry 2016;55(3):196–207.

43. Jensen PS, Youngstrom EA, Steiner H, et al. Consensus report on impulsive aggression as a symptom across diagnostic categories in child psychiatry: implications for medication studies. J Am Acad Child Adolesc Psychiatry 2007;46(3): 309–22.

44. Waxmonsky J, Pelham WE, Gnagy E, et al. The efficacy and tolerability of methylphenidate and behavior modification in children with attention-deficit/hyperactivity disorder and severe mood dysregulation. J Child Adolesc Psychopharmacol 2008;18(6):573–88.

45. Leibenluft E. Severe mood dysregulation, irritability, and the diagnostic boundaries of bipolar disorder in youths. Am J Psychiatry 2011;168(2):129–42.

46. Scheffer RE, Kowatch RA, Carmody T, et al. Randomized, placebo-controlled trial of mixed amphetamine salts for symptoms of comorbid ADHD in pediatric bipolar disorder after mood stabilization with divalproex sodium. Am J Psychiatry 2005; 162(1):58–64.

47. Findling RL, Short EJ, McNamara NK, et al. Methylphenidate in the treatment of children and adolescents with bipolar disorder and attention-deficit/hyperactivity disorder. J Am Acad Child Adolesc Psychiatry 2007;46(11): 1445–53.

48. Viktorin A, Rydén E, Thase ME, et al. The risk of treatment-emergent mania with methylphenidate in bipolar disorder. Am J Psychiatry 2017;174(4):341–8.

49. Pozzi M, Carnovale C, Peeters GG, et al. Adverse drug events related to mood and emotion in paediatric patients treated for ADHD: a meta-analysis. J Affect Disord 2018;238:161–78.

50. Stuckelman ZD, Mulqueen JM, Ferracioli-Oda E, et al. Risk of irritability with psychostimulant treatment in children with ADHD: a meta-analysis. J Clin Psychiatry 2017;78(6):e648–55.

51. Childress AC, Arnold V, Adeyi B, et al. The effects of lisdexamfetamine dimesylate on emotional lability in children 6 to 12 years of age with ADHD in a double-blind placebo-controlled trial. J Atten Disord 2014;18(2):123–32.

52. Froehlich TE, Brinkman WB, Peugh JL, et al. Pre-existing comorbid emotional symptoms moderate short-term methylphenidate adverse effects in a randomized trial of children with attention-deficit/hyperactivity disorder. J Child Adolesc Psychopharmacol 2020;30(3):137–47.

53. Faedda GL, Baldessarini RJ, Glovinsky IP, et al. Treatment-emergent mania in pediatric bipolar disorder: a retrospective case review. J Affect Disord 2004;82(1): 149–58.

54. Scotto Rosato N, Correll CU, Pappadopulos E, et al. Treatment of maladaptive aggression in youth: CERT guidelines II. Treatments and ongoing management. Pediatrics 2012;129(6):e1577–86.

55. Sultan RS, Wang S, Crystal S, et al. Antipsychotic treatment among youths with attention-deficit/hyperactivity disorder. JAMA Netw open 2019;2(7):e197850.

56. Cortese S, Novins DK. Why JAACAP published an" Inconclusive" trial: optimize, optimize, optimize psychostimulant treatment. J Am Acad Child Adolesc Psychiatry 2021;60(2):213–5.

57. Owens EB, Hinshaw SP, Kraemer HC, et al. Which treatment for whom for ADHD? Moderators of treatment response in the MTA. J Consult Clin Psychol 2003;71(3): 540–52.

58. Farmer CA, Brown NV, Gadow KD, et al. Comorbid symptomatology moderates response to risperidone, stimulant, and parent training in children with severe aggression, disruptive behavior disorder, and attention-deficit/hyperactivity disorder. J Child Adolesc Psychopharmacol 2015;25(3):213–24.
59. Rothenberg WA, Weinstein A, Dandes EA, et al. Improving child emotion regulation: effects of parent–child interaction-therapy and emotion socialization strategies. J Child Fam Stud 2019;28(3):720–31.
60. Biederman J, Spencer TJ, Newcorn JH, et al. Effect of comorbid symptoms of oppositional defiant disorder on responses to atomoxetine in children with ADHD: a meta-analysis of controlled clinical trial data. Psychopharmacology 2007;190(1):31–41.
61. Moukhtarian TR, Cooper RE, Vassos E, et al. Effects of stimulants and atomoxetine on emotional lability in adults: a systematic review and meta-analysis. Eur Psychiatry 2017;44:198–207.
62. Newcorn JH, Huss M, Connor DF, et al. Efficacy of guanfacine extended release in children and adolescents with attention-deficit/hyperactivity disorder and co-morbid oppositional defiant disorder. J Dev Behav Pediatr 2020;41(7):565–70.
63. Findling RL, McBurnett K, White C, et al. Guanfacine extended release adjunctive to a psychostimulant in the treatment of comorbid oppositional symptoms in children and adolescents with attention-deficit/hyperactivity disorder. J Child Adolesc Psychopharmacol 2014;24(5):245–52.
64. Connor DF, Findling RL, Kollins SH, et al. Effects of guanfacine extended release on oppositional symptoms in children aged 6–12 years with attention-deficit hyperactivity disorder and oppositional symptoms. CNS drugs 2010;24(9):755–68.
65. Waschbusch DA, Pelham WE Jr, Waxmonsky J, et al. Are there placebo effects in the medication treatment of children with attention-deficit hyperactivity disorder? J Dev Behav Pediatr 2009;30(2):158–68.
66. Fossum S, Handegard BH, Martinussen M, et al. Psychosocial interventions for disruptive and aggressive behaviour in children and adolescents: a meta-analysis. Eur Child Adolesc Psychiatry 2008;17(7):438–51.
67. Waxmonsky JG, Baweja R, Bansal PS, et al. A review of the evidence base for psychosocial interventions for the treatment of emotion dysregulation in children and adolescents. Child Adoles Psychiatr Clin N Am 2021;30(3):573–94.
68. Jensen PS, Hinshaw SP, Kraemer HC, et al. ADHD comorbidity findings from the MTA study: comparing comorbid subgroups. J Am Acad Child Adolesc Psychiatry 2001;40(2):147–58.
69. Pelham WE, Burrows-MacLean L, Gnagy EM, et al. A dose-ranging study of behavioral and pharmacological treatment in social settings for children with ADHD. J Abnorm Child Psychol 2014;42(6):1019–31.
70. Waxmonsky JG, Baweja R, Liu G, et al. A commercial insurance claims analysis of correlates of behavioral therapy use among children with ADHD. Psychiatr Serv 2019;70(12):1116–22.
71. Loy JH, Merry SN, Hetrick SE, et al. Atypical antipsychotics for disruptive behaviour disorders in children and youths. Cochrane Database Syst. Rev. 9, CD008559 2017.
72. Verhaegen AA, Van Gaal LF. Drug-induced obesity and its metabolic consequences: a review with a focus on mechanisms and possible therapeutic options. J Endocrinol Invest 2017;40(11):1165–74.
73. Gadow KD, Brown NV, Arnold LE, et al. Severely aggressive children receiving stimulant medication versus stimulant and risperidone: 12-month follow-up of the TOSCA trial. J Am Acad Child Adolesc Psychiatry 2016;55(6):469–78.

74. Rizzo R, Pavone P. Aripiprazole for the treatment of irritability and aggression in children and adolescents affected by autism spectrum disorders. Expert Rev Neurother 2016;16(8):867–74.
75. Sikich L, Frazier JA, McClellan J, et al. Double-blind comparison of first-and second-generation antipsychotics in early-onset schizophrenia and schizo-affective disorder: findings from the treatment of early-onset schizophrenia spectrum disorders (TEOSS) study. Am J Psychiatry 2008;165(11):1420–31.
76. Geller B, Luby JL, Joshi P, et al. A randomized controlled trial of risperidone, lithium, or divalproex sodium for initial treatment of bipolar I disorder, manic or mixed phase, in children and adolescents. Arch Gen Psychiatry 2012;69(5):515–28.
77. Redden L, DelBello M, Wagner KD, et al. Long-term safety of divalproex sodium extended-release in children and adolescents with bipolar I disorder. J Child Adolesc Psychopharmacol 2009;19(1):83–9.
78. Masi G, Milone A, Manfredi A, et al. Effectiveness of lithium in children and adolescents with conduct disorder. CNS drugs 2009;23(1):59–69.
79. Henry CA, Zamvil LS, Lam C, et al. Long-term outcome with divalproex in children and adolescents with bipolar disorder. J Child Adolesc Psychopharmacol 2003;13(4):523–9.
80. Campbell M, Adams PB, Small AM, et al. Lithium in hospitalized aggressive children with conduct disorder: a double-blind and placebo-controlled study. J Am Acad Child Adolesc Psychiatry 1995;34(4):445–53.
81. Rifkin A, Karajgi B, Dicker R, et al. Lithium treatment of conduct disorders in adolescents. Am J Psychiatry 1997;154(4):554–5.
82. Vitiello B, Riddle MA, Yenokyan G, et al. Treatment moderators and predictors of outcome in the treatment of early age mania (TEAM) study. J Am Acad Child Adolesc Psychiatry 2012;51(9):867–78.
83. Shine B, McKnight RF, Leaver L, et al. Long-term effects of lithium on renal, thyroid, and parathyroid function: a retrospective analysis of laboratory data. Lancet 2015;386(9992):461–8.
84. McGough J. Characterization and sequential pharmacotherapy of severe mood dysregulation. ClinicalTrials. gov Identifier: NCT01714310; 2021.
85. Baker M, Carlson GA. What do we really know about PRN use in agitated children with mental health conditions: a clinical review. Evid Based Ment Health 2018;21(4):166–70.

Attention Deficit Hyperactivity Disorder Medications and Sleep

Mark A. Stein, PhD[a],*, Courtney Zulauf-McCurdy, PhD[b],
Lourdes M. DelRosso, MD, PhD[c]

KEYWORDS

- Sleep disorders • ADHD • Insomnia • Stimulants

KEY POINTS

- Sleep problems are common and often increase when initiating pharmacotherapy.
- Delayed sleep onset/insomnia is associated with stimulants although daytime sleepiness is associated with nonstimulants.
- Younger children and adolescents are most vulnerable to adverse sleep effects, but sleep problems occur in all age groups.
- Wide variability in severity and duration of sleep effects, but most effects are mild and improve over time.
- Interventions include changing dose schedules, formulations, behavioral interventions, and adding a sleep-promoting agent.

INTRODUCTION

After Charles Bradley's serendipitous discovery of the therapeutic benefit of an amphetamine (AMP), Benzedrine, in children with behavioral problems, he also described the adverse and variable initial impact on sleep in a subset of children, noting "6 of the 30 children's nocturnal sleep was mildly disturbed, as evidenced by a delay in the time of falling asleep for the first night or two. One patient remained awake to a late hour for four nights".[1] Although Benzedrine is no longer used, there are now numerous AMP, methylphenidate (MPH), and nonstimulant medications approved for the treatment of Attention Deficit Hyperactivity Disorder (ADHD).

In the past few years, research on the intersection of ADHD medications and sleep problems has intensified.[2] Moreover, the prevalence of sleep problems in individuals with ADHD appears to be on the rise.[3] This may reflect more attention to or accuracy in measuring sleep, as well as the tendency to treat ADHD with longer-acting agents or dosing schedules for longer periods.

[a] Pediatrics, University of Washington, Seattle, WA, USA; [b] University of Washington, SMART Center, Building 29, 6200 NE 74th Street, Suite 100, Seattle, WA 98115, USA; [c] Seattle Children's Hospital Sleep Center, 1231 116th Avenue, NE Suite 385, Bellevue, WA 98004, USA
* Corresponding author. Seattle Children's Hospital, Box 5371, Seattle, WA 98105.
E-mail address: mstein42@uw.edu

Child Adolesc Psychiatric Clin N Am 31 (2022) 499–514
https://doi.org/10.1016/j.chc.2022.03.006
1056-4993/22/© 2022 Elsevier Inc. All rights reserved.
childpsych.theclinics.com

This article is focused on describing the literature on ADHD medications and sleep. We will first define common sleep problems, discuss the importance of screening for sleep disorders in ADHD, and review methodological issues related to measuring sleep. We then summarize what has been learned about ADHD medications and sleep effects across the lifespan, before discussing clinical management and several new directions.

PREVALENCE OF SLEEP PROBLEMS IN ADHD

Commonly, children with ADHD and comorbid behavioral problems have increased activity levels throughout the day and evening, are easily distracted from task performance, and have difficulty "shutting down" their brain, hence are more likely to have worse sleep hygiene and a higher prevalence of sleep disorders. Sleep problems in youth with ADHD are reported to be in the range of 25% to 55%.[4–7] Moderate-to-severe sleep problems occur at least once a week in 19.3% of the clinic-referred children with ADHD, 13.3% of the psychiatric controls, and 6.2% of the pediatric controls according to parents.[8] Overall when sleep is assessed using rating scales, sleep diaries, or questionnaires, children with ADHD display higher rates of bedtime resistance, sleep onset difficulties, night awakenings, morning awakenings, sleep-disordered breathing, and daytime sleepiness relative to youth without ADHD.[9]

In addition to these commonly recognized sleep problems, restless legs syndrome (RLS) can be found in up to 44% of children with ADHD[10,11] and restless sleep disorder in up to 10%.[12] In an ADHD population referred for sleep evaluations, 80% of parents of children with ADHD were concerned that their children's sleep was restless. In the majority of these children, an underlying sleep diagnosis (such as obstructive sleep apnea, periodic leg movement disorder, restless sleep disorder, or RLS) was found after polysomnography (PSG).[13]

It is very important to accurately evaluate sleep patterns and problems before medication initiation to rule out primary sleep disorders that mimic or exacerbate ADHD symptoms and to serve as a baseline. Sleep logs and diaries are often used to identify sleep patterns and can be used before and after treatment. The clinical interview is crucial to diagnose specific sleep disorders such as RLS, insomnia, and parasomnias.[14] Standardized questionnaires can be used to screen for sleep disorders, such as the *BEARS*, which screens for *B*edtime, *E*xcessive sleepiness, *A*wakenings during the night, *R*egularity of sleep, and *S*noring.[15] Other commonly used questionnaires include the Pediatric Sleep Questionnaire, which screens for sleep-disordered, breathing, sleepiness and behavior,[16] and the Children's Sleep Habits Questionnaire (CSHQ).[17] The CSHQ has eight subscales including circadian delay, parasomnias, breathing, bedtime resistance, daytime sleepiness, and nocturnal awakenings.

In terms of objective evaluations, PSG is considered the "gold standard" to diagnose sleep disorders such as obstructive sleep apnea. PSG has a great utility in research because it can reliably document brain activity patterns, body movements, arousals, and homeostatic indicators. The American Academy of Sleep Medicine has published guidelines on indications of PSG. PSG is indicated any time that sleep-disordered breathing is suspected, in cases of refractory insomnia, and when there is suspicion of periodic leg movement disorder or atypical parasomnias. Another test, the multiple sleep latency test (MSLT) is used to assess for daytime sleepiness[18] and consists of five daytime nap opportunities. Studies using MSLT have demonstrated that children with ADHD are sleepier during the day and have slower reaction times.[19]

Actigraphy is less invasive than PSG and a more ecologically valid method for recording motor activity by means of small, computerized, watch-like devices worn on the wrist. Actigraphy provides an objective measure of body movements that provide a reliable estimate of several sleep parameters, including sleep duration and sleep onset latency (SOL). Actigraphy is particularly indicated when insufficient sleep or circadian disorders are suspected and allows monitoring for several days or even weeks in the home setting. Actigraphy can also provide information on night-to-night variability, a significant characteristic of ADHD youth who are taking stimulants.

Fig. 1 is an example of an actigraphy download from a teenager with ADHD. We can appreciate an inconsistent bedtime, with sleep occurring past midnight on some evenings. Such a pattern can lead to difficulty getting up the next morning and a delayed sleep phase disorder. The parents of children with ADHD could benefit from education on the importance of a bedtime routine including how to time medication to allow for a

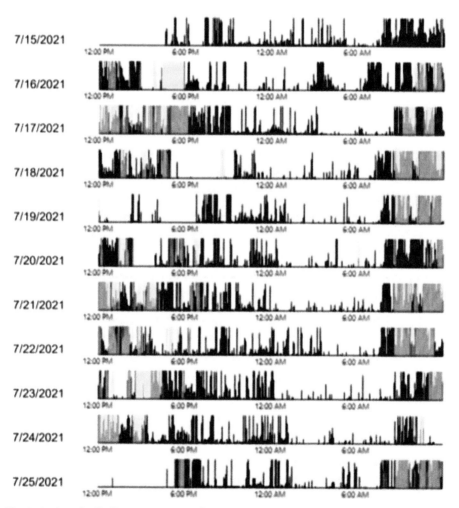

Fig. 1. Actigraphy findings on a teen with ADHD on stimulant medication. Findings show an inconsistent bedtime. Most night bedtime is past midnight consistent with a delayed sleep–wake circadian phase. There is also nocturnal awakening consistent with sleep maintenance insomnia.

bedtime of approximately 9 to 10 PM Adolescents need to sleep approximately 9 hours a night, and school-age children (7–12 year old) need approximately 10 hours of sleep at night. The morning awakening time, school schedule, and social demands (eg, sports, homework, peer interactions) need to be included in the planning for adequate sleep opportunities. Insufficient sleep has also been associated with worsening of ADHD; therefore, actigraphy and sleep diaries can be useful tools to assess sleep latency and calculate total sleep time.[20] Although commercial wearable devices are widely available, they should be used cautiously as most are not validated against the gold standard for sleep and sleep stage detection.[21]

The interrelationships between ADHD and sleep disorders, mutually exacerbating conditions, are further complicated by the use of medications to treat ADHD, which also impact sleep.[22] Research results often vary from study to study based on how and when sleep is measured,[23–25] with subjective and objective measures providing valuable, but different information (see references [9,26–28]). For instance, subjective evaluations based on self-, parent-, or observer-report can provide information about sleep initiation and maintenance, insomnia, sleep quantity and quality, and perceived time of awakening. Subjective reports, such as clinical interviews, sleep questionnaires, and diaries, can also capture summary observations over an extended time period in a naturalistic context and can reveal important aspects of clinically meaningful perceptions of sleep that may differ from objective assessments (such as those using PSG and actigraphy).

METHODOLOGICAL ISSUES IN CLINICAL TRIALS

Much of what is known about ADHD medications and their effects on sleep is based on reports of adverse events from short-term efficacy studies.[3,24,29] Most medication studies are relatively short term (ie, <7 weeks) and thus primarily measure acute effects. Due to a paucity of longitudinal data, less is known about intermediate and long-term effects on sleep.[30] There are also few comparative efficacy studies, as the majority of studies compare an active medication with a placebo (ie, basic efficacy). A recent meta-analysis of 35 studies of MPH formulations found that a wide range of study designs and sample features predicted the relative risk of insomnia, including the type of formulation, number of doses per day, age, sex, percentage of stimulant responders enrolled, year of study, number of sites, and type-of-rater.[3] Indeed, methodological differences between studies and samples present a significant challenge in evaluating the clinical implications of these studies.

One methodological factor that may influence results is ascertainment bias, which can occur when studies only include patients who complete long-term follow-up or if they exclude patients with negative prior medication history, resulting in samples enriched for positive responders. Studies that include stimulant naïve patients are useful for evaluating the impact of medication that is not confounded by prior medication history. On the other hand, these studies are less generalizable to older youth or those with complex medication histories. A second factor is the adequacy of the medication trial and how and when it is delivered. Titration, dose, and dosing strategies also impact findings. Fixed-dose or dose-response studies may provide more distinct information on the effects of medication, for example,[31] although flexible dosing may be more similar to usual care.

In one of the few longer-term studies of stimulant naive youth with ADHD, children on a waiting list were randomly assigned to immediate-release MPH or placebo for 16 weeks.[25] In contrast to findings from many short-term studies, MPH did not negatively affect sleep parameters measured at 8 weeks of treatment relative to placebo.

When sleep was measured a week after medication was discontinued (after 16 weeks of treatment), sleep efficiency was improved in the MPH group. This provocative finding requires replication but suggests that sleep problems are much more prevalent when first initiating treatment compared with after 8 weeks of treatment or after medication is discontinued.

STIMULANTS AND SLEEP PROBLEMS

Methylphenidate. Delayed sleep onset, typically defined as greater than 30 minutes, or insomnia are frequent adverse events associated with MPH,[22,32,33] the most common medication used to treat ADHD in children. In a recent meta-analysis of nine randomized stimulant trials that used objective measures of sleep in 246 children with ADHD,[34] stimulant treatment was associated with longer sleep latencies, worse sleep efficiency, and shorter sleep duration. The authors highlighted the importance of weighing the cognitive and behavioral benefits of stimulant treatment to the adverse impact on sleep. Similarly, Faraone and colleagues[3] found that children receiving MPH were at a 60% greater risk for sleep problems compared with children receiving placebo. The greatest relative risks were seen with longer-acting preparations, such as osmotic-release oral system, transdermal system, and MPH hydrochloride controlled-release.

There are also several studies that have used PSG in children with ADHD who were receiving MPH. For example,[35] compared 53 children taking stimulants, 34 children with ADHD who were not taking stimulants, and 53 controls and found no differences in sleep architecture. However, the rates of insomnia were not reported, children were not randomized to treatment, and children who may have discontinued medication may not have been identified, effecting the results that can be drawn from this study. MPH has been found to reduce total sleep time and reduce sleep efficiency but not alter sleep architecture in children diagnosed with ADHD.[36]

Amphetamine. Relative to MPH, there are far fewer studies of AMP effect on sleep. AMP is associated with longer and more variable pharmacokinetic profiles (eg,[37] compared with MPH).[38] conducted a double-blind, forced dose, parallel-group study in which 290 children received either Lisdexamfetamine (LDX), an AMP prodrug, or a placebo for 4 weeks. More than half of the sample was stimulant naïve. Insomnia was the second most common, spontaneously reported adverse event after decreased appetite, and it occurred in approximately 15% of those prescribed LDX compared with only 2% of those taking the placebo. In another study comparing LDX and mixed AMP salts,[39] reports of insomnia were most common during the first week of treatment for both stimulants.

Examining sleep outcomes in more detail,[40] used parent ratings, actigraphy, and PSG to evaluate the sleep effects of LDX in 24 children with ADHD (6–12 years of age). Other than fewer nighttime awakenings in the LDX group, there were no significant differences between LDX and placebo. Although not statistically significant, latency to persistent sleep during PSG, was approximately 10 minutes longer for the LDX group compared with placebo controls. The small sample size, flexible dosing titration period, time to habituation to medication before assessment of sleep effects, and exclusion of subjects with a history of adverse or nonresponse to AMP may have led to a bias toward failing to find an effect on sleep.[41]

In one of the few comparative effectiveness studies of frequently used AMP and MPH stimulants, Stein and colleagues[31] used a placebo, controlled, crossover design to compare three dose levels of ER-mixed AMP salts with ER dexmethylphenidate and a placebo in 56 youth (30% stimulant naïve). Parent ratings of severe insomnia were significantly higher for Mixed amphetamine salts extended release (ER-MAS) at the 10 mg dose level. However, at the higher dose levels, there was no drug-related difference in the percentage of youth with severe insomnia. Using actigraphy, higher doses were associated with later sleep start time and shorter actual sleep duration for both stimulants.[42]

Nonstimulants. Atomoxetine (ATX) was the first nonstimulant approved by the Food and Drug Administration (FDA) for ADHD. Somnolence, or the state of feeling drowsy, has been found to be an adverse event with ATX for children,[43] especially during the early stages of a trial period or if titration is done too rapidly.[44] Whereas, for adults, insomnia is a more common side effect of nonstimulants. In another comparative efficacy study, a study[45] found that ATX was associated with more frequent night awakenings, although MPH was associated with a greater incidence of insomnia and increased SOL in adults. Residual daytime somnolence seen in children can be minimized by dividing doses or taking ATX in the evening although daytime efficacy may be decreased.[44]

The alpha 2 agonists, clonidine and guanfacine, are other nonstimulants approved to treat ADHD as monotherapy or in combination with a stimulant. They have also been used off-label to treat insomnia. Few studies[46,47] conducted a chart review and found that low-dose clonidine had a beneficial effect on sleep disturbance in youth with ADHD at baseline.

The extended-release formulations of alpha-2 agonists have been found to be associated with somnolence, sedation, and fatigue in 20% to 40% of youth with ADHD when used as monotherapy.[48] Guanfacine has also been associated with increased wakefulness after sleep onset.[49] Although somnolence, sedation, and fatigue are significantly improved when coadministered with a stimulant, they still occur in 15% to 20% of children, especially at the beginning of a trial or during dose titration.[50,51]

SELECT POPULATIONS

Preschoolers. The preschool period is a time of marked changes in sleep routines and expectations as attending school for the first time encourages families to develop a more consistent sleep schedule. What is known about ADHD and sleep in school-age children cannot necessarily be applied to preschoolers (eg,[52] due to unique developmental and environmental factors during this time). *Difficulty initiating sleep* is the most common reported sleep problem in preschoolers with ADHD. Parents often struggle with their preschool children over bedtime, and in the past, this has been largely interpreted as bedtime resistance or behavioral insomnia. However, bedtime resistance in preschoolers with ADHD may be a behavioral manifestation of difficulty with circadian rhythm.[53–55] A recent medical records study of 497 children with ADHD under the age of 6 compared those being treated with stimulants to alpha agonists.[56] Although difficulty sleeping was more common in the stimulant treated group (21% vs 11%), daytime sleepiness was more common in those treated with alpha 2 agonists (38%) compared with only 3% for those treated with stimulants.

Stimulant medication trials in preschool children with ADHD have consistently found a relatively attenuated benefit to risk ratio compared with school-aged children.[57–59] In general, stimulant usage at a younger age is associated with more frequent side effects, including irritability, decreased appetite, and sleep problems. Moreover, findings of adverse effects, such as sleep disturbances, are complicated by families discontinuing clinical trials. For instance, in a recent study of 90 preschool-age children with ADHD,[60] 287 treatment-related side effects were reported in 65 children but only 10 (all of which discontinued) were reported as severe (eg, insomnia, aggression, decreased appetite). During the 1-year follow-up, 40% of the children treated with stimulants dropped out for reasons other than adverse effects. However, this is not an unusual number of drop-outs in a long-term study.

A recent pilot study using both objective and subjective measures found increased motor activity during sleep and more night-to-night variability in sleep duration among preschoolers with ADHD.[61] Other sleep disorders that affect this age group, such as behavioral insomnia of childhood, combined with difficulty initiating sleep, and bedtime resistance can further complicate ADHD and its treatment.[22]

Adolescents. The adolescent period is marked by significant biological, physiologic, and social changes.[62,63] During adolescence, dopamine levels peak in various brain regions although serotonin decreases to adult levels by the age of 14. Norepinephrine levels reach the lowest at the onset of puberty, after which they tend to increase until the age of 40 to 60 years.[64] Similarly adrenergic receptors decline during the young adult years. There are also important sleep-related changes during the adolescence period as evidenced by electroencephalography. Slow-wave sleep (N3) decreases by more than 60% between the ages of 10 and 20 years.[65,66] This decline in N3 parallels a decline in sleep homeostatic pressure, which has important implications when evaluating adolescents for sleep delay. Furthermore, during adolescence, neuronal connections reorganize, unused synapses are eliminated, and maturation of cognitive functions occur, although asynchronously in different brain areas, therefore not all adolescents of the same age will have the same level of development in attention or executive function.[5] Although adolescents are faced with substantial increases in academic and social demands,[67] the ability to undertake new challenges is highly impacted by neurocognitive functioning and ADHD symptoms, which are also closely associated with sleep quality.[68]

Eighth-grade adolescents with ADHD who used stimulant medication reported more sleep–wake problems and longer SOL on school nights using a diary compared with peers without ADHD ($N = 140$).[2] As in children, initiation of a stimulant or dose changes was associated with delayed sleep onset. For example, a study[69] found that 4% of 171 adolescents (13–18 years of age) treated with once-daily Osmotic-release oral system (OROS) MPH-reported insomnia as an adverse effect. It is unclear how many youth were previously treated with MPH, but subjects with an adverse response were excluded from participation.

In addition to insomnia, inadequate sleep duration, and poor sleep efficiency, adolescents with ADHD are at high risk for a delayed sleep–wake phase, which involve a shift in the sleep–wake cycle such that the adolescent going to bed late and sleeping in late (see **Fig. 1**), sometimes to the point of day/night reversal. For example, as reported by [2] adolescents with ADHD were more likely than adolescents without ADHD to obtain insufficient sleep on school days (per diary) and weekends (per diary and actigraphy). Moreover, adolescents with ADHD were also more likely to report falling asleep in class and having stayed up all night at least twice in the previous 2 weeks (14% and 5% reported all-nighters for ADHD and comparison, respectively). Disruptions in circadian rhythm can have a devastating effect on school performance. Delayed sleep–wake phase disorder is of particular importance in that it has become a cultural norm to stay out late on the weekends, sleep late into the afternoon on Saturday and Sunday, and then try to shift back to a normal school schedule by Monday. Should a delayed sleep phase be present, treatment should center on rigorous maintenance of routine sleep and wake times, including no more than an hour difference on nonschool days.

Adults. Although sleep is far less studied in adults with ADHD compared with children, comorbidity of ADHD and sleep disorders is common in adults. In a sample of adults with ADHD, 44.4% of patients met the criteria for insomnia disorder according to the Diagnostic and Statistical Manual of Mental Disorders, Fifth edition (DSM-5) and 63.9% had insomnia symptoms.[70] Higher ADHD severity, psychiatric comorbidity, and fewer months of stable ADHD treatment were independently related to a higher prevalence of insomnia although longer periods of stable treatment were associated with lower rates of insomnia. Regardless of the presence or absence of insomnia, adults with ADHD have been found to have delayed sleep time and wake up time with a late onset of dim light melatonin secretion.[71]

In contrast to studies of stimulants in children, in adults, there is a mixed picture. In several clinical trials, AMP formulations (the typical duration of action of 12–16 hours) have been shown to not affect sleep based on subjective sleep measures in adults with ADHD.[72,73] For example, a study[72] analyzed two large randomized, double-blind placebo-controlled trials of LDX and extended-release mixed AMP salts for shifts from good sleep at baseline to poor sleep and found no significant difference between drug and placebo. In another adult ADHD trial, one-third of stimulant-treated patients showed improvements in sleep efficiency.[74] Similarly, Sobanski and colleagues[75–77] reported improvement in sleep onset and sleep maintenance according to subjective and objective measures although total sleep time decreased.

As of yet, we do not have dose–response or fixed–dose studies of medication effects on sleep in representative samples of adults with ADHD. Nonetheless, these early reports suggest that the effects of stimulants on sleep in adults and children may differ significantly, and that children's sleep may be more sensitive to stimulant effects.[41]

MANAGEMENT OF CO-OCCURRING SLEEP AND ADHD

According to Sengal and colleagues[45] (2006), "Avoiding adverse effects on sleep may represent a considerable advantage for the clinician in developing effective ADHD treatment strategies". Dose adjustments to minimize total daily medication burden, plus environmental or sleep hygiene interventions are recommended as first-line treatment in the child with stimulant-induced or exacerbated insomnia that persists beyond a few days (**Fig. 2**). Often, adverse sleep effects from medications for ADHD decrease by adjusting the dose and/or timing, as well as other strategies aimed at optimizing sleep before initiation of and throughout treatment (see reference[78]).

Improving sleep hygiene and establishing a consistent bedtime schedule with structured routines, avoidance of electronics and caffeine, and keeping a sleep-promoting bedroom environment with respect to temperature, light, and noise can reduce SOL. Short-term behavioral interventions, such as the Sleeping Sound with ADHD program,[79] have demonstrated efficacy in reducing moderate to severe sleep problems in a sample where approximately 80% of children were receiving stimulants.[80] Nonetheless, 28%–35% in the treatment group still displayed sleep problems highlighting the need for multimodal interventions targeting sleep and ADHD symptoms.

Environmental and behavioral interventions remain the foundation for most successful sleep interventions. Focus on the maintenance of routine sleep onset and wake times even on nonschool days should also be included. Optimizing the sleep environment not just in the child's bedroom, but for the whole household/family, is critical. Other recommendations include having positive and consistent bedtime routines. In fact, using sticker charts, sleep fairies, and other reward methods can help to establish a positive bedtime environment and have been shown to be effective in the treatment of behavioral sleep problems in children.[81,82] Incidentally, the use of weighted blankets has also been reported to be beneficial in some children with ADHD.[83]

Melatonin. Melatonin, a commercially available supplement, is often used to treat insomnia.[84] More commonly, melatonin is used as a hypnotic, with doses of 1–6 mg.

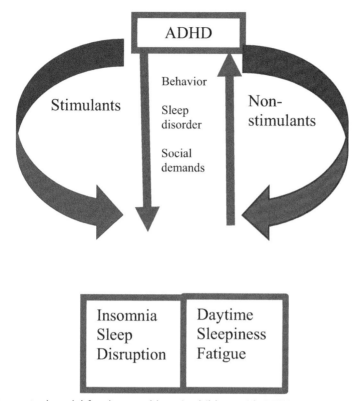

Fig. 2. Conceptual model for sleep problems in children with ADHD.

administered 30–60 minutes before desired sleep onset time. In cases of stimulant-induced or exacerbated insomnia that neither improves after several weeks nor is responsive to environmental and behavioral interventions, adding melatonin for the short term can be helpful. Melatonin is commonly used in children, for example, in the [80] trial of behavioral treatment conducted in Australia, 32.8% of children in the intervention group and 36.9% of children in the control group were receiving melatonin.[80] There are now several well-controlled melatonin studies. Van der Heijden and colleagues[85] (2007) found that 3 to 6 mg. of melatonin was superior to placebo in reducing SOL and that subsequently sleep hygiene improved. Similarly, a study[86] found that the mean sleep latency and total sleep disturbance scores were reduced in the melatonin group while the scores increased in the placebo group.

Weiss and colleagues[87] (2006) evaluated the impact of sleep hygiene procedures (eg, keeping a consistent sleep schedule, turning electronics off, discontinuing naps, and caffeinated beverage) and melatonin in a sample of children taking stimulant medication who also had a sleep latency of greater than 60 minutes. After sleep hygiene procedures, 15% of patients were sleep hygiene "responders," although the average SOL after sleep hygiene training was still quite long (73 minutes), as determined by actigraphy. The remaining patients who did not respond to sleep hygiene training were then randomized to receive either 5 mg of melatonin or placebo. Melatonin was well tolerated and statistically superior to placebo. The most effective treatment was a combination melatonin/sleep hygiene. Subjects were followed over time and eventually had complete normalization of sleep.

> **Box 1**
> **Recommended strategies for sleep problems in children with ADHD and medication**
>
> 1. Obtain thorough sleep history and rule out a primary sleep disorder
> 2. Treat primary sleep disorder if present (restless legs syndrome, obstructive sleep apnea)
> 3. Monitor sleep with sleep diaries or actigraphy at baseline and throughout medication trial
> 4. Encourage sleep hygiene
> 5. If sleep-onset latency or insomnia persists, consider reducing the dose of stimulants and observe
> 6. Consider adding melatonin, switching formulations, or combining with a nonstimulant

Typically, melatonin is well tolerated. Reported side effects include diarrhea, headache, enuresis, dizziness, nausea, and sleepiness. However, there are only a few long-term studies (up to 10 years) of melatonin at this time.[88] Given the evidence for melatonin and the benign side effect profile with widespread usage, melatonin may be recommended along with re-evaluation of ADHD medication dose and formulation and sleep hygiene strategies for ADHD medication-induced sleep problems (**Box 1**). However, despite the potential benefits, challenges exist to the effective use of melatonin, including wide variation in the potency and time course of melatonin formulation as the FDA does not regulate over-the-counter melatonin content,[89] allowing for the potential presence of contaminants.[90] Therefore, clinicians should be ready to speak to their patients about how to safely identify and use melatonin.

Other medications. Other medications for insomnia in children with ADHD have not been thoroughly studied. Limited evidence based on observational case series or retrospective chart reviews support the use of clonidine for sleep onset symptoms.[47,91] A single randomized controlled trial on Eszopiclone low dose (1 mg) versus high dose (3 mg) did not show improvement in sleep latency and demonstrated an 11% discontinuation rate due to side effects (eg, headache, dysgeusia, and dizziness).[92] Several potential areas of future research in children with ADHD and sleep disruption include orexin agonists (currently under development) and iron supplementation.

Several studies suggest a link between iron deficiency and ADHD.[93] Iron supplementation has been very successful in the treatment of RLS and restless sleep disorder in children.[94] The pathophysiology involves iron in the production of dopamine in areas of the brain involved in motor control (substantia nigra).

In summary, there is little evidence for sleep medications in children with ADHD. Although stimulants can decrease sleep latency, the opposite is usually true for nonstimulants (eg, ATX has been shown to increase somnolence). Although the effects of nonstimulants on fatigue and somnolence may be minimized with evening administration, although daytime efficacy for ADHD may be decreased, combined use of a stimulant and nonstimulant (eg, alpha2s, ATX) treatment may be helpful and optimal.

SUMMARY

Sleep disorders are common in individuals with ADHD both during and before pharmacologic intervention. If symptoms of a primary sleep disorder, such as obstructive sleep apnea, are present, it is important to further evaluate or refer to a sleep center. Insomnia and delays in latency to sleep onset greater than 30 minutes, either new onset or an exacerbation of prior sleep difficulties, are one of the most common adverse effects of stimulant medications and have been most studied in school-age-children with ADHD. With the advent of more long-acting stimulant medications and the awareness that ADHD impacts afternoon and evening behavior, more children are being treated for longer periods and with higher total daily doses compared with treatment with immediate-release formulations. Effects on sleep latency are most pronounced during initiation of a new medication and after dose changes. Although higher and later doses are associated with a greater impact on sleep, only a minority of children with ADHD (<20%) display persistent or severe sleep effects. First-line treatments for sleep concerns are behavioral and environmental treatments focused on improving sleep hygiene. If problems persist, melatonin may be added under the guidance of a professional.

Variable dosing schedules can also contribute to circadian rhythm disturbances, such as administration on school days only or markedly different weekend and week-day schedules, which are common in adolescents. Adolescents are also at the highest risk for medication nonadherence, further contributing to night-to-night variability. Consequently, they are at heightened risk for delayed sleep–wake phase disorder and resultant daytime sleepiness when having to wake up earlier than their circadian schedule.

Children who take stimulants may experience fewer nighttime waking and may be more difficult to arouse in the morning. However, nonstimulants can affect sleep in different ways than stimulants, with somnolence seen as a common side effect. Clinical evaluation related to the start of medication and the timing of titration, in addition to counseling related to the timing of daily use, may lessen the negative effects of ADHD medication on sleep.

CLINICS CARE POINTS

1. Screen for sleep disorders that can mimic and coexist in children with ADHD before initiating pharmacotherapy and monitor throughout the medication trial.

2. Stimulant medications can adversely affect sleep latency, duration, and efficiency but also may decrease night awakenings although nonstimulants can increase daytime sleepiness.

3. Nonstimulants can contribute to daytime sleepiness despite being important for this population.

4. For the majority of ADHD youth, effects of ADHD medications on sleep tend to occur when initiating medication trial, during escalating dose titration, or with multiple doses used to extend the stimulant duration of action on ADHD symptoms

5. Chronic sleep deprivation can also occur, and night-to-night variability (eg, medication on school days) can adversely affect circadian rhythms, especially in adolescents.

ACKNOWLEDGMENTS

The authors are grateful to Dr. Margaret Weiss for her thoughtful review and suggestions.

REFERENCES

1. Bradley C. The behavior of young children receiving Benzedrine. Am J Psychiatry 1937;94:577–85.
2. Becker SP, Langberg JM, Eadeh HM, et al. Sleep and daytime sleepiness in adolescents with and without ADHD: differences across ratings, daily diary, and actigraphy. J Child Psychol Psychiatry 2019;60(9):1021–31.

3. Faraone SV, Po MD, Komolova M, et al. Sleep-associated adverse events during methylphenidate treatment of attention-deficit/hyperactivity disorder: a meta-analysis. J Clin Psychiatry 2019;80(3). https://doi.org/10.4088/JCP.18r12210.

4. Hodgkins P, Setyawan J, Mitra D, et al. Management of ADHD in children across Europe: patient demographics, physician characteristics and treatment patterns. Eur J Pediatr 2013;172(7):895–906.

5. Huttenlocher PR. Synaptic density in human frontal cortex - developmental changes and effects of aging. Brain Res 1979;163(2):195–205.

6. Owens JA. The ADHD and sleep conundrum: a review. J Dev Behav Pediatr 2005;26(4):312–22.

7. Sung V, Hiscock H, Sciberras E, et al. Sleep problems in children with attention-deficit/hyperactivity disorder: prevalence and the effect on the child and family. Arch Pediatr Adolesc Med 2008;162(4):336–42.

8. Stein MA. Unravelling sleep problems in treated and untreated children with ADHD. J Child Adolesc Psychopharmacol 1999;9(3):157–68.

9. Cortese S, Faraone SV, Konofal E, et al. Sleep in children with attention-deficit/hyperactivity disorder: meta-analysis of subjective and objective studies. J Am Acad Child Adolesc Psychiatry 2009;48(9):894–908. Available at. http://www.ncbi.nlm.nih.gov/entrez/query.fcgi?cmd=Retrieve&db=PubMed&dopt=Citation&list_uids=19625983.

10. Picchietti MA, Picchietti DL. June). Restless legs syndrome and periodic limb movement disorder in children and adolescents. Semin Pediatr Neurol 2008; 15(No. 2):91–9. WB Saunders.

11. Pitzer M. The development of monoaminergic neurotransmitter systems in childhood and adolescence. Int J Dev Neurosci 2019;74:49–55.

12. Wajszilber D, Santiseban JA, Gruber R. Sleep disorders in patients with ADHD: impact and management challenges. Nat Sci Sleep 2018;10:453.

13. Kapoor V, Ferri R, Stein MA, et al. Restless sleep disorder in children with attention-deficit/hyperactivity disorder. J Clin Sleep Med 2021;17(4):639–43.

14. Taylor DJ, Wilkerson AK, Pruiksma KE, et al. Reliability of the structured clinical interview for DSM-5 sleep disorders module. J Clin Sleep Med 2018;14(3):459–64.

15. Owens and Dalzell 2005.

16. Chervin et al., 2000.

17. Owens JA, Spirito A, McGuinn M. The Children's Sleep Habits Questionnaire (CSHQ): psychometric properties of a survey instrument for school-aged children. Sleep 2000;23(8):1043–51.

18. Biggs SN, Lushington K, van den Heuvel CJ, et al. Inconsistent sleep schedules and daytime behavioral difficulties in school-aged children. Sleep Med 2011; 12(8):780–6.

19. Lecendreux M, Konofal E, Bouvard M, et al. Sleep and alertness in children with ADHD. J Child Psychol Psychiatry 2000;41(6):803–12. Available at: http://www.ncbi.nlm.nih.gov/pubmed/11039692.

20. Floros O, Axelsson J, Almeida R, et al. Vulnerability in Executive Functions to Sleep Deprivation Is Predicted by Subclinical Attention-Deficit/Hyperactivity Disorder Symptoms. Biol Psychiatry Cogn Neurosci Neuroimaging 2021;6(3):290–8.

21. Rentz LE, Ulman HK, Galster SM. Deconstructing commercial wearable technology: contributions toward accurate and free-living monitoring of sleep. Sensors (Basel) 2021;21(15). https://doi.org/10.3390/s21155071.

22. Stein MA, Weiss M, Hlavaty L. ADHD treatments, sleep, and sleep problems: complex associations. Neurotherapeutics 2012;9(3):509–17.

23. Chin WC, Huang YS, Chou YH, et al. Subjective and objective assessments of sleep problems in children with attention deficit/hyperactivity disorder and the effects of methylphenidate treatment. Biomed J 2018;41(6):356–63.

24. Cortese S, Panei P, Arcieri R, et al. Safety of methylphenidate and atomoxetine in children with attention-deficit/hyperactivity disorder (ADHD): data from the Italian National ADHD Registry. CNS drugs 2015;29(10):865–77.

25. Solleveld MM, Schrantee A, Baek HK, et al. Effects of 16 Weeks of methylphenidate treatment on actigraph-assessed sleep measures in medication-naive children with ADHD. Front Psychiatry 2020;11:82.

26. Hvolby A. Associations of sleep disturbance with ADHD: implications for treatment. Atten Defic Hyperact Disord 2015;7(1):1–18.

27. Rechtschaffen A. Polygraphic aspects of insomnia. In: Encephalography. 1967. Bologna: p. 109–25.

28. Stein MA, Blondis TA, Schnitzler ER, et al. Methylphenidate dosing: twice daily versus three times daily. Pediatrics 1996;98(4 Pt 1):748–56. Available at: http://www.ncbi. nlm.nih.gov/entrez/query.fcgi?cmd=Retrieve&db=PubMed&dopt=Citation&list_ uids=8885956.

29. De Crescenzo F, Licchelli S, Ciabattini M, et al. The use of actigraphy in the monitoring of sleep and activity in ADHD: a meta-analysis. Sleep Med Rev 2016; 26:9–20.

30. Becker SP, Langberg JM, Eadeh HM, et al. Sleep and daytime sleepiness in adolescents with and without ADHD: Differences across ratings, daily diary, and actigraphy. Journal of Child Psychology and Psychiatry 2019;60(9):1021–31.

31. Stein MA, Waldman ID, Charney E, et al. Dose effects and comparative effectiveness of extended release dexmethylphenidate and mixed amphetamine salts. J Child Adolesc Psychopharmacol 2011;21(6):581–8.

32. Storebø OJ, Ramstad E, Krogh HB, et al. Methylphenidate for children and adolescents with attention deficit hyperactivity disorder (ADHD). Cochrane Database Syst Rev 2015;11:CD009885.

33. Storebø OJ, Pedersen N, Ramstad E, et al. Methylphenidate for attention deficit hyperactivity disorder (ADHD) in children and adolescents–assessment of adverse events in non-randomised studies. Cochrane Database Syst Rev 2018;(5):CD012069.

34. Kidwell KM, Van Dyk TR, Lundahl A, et al. Stimulant medications and sleep for youth with ADHD: a meta-analysis. Pediatrics 2015;136(6):1144–53.

35. O'Brien et al. (2003).

36. Galland BC, Tripp EG, Taylor BJ. The sleep of children with attention deficit hyperactivity disorder on and off methylphenidate: a matched case-control study. J Sleep Res 2010;19(2):366–73.

37. McGough JJ, Biederman J, Greenhill LL, et al. Pharmacokinetics of SLI381 (ADDERALL XR), an extended-release formulation of Adderall. J Am Acad Child Adolesc Psychiatry 2003;42(6):684–91.

38. Biederman J, Krishnan S, Zhang Y, et al. Efficacy and tolerability of lisdexamfetamine dimesylate (NRP-104) in children with attention-deficit/hyperactivity disorder: a phase III, multicenter, randomized, double-blind, forced-dose, parallel-group study. Clin Ther 2007;29(3):450–63.

39. Biederman J, Boellner SW, Childress A, et al. Lisdexamfetamine dimesylate and mixed amphetamine salts extended-release in children with ADHD: a double-blind, placebo-controlled, crossover analog classroom study. Biol Psychiatry 2007;62(9):970–6.

40. Giblin and Strobel 2011.

41. Diaz-Roman et al., 2018.
42. Santisteban JA, Stein MA, Bergmame L, et al. Effect of extended-release dexmethylphenidate and mixed amphetamine salts on sleep: a double-blind, randomized, crossover study in youth with attention-deficit hyperactivity disorder. CNS drugs 2014;28(9):825–33.
43. Yildiz O, Cakin-Memik N, Agauglu B. Quality of life in children with (attention-deficit hyperactivity disorder): a cross-sectional study/Dikkat eksikligi hiperaktivite bozuklugu tanili cocuklarda yasam kalitesi: kesitsel bir calisma. Arch Neuropsychiatry 2010;47(4):314–9.
44. Block SL, Williams D, Donnelly CL, et al. Post hoc analysis: early changes in ADHD-RS items predict longer term response to atomoxetine in pediatric patients. Clin Pediatr 2010;49(8):768–76.
45. Sangal RB, Owens J, Allen AJ, et al. Effects of atomoxetine and methylphenidate on sleep in children with ADHD. Sleep 2006;29(12):1573–85. Available at: http://www.ncbi.nlm.nih.gov/pubmed/17252888.
46. Wilens TE, Biederman J, Spencer TJ. Clonidine for sleep disturbances associated with attention-deficit hyperactivity disorder. J Am Acad Child Adolesc Psychiatry 1994;33(3):424–6.
47. Prince JB, Wilens TE, Biederman J, et al. Clonidine for sleep disturbances associated with attention-deficit hyperactivity disorder: a systematic chart review of 62 cases. J Am Acad Child Adolesc Psychiatry 1996;35(5):599–605.
48. Daviss WB, Patel NC, Robb AS, et al. Clonidine for attention-deficit/hyperactivity disorder: II. ECG changes and adverse events analysis. Journal of the American Academy of Child & Adolescent Psychiatry 2008;47(2):189–98.
49. Rugino TA. Effect on primary sleep disorders when children with ADHD are administered guanfacine extended release. Journal of attention disorders 2018; 22(1):14–24.
50. Kollins SH, Jain R, Brams M, et al. Clonidine extended-release tablets as add-on therapy to psychostimulants in children and adolescents with ADHD. Pediatrics 2011;127(6):e1406–13.
51. Faraone SV, Glatt SJ. Effects of extended-release guanfacine on ADHD symptoms and sedation-related adverse events in children with ADHD. J attention Disord 2010;13(5):532–8.
52. Charach A, Carson P, Fox S, et al. Interventions for preschool children at high risk for ADHD: a comparative effectiveness review. Pediatrics 2013;131(5):e1584–e1604.
53. Van der Heijden KB, Smits MG, Gunning WB. Sleep hygiene and actigraphically evaluated sleep characteristics in children with ADHD and chronic sleep onset insomnia. Journal of sleep research 2006;15(1):55–62.
54. Van der Heijden KB, Smits MG, Someren EJV, et al. Idiopathic chronic sleep onset insomnia in attention-deficit/hyperactivity disorder: A circadian rhythm sleep disorder. Chronobiology international 2005;22(3):559–70.
55. Van her Heijden, Smits, Van Someren, Ridderinkof, & Gunning, 2007
56. Harstad E, Shults J, Barbaresi W, et al. alpha2-Adrenergic agonists or stimulants for preschool-age children with attention-deficit/hyperactivity disorder. JAMA 2021;325(20):2067–75.
57. Ghuman JK, Aman MG, Lecavalier L, Riddle MA, Gelenberg A, Wright R, Fort C. Randomized, placebo-controlled, crossover study of methylphenidate for attention-deficit/hyperactivity disorder symptoms in preschoolers with developmental disorders. Journal of child and adolescent psychopharmacology 2009;19(4):329–39.

58. Greenhill et al., 2005.
59. Lee SS, Falk AE, Aguirre VP. Association of comorbid anxiety with social functioning in school-age children with and without attention-deficit/hyperactivity disorder (ADHD). Psychiatry research 2012;197(1-2):90–6.
60. Childress et al., 2021.
61. Melegari MG, Vittori E, Mallia L, Devoto A, Lucidi F, Ferri R, Bruni O. Actigraphic sleep pattern of preschoolers with ADHD. Journal of Attention Disorders 2020; 24(4):611–24.
62. Colrain IM, Baker FC. Changes in sleep as a function of adolescent development. Neuropsychology review 2011;21(1):5–21.
63. Darchia N, Cervena K. The journey through the world of adolescent sleep. Reviews in the Neurosciences 2014;25(4):585–604.
64. Abd-Allah NM, Hassan FH, Esmat AY, et al. Age dependence of the levels of plasma norepinephrine, aldosterone, renin activity and urinary vanillylmandelic acid in normal and essential hypertensives. Biol Res 2004;37(1):95–106.
65. Feinberg I, Campbell IG. Sleep EEG changes during adolescence: an index of a fundamental brain reorganization. Brain Cogn 2010;72(1):56–65.
66. Floros O, Axelsson J, Almeida R, et al. Vulnerability in executive functions to sleep deprivation is predicted by subclinical attention-deficit/hyperactivity disorder symptoms. Biol Psychiatry Cogn Neurosci Neuroimaging 2021;6(3):290–8.
67. Crockett LJ, Crouter AC. Pathways through adolescence: Individual development in relation to social contexts. Psychology Press 2014.
68. Carskadon MA. Sleep in adolescents: the perfect storm. Pediatric Clinics 2011;58(3):637–47.
69. McGough J, McCracken J, Swanson J, et al. Pharmacogenetics of methylphenidate response in preschoolers with ADHD. J Am Acad Child Adolesc Psychiatry 2006;45(11):1314–22.
70. Fadeuilhe C, Daigre C, Richarte V, et al. Insomnia disorder in adult attention-deficit/hyperactivity disorder patients: clinical, comorbidity, and treatment correlates. Front Psychiatry 2021;12:663889.
71. Snitselaar MA, Smits MG, van der Heijden KB, et al. Sleep and circadian rhythmicity in adult ADHD and the effect of stimulants. J Atten Disord 2017;21(1): 14–26.
72. Surman CB, Roth T. Impact of stimulant pharmacotherapy on sleep quality: post hoc analyses of 2 large, double-blind, randomized, placebo-controlled trials. The Journal of clinical psychiatry 2011;72(7):8683.
73. Brams, Matthew, et al. 2011.
74. Surman CB, Adamson JJ, Petty C, et al. Association between attention-deficit/hyperactivity disorder and sleep impairment in adulthood: evidence from a large controlled study. The Journal of clinical psychiatry 2009;70(11):1483.
75. Boonstra AM, Kooij JJ, Oosterlaan J, et al. Hyperactive night and day? Actigraphy studies in adult ADHD: a baseline comparison and the effect of methylphenidate. Sleep 2007;30:433–42.
76. Roth T, Zinsenheim J. Sleep in adults with ADHD and the effects of stimulants. Prim Psychiatry 2009;16:32–7.
77. Sobanski E, Schredl M, Kettler N, et al. Sleep in adults with attention deficit hyperactivity disorder (ADHD) before and during treatment with methylphenidate: a controlled polysomnographic study. Sleep 2008;31(3):375–81. Available at: http://www.ncbi.nlm.nih.gov/pubmed/18363314.

78. Cortese S, Newcorn JH, Coghill D. A practical, evidence-informed approach to managing stimulant-refractory attention deficit hyperactivity disorder (ADHD). CNS Drugs 2021;35(10):1035–51.
79. Sciberras E, Efron D, Gerner B, et al. Study protocol: the sleeping sound with attention-deficit/hyperactivity disorder project. BMC Pediatr 2010;10:101.
80. Hiscock H, Mulraney M, Heussler H, et al. Impact of a behavioral intervention, delivered by pediatricians or psychologists, on sleep problems in children with ADHD: a cluster-randomized, translational trial. J Child Psychol Psychiatry 2019;60(11):1230–41.
81. Delemere E, Dounavi K. Parent-implemented bedtime fading and positive routines for children with autism spectrum disorders. J Autism Dev Disord 2018; 48(4):1002–19.
82. Díaz-Román A, Mitchell R, Cortese S. Sleep in adults with ADHD: systematic review and meta-analysis of subjective and objective studies. Neurosci Biobehavioral Rev 2018;89:61–71.
83. Larsson I, Aili K, Nygren JM, et al. Parents' experiences of weighted blankets' impact on children with attention-deficit/hyperactivity disorder (ADHD) and sleep problems—a qualitative study. Int J Environ Res Public Health 2021;18(24): 12959.
84. Masi G, Fantozzi P, Villafranca A, et al. Effects of melatonin in children with attention-deficit/hyperactivity disorder with sleep disorders after methylphenidate treatment. Neuropsychiatr Dis Treat 2019;15:663.
85. der HEIJDEN KBV, Smits MG, Van Someren EJ, et al. Effect of melatonin on sleep, behavior, and cognition in ADHD and chronic sleep-onset insomnia. J Am Acad Child Adolesc Psychiatry 2007;46(2):233–41.
86. Mohammadi MR, Mostafavi SA, Keshavarz SA, et al. Melatonin effects in methylphenidate treated children with attention deficit hyperactivity disorder: a randomized double blind clinical trial. Iranian J Psychiatry 2012;7(2):87.
87. Weiss MD, Wasdell MB, Bomben MM, et al. Sleep hygiene and melatonin treatment for children and adolescents with ADHD and initial insomnia. J Am Acad Child Adolesc Psychiatry 2006;45:512–9.
88. Andersen LPH, Gögenur I, Rosenberg J, et al. The safety of melatonin in humans. Clin Drug Invest 2016;36(3):169–75.
89. Owens JA, Moturi S. Pharmacologic treatment of pediatric insomnia. Child Adolesc Psychiatr Clin N Am 2009;18(4):1001–16.
90. Grigg-Damberger MM, Ianakieva D. Poor quality control of over-the-counter melatonin: what they say is often not what you get. J Clin Sleep Med 2017; 13(2):163–5.
91. Anand S, Tong H, Besag F, et al. Safety, tolerability and efficacy of drugs for treating behavioural insomnia in children with attention-deficit/hyperactivity disorder: a systematic review with methodological quality assessment. Pediatr Drugs 2017;19(3):235–50.
92. Sangal RB, Blumer JL, Lankford DA, et al. Eszopiclone for insomnia associated with attention-deficit/hyperactivity disorder. Pediatrics 2014;134(4):e1095–103.
93. East PL, Doom JR, Blanco E, et al. Iron deficiency in infancy and sluggish cognitive tempo and ADHD symptoms in childhood and adolescence. J Clin Child Adolesc Psychol 2021;1–12.
94. Joseph V, Nagalli S. Periodic limb movement disorder. StatPearls; 2021.

ADHD and Substance Use Disorders in Young People
Considerations for Evaluation, Diagnosis, and Pharmacotherapy

Daria Taubin, BA[a], Julia C. Wilson, BA[a],
Timothy E. Wilens, MD[b,c,d],*

KEYWORDS

- Attention-deficit/hyperactivity disorder • ADHD • Substance use disorder • SUD
- Comorbidity • Pharmacotherapy • Treatment

KEY POINTS

- There is a bidirectional overlap of attention-deficit/hyperactivity disorder (ADHD) and substance use disorders (SUDs), with shared risk factors as well as similar underlying neurobiology
- Early pharmacotherapy for ADHD reduces the risk of subsequent nicotine and other SUDs
- Treatment of ADHD needs to be considered in individuals with comorbid SUD, though potential symptom overlap between ADHD and SUD can make accurate diagnosis challenging
- Medication-based treatment of ADHD in individuals with SUD includes both nonstimulants and stimulants, and may result in improved outcomes of retention, ADHD, and SUD
- The nonmedical use of stimulants continues to be problematic, particularly in college students, and those with SUD

INTRODUCTION

Among young people with attention-deficit/hyperactivity disorder (ADHD), addictive disorders are among the most feared comorbidities by patients, clinicians, and families. When left untreated, it is estimated that up to 50% of individuals with ADHD will manifest

[a] Pediatric Psychopharmacology Program, Division of Child and Adolescent Psychiatry, Massachusetts General Hospital, Warren Building 628B, 55 Fruit Street, Boston, MA 02114, USA; [b] Division of Child and Adolescent Psychiatry, Child Psychiatry Service, Massachusetts General Hospital, 55 Fruit Street, YAW 6A, Boston, MA 02114, USA; [c] Center for Addiction Medicine, Massachusetts General Hospital, Boston, MA 02114, USA; [d] Massachusetts General Hospital, and Harvard Medical School, Boston, MA 02114, USA
* Corresponding author. Child Psychiatry Service, Massachusetts General Hospital, 55 Fruit Street, YAW 6A, Boston, MA 02114.
E-mail address: twilens@mgh.harvard.edu

Child Adolesc Psychiatric Clin N Am 31 (2022) 515–530
https://doi.org/10.1016/j.chc.2022.01.005
1056-4993/22/© 2022 Elsevier Inc. All rights reserved.
childpsych.theclinics.com

a substance use disorder (SUD) at some point in their lives.[1-3] Individuals with ADHD and comorbid SUD experience significantly greater impairment in both their SUD and ADHD.[2,4,5] Given the high prevalence and impairment associated with this comorbidity, a thorough understanding of the bidirectional overlap between ADHD and SUD, coupled with diagnostic and treatment recommendations, is necessary.[6] In the following sections, we highlight the identification, diagnoses, and treatment of young people with ADHD and SUD, with a focus on pharmacotherapeutic interventions.

DISCUSSION
Prevalence of SUD

Epidemiologic data demonstrate that SUD is highly prevalent among youth and adult populations. It is estimated that 10% of adolescents and between 20% and 30% of adults will meet the criteria for a SUD in their lifetime.[7] Indeed, according to 2018 data from SAMHSA, over 20 million people in the United States met the criteria for a SUD in the past year, representing approximately 7.4% of the overall population ages 12 years and older. Broken down across age groups, 3.7% of adolescents ages 12 to 17 years, 15% of young adults ages 18 to 25 years, and 6.6% of adults ages 26 years and older met criteria for a past year SUD.[8]

Individuals with SUD experience impairments across multiple domains, including academics, occupation, suicidality, and risky behavior.[9] SUD is also associated with extensive comorbid psychopathologies, such as mood disorders, anxiety disorders, and ADHD.[1] Given that almost half of SUD onsets during childhood and three-quarters by age 26, it is imperative to consider childhood antecedents that may influence SUD risk.[10] One important developmental risk factor for SUD is ADHD.

Risk of Nicotine, SUD, and Behavioral Addictions in ADHD

There is substantial literature documenting the high rates of substance use and use disorders in both adults and adolescents with ADHD.[11,12] Research has demonstrated that youth with ADHD are 2 to 3 times more likely to develop cigarette smoking, nicotine use, and/or SUD than peers,[11,13] with some samples even reporting a sixfold risk for SUD in adolescents with ADHD.[14] Overall, ADHD symptoms have been shown to predict tobacco, alcohol, and cannabis use in young adults.[15] Indeed, in a systematic review of smoking behavior in youth by van Amsterdam and colleagues, 40% of individuals with ADHD reported using tobacco, compared with only 28% of controls. Moreover, adolescents with ADHD were at higher risk of earlier initiation of nicotine use, nicotine dependence, and lower remission rates from quitting smoking.[16]

More recently, research has demonstrated that ADHD is also a risk factor for e-cigarette use.[17,18] For instance, in a sample of 9th graders who reported never using tobacco, ADHD symptoms at baseline predicted initiation of e-cigarette use by the time participants reached 11th grade.[19] Similarly, ADHD symptoms in high school have been shown to predict e-cigarette use in college.[20] These findings with nicotine are entirely consistent with work showing a link between ADHD and an earlier initiation of substance use/use disorders.[2] These findings are especially concerning given that early-onset SUD has been linked to a greater impairment overall.[9]

ADHD has also been linked to several behavioral addictions, including Internet, gaming, and gambling addictions.[21-23] In a sample of children ages 8 to 16 years, 56% of those with ADHD met the criteria for Internet addiction, compared with 12% of those without ADHD.[22] This higher risk of Internet addiction in ADHD has also been documented in older adolescent samples,[21] as well as in college-aged youth.[24] In further support of this association, Schoenmacker and colleagues previously demonstrated that in patients with ADHD, symptom severity serves as a risk factor for Internet addiction.[25]

Several aspects of ADHD may influence the link between ADHD and Internet/gaming addiction. For example, Yen and colleagues found that symptoms of impulsivity and hostility in young adults ages 20 to 30 years partially mediated the relationship between ADHD and Internet gaming disorder.[23] Other research has indicated that inattentive symptoms may be associated with problematic video game play.[26] Relatedly, in one sample of adults seeking treatment for gambling addiction (in which 43% of participants met criteria for ADHD), both a history of childhood ADHD symptoms and the presence of ADHD symptoms persisting into adulthood were associated with more severe gambling addiction.[27] These aggregate findings highlight the need to query about Internet-related use and further examine potential impulsivity and mood dysregulation that may be contributing to overuse and/or behavioral addictions.

ADHD in SUD

ADHD is a frequently observed comorbid disorder in adolescents and adults with SUD. For instance, in the older Cannabis Youth Treatment Study, 38% of the 600 adolescent participants self-reported experiencing ADHD, making it the second most common comorbidity observed in the sample.[3] Moreover, a retrospective medical record review conducted by our group revealed that over 50% of adolescents and young adults receiving outpatient treatment for SUD have ADHD.[28] Rates of ADHD in adults with SUD also appear to be higher than population rates. For instance, a review by van der Burg and colleagues found that 15% to 25% of adult SUD patients have been diagnosed with ADHD.[29] In justice-involved populations, these rates may be even higher. For example, in one sample of incarcerated individuals engaged in medication treatment for opioid use disorder, over 50% had a history of childhood ADHD.[30]

Despite these consistent findings, co-occurring ADHD in individuals with SUD continues to be underidentified. For example, in one sample of adults in treatment for SUD, among the over one-third of patients who met criteria for ADHD, more than two-thirds had no previous ADHD diagnosis.[31] Clearly, SUD populations represent an area of need for diagnostic evaluation for ADHD, ultimately leading to potential pharmacologic and behavioral interventions.

Linking ADHD and SUD

Prior work has proposed several possible explanations for the link between ADHD and SUD, including biologic, psychosocial, and familial/genetic connections.[32] Both ADHD and SUD are thought to be associated with impairments in the dopamine system,[9] as well as abnormal functioning of the striatum.[33–35] Data suggest that SUD and ADHD both arise from abnormalities in the brain's reward system, that is thought to be connected to dopaminergic functioning,[36] or from a reduced ability of the prefrontal cortex to dampen abnormal reward system functioning.[35]

There is also evidence for a genetic link between ADHD and SUD. Our group has demonstrated a higher risk for SUD and ADHD in first-degree family members of patients with SUD and ADHD. Data from 2 case-controlled family studies of youth with ADHD indicated that ADHD in probands predicted SUD in relatives, irrespective of proband SUD status.[37] In addition, work by Wimberley and colleagues using polygenic risk scores demonstrated that genetic risk for ADHD was associated with higher rates of SUD in patients with ADHD.[38]

Another common theory connecting SUD and ADHD is the "self-medication hypothesis," which argues that individuals with ADHD use drugs and alcohol to alleviate or manage ADHD symptoms.[39] Literature in support of this hypothesis includes work by Manni and colleagues, who showed that patients with ADHD and cocaine use disorder receiving methylphenidate and atomoxetine treatment demonstrated significant reductions in their cocaine use following treatment. This decrease in cocaine use was correlated with significant improvement in ADHD symptoms.[40] However, the overall literature on the self-medication theory remains mixed. For example, van Amsterdam and colleagues note in a review that in a sample of smokers with ADHD, nicotine use was not correlated with improvement of ADHD symptoms, suggesting that in this case, substance use was not serving a self-medication role.[16] Our group previously failed to show differences in endorsements of self-medication using the Drug Use Severity Index in young people with ADHD compared to non-ADHD controls.[41] Similarly, other work has suggested that individuals who report nonmedical use of prescription stimulants do not differ from controls in objective measures of impulsivity and inattention,[42] further calling into question the notion that substance misuse is motivated by a need to "self-medicate" problematic symptoms. Given these complex findings, it is evident that further exploration of biological systems and psychological mechanisms in individuals with ADHD and SUD is necessary to better understand the etiology(ies) of this comorbidity.

Does Earlier Treatment of ADHD Mitigate Subsequent SUD?

One of the most common questions posed by parents of youth being considered for stimulant pharmacotherapy for ADHD is the query of the effect of early stimulant treatment on increasing the risk for nicotine use and SUD. In contrast to the directionality of the question, medication-based treatment of ADHD appears to have a protective effect on later nicotine use and SUD in ADHD.[43–45] A recent review of the literature from our group demonstrated that stimulant treatment of ADHD was associated with a *decreased* risk for SUD.[46] Results from several prospective medication trials of stimulant treatment in ADHD samples support this finding. In a large Swedish registry sample, an over 30% reduction in SUD for individuals in stimulant treatment was reported at 3-year follow-up.[44] Similarly, in a sample of over 3 million adolescents and adults in the United States, a 35% reduction in substance-related events (substance-related emergency department visits) was observed in men taking medication for ADHD.[43] In Chang and colleagues' sample, the risk of SUD was found to reduce by 13% for each year a person was receiving stimulant treatment.[44] This is in line with McCabe and colleagues' finding that earlier onset and longer duration of stimulant treatment appears to be linked to a greater reduction in SUD risk.[47] In the McCabe study, early and sustained stimulant treatment was associated with the greatest reduction in substance use in high school. Finally, our group has previously shown in a longitudinal, case-controlled study of youth with ADHD that pharmacotherapy was related not only to reduced cigarette smoking but also reduced SUD through adolescence.[45] Of interest, the aggregate literature converges in findings independent of whether they originated from treated compared with untreated individuals with ADHD (between-group comparisons), or in examining periods of individuals with ADHD receiving versus not receiving medications (within-group comparisons), furthering the notion of the importance of ongoing treatment of ADHD through the ages of risk for SUD including late adolescence through young adulthood. Two large studies also support the efficacy of early initiation of medication for ADHD (before age 9 years) in most optimally mitigating the ultimate risk for nicotine and SUD.[44,47]

Diagnostic Considerations of ADHD and SUD

Screening for and diagnosing ADHD in SUD populations has been named a priority on the international level.[48] However, diagnosing ADHD in context with SUD may be challenging because of potential overlap between symptoms of both disorders (including inattention, hyperactivity, and impulsivity),[49] the possibility that current substance use may worsen existing ADHD symptoms,[50] and the risk of intoxication and withdrawal symptoms in SUD populations obfuscating the diagnosis of ADHD.[48] Given these challenges, if possible, before establishing a diagnosis of ADHD, we recommend a period of abstinence or reduced substance use in patients with active SUD. For instance, it is not recommended to diagnose ADHD during early withdrawal phases of SUD in a detoxification setting.

Accurately diagnosing adolescents and young adults with ADHD requires the review of past performance, testing and medical review, as well as consideration of self and observer/parent-reported ADHD rating scales, when available. The diagnosis of ADHD in those with SUD has been validated using retrospective recall of symptoms; with the most consistent issues actually being the underidentification of symptoms and diagnosis in adults with ADHD.[41,51] As in non-SUD groups, the presence of a childhood diagnosis or prominent symptoms of ADHD along with current ADHD symptoms is suggestive of a diagnosis.[52]

Why Treat ADHD in Individuals with SUD?

There are several compelling reasons to treat individuals with SUD for their comorbid ADHD. For instance, individuals with ADHD and SUD experience significant impairments and challenges (**Table 1**). Data suggest that co-occurring ADHD predicts more severe SUD, a longer course of illness, poorer response to SUD treatment, and a greater likelihood of relapse,[2,4,5] as well as more difficulties in social and employment spheres.[4] Recent research has also demonstrated that SUD may be related to more severe ADHD. In a sample of patients with alcohol use disorder (AUD), Coppola & Mondola reported that those with co-occurring ADHD presented with higher levels of impulsivity than those without ADHD, and that higher levels of impulsivity were in turn correlated with higher levels of hazardous and harmful drinking.[4] Similarly, as part of a multisite treatment study in adults with ADHD and AUD, adults who relapsed to alcohol use during any study period experienced immediate worsening of 15 of 18 ADHD symptoms measured on the Adult ADHD Investigator Symptom Rating Scale (AISRS).[50]

Of great importance, treatment of ADHD in SUD does not worsen SUD—nor has misuse of the medication been reported in these closely monitored studies.[40,53] Instead, a growing body of literature suggests that treatment of ADHD in individuals with comorbid SUD is linked to significant improvement in symptoms of one or both disorders,[40,47,54,55] retention in treatment,[56] and reduced risk of later worsening of SUD.[44] For example, using a naturalistic sample derived from an outpatient SUD

Table 1	
Impairments in co-occurring ADHD and SUD	
Impact of ADHD on SUD	**Impact of SUD on ADHD**
More severe SUD	Worsening of overall ADHD symptoms
Earlier-onset, and longer duration of SUD	Increased impulsivity
Poorer response to nicotine and SUD treatment Poorer retention in treatment Greater likelihood of relapse to SUD	Reduced efficacy of standard pharmacotherapy for ADHD
Challenges in social life and employment	

treatment clinic, we recently showed clinically and significantly improved retention in SUD care when ADHD was treated pharmacologically.[56] Interestingly, the apparent half-life of treatment increased from 9 months (untreated) to 36 months (treated; **Fig. 1**). Stimulants were significantly more effective on retention compared with non-stimulants. Moreover, ADHD pharmacotherapy was associated with an almost fivefold decrease in attrition in the first 90 days of treatment compared with those not receiving treatment for their ADHD.[56] Given the critical importance of engagement and retention in treatment for SUD outcomes, treating ADHD has a profound influence on the likelihood of sustained success for SUD outcomes.

Relatedly, studies have demonstrated that treating ADHD symptoms early in the course of SUD treatment may be related to better treatment outcomes.[53,56] Levin and colleagues evaluated the temporal relationship between improvement in ADHD symptoms and achievement of abstinence in those receiving methadone treatment for opioid use disorder with combined cocaine addiction and ADHD. Patients who experienced both improvements in ADHD and cocaine abstinence were more likely to improve in ADHD symptoms before achieving cocaine abstinence, rather than after. In addition, more patients had improved ADHD symptoms without achieving cocaine abstinence, compared with the number of patients who achieved cocaine abstinence without improved ADHD symptoms, suggesting that early treatment of ADHD may improve SUD outcomes.[53]

Treatment of ADHD and SUD

Treatment of adolescents and adults with ADHD and SUD should follow a careful diagnostic workup and requires both psychotherapy and pharmacotherapy. Some have suggested treatment with cognitive behavioral therapies (CBT), focusing first on

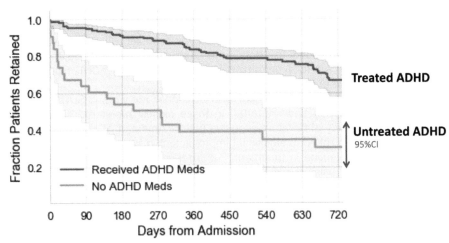

Fig. 1. Kaplan-Meier retention curves: ADHD pharmacotherapy versus no ADHD medication. Vertical axis depicts proportion of patients retained in treatment. Horizontal axis depicts days in treatment after admission. Shaded area around each curve represents the 95%-CI. Sample size: Untreated ADHD: N = 32; Treated ADHD: N = 171. Individuals were considered as receiving early treatment if they received ADHD pharmacotherapy with the first 90 days of admission. (*From* Kast KA, Rao V, Wilens TE. Pharmacotherapy for Attention-Deficit/Hyperactivity Disorder and Retention in Outpatient Substance Use Disorder Treatment: A Retrospective Cohort Study. J Clin Psychiatry. 82(2), 82(2):20m13598. 2021. Copyright 2021. Physicians Postgraduate Press. Reprinted with permission. with permission.)

SUD and later ADHD.[57] There is well-documented evidence supporting the efficacy of CBT in treating SUD (see Carroll[58]; Magill & Ray[59] for a review). In addition, Safren and colleagues previously demonstrated that a course of 3 to 6 modules of motivational interviewing and skill-based individual sessions of CBT was effective in significantly reducing ADHD symptoms, as well as anxiety and depression, and was well tolerated by participants.[60] Research has also found support for the efficacy of group sessions of CBT in reducing ADHD symptoms in adult patients.[61] CBT also appears to be effective at addressing ADHD symptoms in dually diagnosed populations, including those with SUD and ADHD.[62] Van Emmerik-van Ootmerssen and colleagues have reported that integrated CBT treatment of both ADHD and SUD successfully reduced ADHD symptoms in dually diagnosed populations[62]; however, less is known about the impact on SUD in this group.

Clinicians engaging in pharmacotherapy of SUD in ADHD should consider the use of both nonstimulants and stimulants. Although early work examining the efficacy of pharmacotherapy in treating ADHD + SUD found that it was minimally effective in treating ADHD and/or SUD,[63] outcomes from more recent studies using higher doses of medication and dimensional SUD are more promising.

Nonstimulant Pharmacotherapy. Individuals with ADHD and SUD, particularly those at higher risk for stimulant misuse or diversion (see below) may be considered for a nonstimulant medication as the first line of treatment for ADHD.[5,49] Nonstimulants that have demonstrated efficacy in the treatment of ADHD, SUD, and comorbid conditions include bupropion, atomoxetine, and tricyclic antidepressants.[4,5,64,65]

Atomoxetine is one of the most popular nonstimulant medications used in SUD populations because of its demonstrated effectiveness and relative lack of abuse liability.[4,5,65] In an open-label trial, Coppola and Mondola showed that atomoxetine in patients with co-occurring AUD and ADHD significantly reduced symptoms of impulsivity in those patients. Importantly, greater alcohol consumption did not influence treatment effects at both 8 and 12 weeks.[4] Similarly, in a controlled trial, atomoxetine was effective in reducing ADHD symptoms and episodes of heavy drinking and obsessiveness related to alcohol; but not relapse, in patients with AUD.[64] Of interest, the effect in reducing episodes of heavy drinking was similar to the effect noted in studies of naltrexone.

Other nonstimulant medications that have been used to treat ADHD in SUD settings include alpha-2 agonists (guanfacine and clonidine), tricyclic antidepressants,[65] and bupropion.[5] A retrospective chart review of patients with ADHD and co-occurring SUD in correctional community treatment taking atomoxetine, guanfacine, clonidine, and tricyclic antidepressants found that individuals treated with one or more of these medications experienced a decrease in ADHD symptoms.[65] Interestingly, individuals with no prior history of stimulant treatment in this sample showed greater improvement, suggesting that nonstimulant treatment may be an especially useful tool in individuals whose ADHD has only been recently identified.[65] The limited sample in this and other comparable studies, as well as the presence of some literature suggesting no effect of nonstimulant treatment on co-occurring ADHD and SUD symptoms,[66] highlights a need for work exploring nonstimulant therapies in SUD populations.[5] Another nonstimulant treatment for ADHD is viloxazine, which has been shown to effectively address ADHD symptoms in children and adolescents[67] and has previously been used to treat symptoms of alcohol misuse in individuals with comorbid depressive disorders.[68] Research is needed to examine the efficacy of this treatment in patients with co-occurring SUD and ADHD.

Stimulant Pharmacotherapy. Stimulant medications are generally safe for individuals with comorbid SUD and continue to be the most effective treatment for ADHD symptoms. A controlled trial conducted by Konstenius and colleagues examined the efficacy of a high dose of extended-release methylphenidate (OROS MPH; mean 108 mg; dosing to 180 mg/d) in treating ADHD and SUD symptoms in formerly incarcerated individuals with ADHD and amphetamine addiction. The researchers reported that MPH improved ADHD, retention in treatment, and reduced misuse of amphetamines compared with placebo.[69] Similarly, a controlled trial conducted by Levin and colleagues demonstrated that 60 and 80 mg of mixed amphetamine salts were effective at reducing symptoms of both ADHD and SUD (cocaine) in patients receiving methadone.[70] More recently, a retrospective study by Manni and colleagues extended this finding, showing that MPH or atomoxetine was associated with a significant improvement in both ADHD and SUD in adults with ADHD and cocaine use disorder.[40]

It is worth noting that there have been some reports of lower than expected efficacy of stimulant pharmacotherapy in both adults and adolescents with comorbid ADHD and SUD.[5,71] Though the immediate cause of this discrepancy remains unclear, it is possible that individuals with co-occurring ADHD and SUD require a higher dose of stimulant medications, such as those used in the Konsentius[69] and Levin[70] studies, to reach a therapeutic effect. Indeed, results from a large Swedish registry study have previously demonstrated that 2 years into treatment, those with comorbid ADHD and SUD were prescribed a 40% higher dose of stimulant medication than those without SUD.[72] Hence, when considering stimulant therapy for adolescents or adults with SUD, prescribers should entertain the very likely need for titration to potentially higher doses which may exceed FDA-approved dosing.

Another consideration for treatment is managing the high risk for cognitive impairment in those in early treatment for SUD. We previously showed that outpatients in SUD treatment had clinically and significantly more impaired executive functioning than historical controls.[73] In a separate sample of adults seeking inpatient SUD treatment, those with co-occurring ADHD receiving stimulant treatment had a 72% lower risk of mild cognitive impairment compared with unmedicated ADHD patients.[74] Interestingly, the risk for mild cognitive impairment did not differ between patients with and without co-occurring ADHD. Given that cognitive impairment has been linked to SUD,[73] these findings demonstrate that along with treating symptoms of ADHD, stimulant medications may also be effective at addressing SUD-related cognitive/executive functioning deficits and require further study.

Tolerability of Medication. Practitioners need to be mindful of potential interactions between substances of misuse and medications for ADHD. Several studies examining the efficacy of atomoxetine treatment in individuals with co-occurring AUD have reported no major concerning side effects of treatment,[64,75] although some increase in fatigue has been noted.[4,64] Similarly, Barkla and colleagues reported no clinically significant adverse effects of stimulant medications used with alcohol or drugs.[76] Carefully conducted adverse effect monitoring during randomized trials of stimulant medications in current substance users has failed to show meaningful adverse effects related to the specific substance of misuse (eg, cocaine, amphetamines).[69,70,77]

Timing of Treatment. Although there is agreement that ADHD should be treated in those with SUD, the precise timing of pharmacotherapy initiation remains unclear. Although there has been consensus that treatment should commence as soon as plausible, best practices for the initiation or reinstatement of pharmacotherapy continue to be debated and may be related to SUD frequency, severity, and diagnostic confidence. For instance, in adolescents with ADHD who are using marijuana infrequently, continued treatment of ADHD is recommended. However, if the adolescent develops a cannabis use disorder, it may be helpful to prioritize the treatment of the SUD and then reintroduce the treatment of the ADHD. In other words, in patients with established ADHD, because of diagnostic confidence, the treatment of the SUD should be considered immediately with the concurrent ADHD pharmacotherapy used on a case-by-case basis. This should be done with the understanding that there may be lower responsivity for ADHD using traditional dosing during periods of active heavy use/dependence,[51] necessitating consideration of higher doses-particularly of stimulants.[69,70]

In cases of diagnostic confusion and/or when other psychiatric comorbidities such as anxiety or mood disorders exist,[78] it is reasonable to sequence treatment to initially address SUD. This can then be followed by reevaluation and consideration of medication for ADHD after some stabilization of the SUD and/or psychiatric comorbidities. However, as reviewed previously, delay in the diagnosis and treatment of ADHD needs to be balanced against an increasing literature suggesting that early ADHD pharmacotherapy enhances engagement and retention of outpatients with ADHD and SUD.[56]

Nonmedical Use of Stimulants

Diversion and nonmedical use of stimulants continues to be an issue of growing concern for clinicians and researchers. On college campuses, rates of stimulant misuse have been reported to range between 8% and 34%[79] and even exceed 50% for those who are members of social fraternities and sororities.[79,80] In a comprehensive review of over 100 studies, Faraone and colleagues found that self-report rates of stimulant misuse are as high as 80% in some population samples, with adverse events most commonly resulting from nonoral administration of stimulants. Performance enhancement is the most frequent self-reported motivator for misuse,[81] though the actual efficacy of nonmedically used stimulants in enhancing cognitive performance in non-ADHD groups is relatively mixed in well-conducted, controlled studies.[32] Despite the negative physical and mental health outcomes associated with stimulant diversion and misuse,[81] evidence suggests that individuals misusing stimulants do not perceive their use as being associated with negative physical or mental health outcomes, and report viewing stimulant misuse as common.[80] Along with the increasingly robust literature demonstrating negative consequences of stimulant misuse, work from our group and others indicates that one-half of individuals who engaged in this behavior met criteria for a SUD, and over one-third met criteria for at least subthreshold stimulant use disorder.[82] Of note, our group has also previously demonstrated that college students with SUDs who endorse nonmedical use of stimulants were more likely to also endorse several other risky behaviors, such as intranasal stimulant use and use of stimulants with other drugs and alcohol.[83] We have also shown that those who misuse stimulants are at higher risk for multiple domains of deficits in executive functioning.[84]

Interestingly, there is an underappreciation by clinicians of the extent of nonmedical use of stimulants, despite survey and epidemiologic evidence of prominent misuse and diversion. In a national sample of practitioners treating young people, 59% reported suspecting that one of their patients with ADHD diverted their stimulant medication in the last 12 months. However, only 39% of physicians reported believing that stimulant diversion among adolescents with ADHD was "common" or "very common."[85] It continues to be recommended that the use of nonstimulants, use of extended-release stimulants, and education and monitoring of the elevated risk for stimulant misuse and diversion be undertaken in young people, particularly older high school and college students. There continues to be a need for research into novel stimulant preparations, such as the recently FDA-approved prodrug serdexmethylphenidate,[86] and stimulants with dissolution properties that negate intravenous or intranasal misuse.[87]

Table 2 Recommendations for treating ADHD in SUD	
Treatment Point	**Recommendation**
Assessment	ADHD screening should be part of standard clinical care in SUD. Nicotine and SUD and behavioral addictions should be part of standard clinical care in ADHD.
Diagnosis	If new diagnosis of ADHD, if possible, maintain a period of abstinence/low SUD use before diagnosing ADHD in SUD.
Treatment	Treat both conditions simultaneously. With more severe SUD, one may need to address SUD before ADHD treatment. Initiate ADHD treatment as soon as possible. Consider CBT, nonstimulants, or extended-release stimulants in higher-risk groups
Stimulant diversion/misuse	Use of nonstimulants, extended-release, and prodrug stimulants. Avoid immediate-release stimulants Educate and monitor closely

Given the high prevalence of nonmedical use of stimulants,[88,89] it is crucial that providers actively engage in strategies to avoid misuse. Several steps can be taken to promote safer prescription of stimulants, including assessment of potential co-occurring SUDs in patients, refraining from overprescribing (creating a reservoir of excess stimulants), monitoring pill counts, and educating patients on the safe storage, ethical, legal, and medical connotations of stimulant misuse.[86] Recently, a novel, 1-hour intervention for primary care providers has shown promise in decreasing risk factors for stimulant diversion in youth with ADHD through a workshop aimed at building provider skills in educating patients about risks of stimulant misuse, medication monitoring, and other risk reduction practices[90] and a randomized controlled trial of the efficacy of this intervention is ongoing.[91]

SUMMARY

Evaluating and treating co-occurring ADHD in SUD populations is a topic of growing importance in the field of psychiatry. Given the high prevalence of this comorbidity, it is crucial that clinicians working in patient groups with ADHD and/or SUD are aware of recommendations for evaluating and treating this group (**Table 2** for a summary of recommendations). Continuing to monitor for nicotine use and SUD while treating children, adolescents, and adults with ADHD is recommended.

CLINICS CARE POINTS

- Evaluating the presence of ADHD should be part of routine screening in adolescents and adults with SUD
- Patients with ADHD should be monitored for nicotine and substance use and use disorders
- Pharmacotherapy of ADHD reduces the subsequent risk for nicotine and substance use disorders
- Treatment for co-occurring ADHD in SUD populations should begin as early as possible in the SUD treatment process, taking into consideration the severity of existing SUD
- Stimulant medications can be safely and effectively used in SUD populations

DISCLOSURE

D. Taubin and J. Wilson have nothing to disclose. Dr T.E. Wilens is Chief, Division of Child and Adolescent Psychiatry and (Co) Director of the Center for Addiction Medicine at Massachusetts General Hospital. He receives grant support from the following sources: NIH (NIDA). Dr Wilens has published a book, Straight Talk About Psychiatric Medications for Kids (Guilford Press), and co/edited books: ADHD in Adults and Children (Cambridge University Press). Dr Wilens is co/owner of a copyrighted diagnostic questionnaire (Before School Functioning Questionnaire) and has a licensing agreement with Ironshore (BSFQ Questionnaire). He is or has been a consultant for 3D Therapy, Vallon, and Ironshore, and serves as a clinical consultant to the US National Football League (ERM Associates), US Minor/Major League Baseball; Gavin Foundation and Bay Cove Human Services.

REFERENCES

1. van Emmerik-van Oortmerssen K, van de Glind G, van den Brink W, et al. Prevalence of attention-deficit hyperactivity disorder in substance use disorder patients: a meta-analysis and meta-regression analysis. Drug Alcohol Depend 2012;122(1–2):11–9.

2. Wilens TE, Biederman J, Mick E, et al. Attention deficit hyperactivity disorder (ADHD) is associated with early onset substance use disorders. J Nerv Ment Dis 1997;185(8):475–82.

3. Dennis M, Godley SH, Diamond G, et al. The Cannabis Youth Treatment (CYT) Study: main findings from two randomized trials. J Subst Abuse Treat 2004; 27(3):197–213.

4. Coppola M, Mondola R. Impulsivity in alcohol-Dependent patients with and without ADHD: the role of atomoxetine. J Psychoactive Drugs 2018;50(4):361–6.

5. Zaso MJ, Park A, Antshel KM. Treatments for adolescents with comorbid ADHD and substance Use disorder: a systematic review. J Atten Disord 2020;24(9): 1215–26.

6. Capusan AJ, Bendtsen P, Marteinsdottir I, et al. Comorbidity of adult ADHD and its Subtypes with substance Use disorder in a large population-based epidemiological study. J Atten Disord 2019;23(12):1416–26.

7. Merikangas KR, McClair VL. Epidemiology of substance use disorders. Hum Genet 2012;131(6):779–89.

8. Substance abuse and mental health Services administration. Key substance use and mental health indicators in the United States: results from the 2018 national survey on drug Use and health. In: Rockville MD, editor. Center for behavioral health Statistics and Quality, substance abuse and mental health Services administration. 2019.

9. Volkow ND, Koob GF, McLellan AT. Neurobiologic Advances from the brain Disease model of addiction. N Engl J Med 2016;374(4):363–71.

10. Compton WM, Thomas YF, Stinson FS, et al. Prevalence, correlates, disability, and comorbidity of DSM-IV drug abuse and dependence in the United States: results from the national epidemiologic survey on alcohol and related conditions. Arch Gen Psychiatry 2007;64(5):566–76.

11. Wilens TE, Martelon M, Joshi G, et al. Does ADHD predict substance-use disorders? A 10-year follow-up study of young adults with ADHD. J Am Acad Child Adolesc Psychiatry 2011;50(6):543–53.

12. Wilens TE, Martelon M, Fried R, et al. Do executive function deficits predict later substance use disorders among adolescents and young adults? J Am Acad Child Adolesc Psychiatry 2011;50(2):141–9.
13. Charach A, Yeung E, Climans T, et al. Childhood attention-deficit/hyperactivity disorder and future substance use disorders: comparative meta-analyses. J Am Acad Child Adolesc Psychiatry 2011;50(1):9–21.
14. Katusic SK, Barbaresi WJ, Colligan RC, et al. Psychostimulant treatment and risk for substance abuse among young adults with a history of attention-deficit/hyperactivity disorder: a population-based, birth cohort study. J Child Adolesc Psychopharmacol 2005;15(5):764–76.
15. Bierhoff J, Haardörfer R, Windle M, et al. Psychological risk factors for alcohol, cannabis, and Various tobacco Use among young adults: a longitudinal analysis. Subst Use Misuse 2019;54(8):1365–75.
16. van Amsterdam J, van der Velde B, Schulte M, et al. Causal factors of increased smoking in ADHD: a systematic review. Subst Use Misuse 2018;53(3):432–45.
17. Xu G, Snetselaar LG, Strathearn L, et al. Association of attention-deficit/hyperactivity disorder with E-cigarette Use. Am J Prev Med 2021;60(4):488–96.
18. Grant JE, Lust K, Fridberg DJ, et al. E-cigarette use (vaping) is associated with illicit drug use, mental health problems, and impulsivity in university students. Ann Clin Psychiatry 2019;31(1):27–35.
19. Goldenson NI, Khoddam R, Stone MD, et al. Associations of ADHD symptoms with smoking and Alternative tobacco Product Use initiation during adolescence. J Pediatr Psychol 2018;43(6):613–24.
20. Dvorsky MR, Langberg JM. Cigarette and e-cigarette use and social perceptions over the transition to college: the role of ADHD symptoms. Psychol Addict Behav 2019;33(3):318–30.
21. Kahraman Ö, Demirci E. Internet addiction and attention-deficit-hyperactivity disorder: effects of anxiety, depression and self-esteem. Pediatr Int 2018;60(6):529–34.
22. Enagandula R, Singh S, Adgaonkar GW, et al. Study of Internet addiction in children with attention-deficit hyperactivity disorder and normal control. Ind Psychiatry J 2018;27(1):110–4.
23. Yen JY, Liu TL, Wang PW, et al. Association between Internet gaming disorder and adult attention deficit and hyperactivity disorder and their correlates: impulsivity and hostility. Addict Behav 2017;64:308–13.
24. Shen Y, Wang L, Huang C, et al. Sex differences in prevalence, risk factors and clinical correlates of internet addiction among Chinese college students. J Affect Disord 2021;279:680–6.
25. Schoenmacker GH, Groenman AP, Sokolova E, et al. Role of conduct problems in the relation between Attention-Deficit Hyperactivity disorder, substance use, and gaming. Eur Neuropsychopharmacol 2020;30:102–13.
26. Panagiotidi M. Problematic video Game play and ADHD Traits in an adult population. Cyberpsychol Behav Soc Netw 2017;20(5):292–5.
27. Brandt L, Fischer G. Adult ADHD is associated with gambling severity and psychiatric comorbidity among treatment-seeking Problem Gamblers. J Atten Disord 2019;23(12):1383–95.
28. Yule AM, Carrellas NW, DiSalvo M, et al. Risk factors for Overdose in young people who received substance Use disorder treatment. Am J Addict 2019;28(5):382–9.
29. van der Burg D, Crunelle CL, Matthys F, et al. Diagnosis and treatment of patients with comorbid substance use disorder and adult attention-deficit and

hyperactivity disorder: a review of recent publications. Curr Opin Psychiatry 2019;32(4):300–6.

30. Silbernagl M, Yanagida T, Slamanig R, et al. Comorbidity Patterns among patients with opioid Use disorder and Problem gambling: ADHD status predicts Class membership. J Dual Diagn 2019;15(3):147–58.

31. Coetzee C, Truter I, Meyer A. Prevalence and characteristics of South African treatment-seeking patients with substance use disorder and co-occurring attention-deficit/hyperactivity disorder. Expert Rev Clin Pharmacol 2020;13(11):1271–80.

32. Wilens TE, Kaminski TA. The co-occurrence of ADHD and substance use disorders. Psychiatr Ann 2018;48(7):328–32.

33. van Wingen GA, van den Brink W, Veltman DJ, et al. Reduced striatal brain volumes in non-medicated adult ADHD patients with comorbid cocaine dependence. Drug Alcohol Depend 2013;131(3):198–203.

34. Tervo-Clemmens B, Quach A, Calabro FJ, et al. Meta-analysis and review of functional neuroimaging differences underlying adolescent vulnerability to substance use. Neuroimage 2020;209:116476.

35. Adisetiyo V, Gray KM. Neuroimaging the neural correlates of increased risk for substance use disorders in attention-deficit/hyperactivity disorder-A systematic review. Am J Addict 2017;26(2):99–111.

36. Regnart J, Truter I, Meyer A. Critical exploration of co-occurring attention-deficit/hyperactivity disorder, mood disorder and substance Use disorder. Expert Rev Pharmacoecon Outcomes Res 2017;17(3):275–82.

37. Yule AM, Martelon M, Faraone SV, et al. Examining the association between attention deficit hyperactivity disorder and substance use disorders: a familial risk analysis. J Psychiatr Res 2017;85:49–55.

38. Wimberley T, Agerbo E, Horsdal HT, et al. Genetic liability to ADHD and substance use disorders in individuals with ADHD. Addiction 2020;115(7):1368–77.

39. Khantzian EJ. The self-medication hypothesis of substance use disorders: a reconsideration and recent applications. Harv Rev Psychiatry 1997;4(5):231–44.

40. Manni C, Cipollone G, Pallucchini A, et al. Remarkable reduction of cocaine Use in dual disorder (adult attention deficit hyperactive disorder/cocaine Use disorder) patients treated with medications for ADHD. Int J Environ Res Public Health 2019;16(20).

41. Faraone SV, Wilens TE, Petty C, et al. Substance use among ADHD adults: Implications of late onset and subthreshold diagnoses. Am J Addict 2007;16(Suppl 1):24–32, quiz 33-24.

42. Looby A, Sant'Ana S. Nonmedical prescription stimulant users experience subjective but not objective impairments in attention and impulsivity. Am J Addict 2018;27(3):238–44.

43. Quinn PD, Chang Z, Hur K, et al. ADHD medication and substance-related problems. Am J Psychiatry 2017;174(9):877–85.

44. Chang Z, Lichtenstein P, Halldner L, et al. Stimulant ADHD medication and risk for substance abuse. J Child Psychol Psychiatry 2014;55(8):878–85.

45. Wilens TE, Adamson J, Monuteaux MC, et al. Effect of prior stimulant treatment for attention-deficit/hyperactivity disorder on subsequent risk for cigarette smoking and alcohol and drug use disorders in adolescents. Arch Pediatr Adolesc Med 2008;162(10):916–21.

46. Boland H, DiSalvo M, Fried R, et al. A literature review and meta-analysis on the effects of ADHD medications on functional outcomes. J Psychiatri Res 2020;123:21–30.

47. McCabe SE, Dickinson K, West BT, et al. Age of onset, duration, and Type of medication therapy for attention-deficit/hyperactivity disorder and substance Use during adolescence: a Multi-cohort national study. J Am Acad Child Adolesc Psychiatry 2016;55(6):479–86.

48. Crunelle CL, van den Brink W, Moggi F, et al. International consensus Statement on screening, diagnosis and treatment of substance Use disorder patients with comorbid attention deficit/hyperactivity disorder. Eur Addict Res 2018;24(1): 43–51.

49. Perugi G, Pallucchini A, Rizzato S, et al. Pharmacotherapeutic strategies for the treatment of attention-deficit hyperactivity (ADHD) disorder with comorbid substance-use disorder (SUD). Expert Opin Pharmacother 2019;20(3):343–55.

50. Wilens TE, Adler LA, Tanaka Y, et al. Correlates of alcohol use in adults with ADHD and comorbid alcohol use disorders: exploratory analysis of a placebo-controlled trial of atomoxetine. Curr Med Res Opin 2011;27(12):2309–20.

51. Wilens TE, Morrison NR. The intersection of attention-deficit/hyperactivity disorder and substance abuse. Curr Opin Psychiatry 2011;24(4):280–5.

52. Faraone SV, Biederman J, Spencer TJ, et al. Diagnosing adult attention deficit hyperactivity disorder: are late onset and subthreshold diagnoses valid? Am J Psychiatry 2006;163(10):1720–9.

53. Levin FR, Choi CJ, Pavlicova M, et al. How treatment improvement in ADHD and cocaine dependence are related to one another: a secondary analysis. Drug Alcohol Depend 2018;188:135–40.

54. Hammerness P, Joshi G, Doyle R, et al. Do stimulants reduce the risk for cigarette smoking in youth with attention-deficit hyperactivity disorder? A prospective, Long-term, open-label study of extended-release methylphenidate. J Pediatr 2013;162(1):22–7.

55. Ginsberg L, Katic A, Adeyi B, et al. Long-term treatment outcomes with lisdexamfetamine dimesylate for adults with attention-deficit/hyperactivity disorder stratified by baseline severity. Curr Med Res Opin 2011;27(6):1097–107.

56. Kast KA, Rao V, Wilens TE. Pharmacotherapy for attention-deficit/hyperactivity disorder and retention in outpatient substance Use disorder treatment: a retrospective cohort study. J Clin Psychiatry 2021;82(2).

57. van Emmerik-van Oortmerssen K, Vedel E, van den Brink W, et al. Integrated cognitive behavioral therapy for patients with substance use disorder and comorbid ADHD: two case presentations. Addict Behav 2015;45:214–7.

58. Carroll KM, Kiluk BD. Cognitive behavioral interventions for alcohol and drug use disorders: through the stage model and back again. Psychol Addict Behav 2017; 31(8):847–61.

59. Magill M, Ray LA. Cognitive-behavioral treatment with adult alcohol and illicit drug users: a meta-analysis of randomized controlled trials. J Stud Alcohol Drugs 2009;70(4):516–27.

60. Safren SA, Otto M, Sprich S, et al. Cognitive-behavioral therapy for ADHD in medication-treated adults with continued symptoms. Beh Res Ther 2005;43(7): 831–42.

61. Solanto MV, Surman CB, Alvir JMJ. The efficacy of cognitive-behavioral therapy for older adults with ADHD: a randomized controlled trial. Atten Defic Hyperact Disord 2018;10(3):223–35.

62. van Emmerik-van Oortmerssen K, Vedel E, Kramer FJ, et al. Integrated cognitive behavioral therapy for ADHD in adult substance use disorder patients: results of a randomized clinical trial. Drug Alcohol Depend 2019;197:28–36.

63. Castells X, Ramos-Quiroga JA, Rigau D, et al. Efficacy of methylphenidate for adults with attention-deficit hyperactivity disorder: a meta-regression analysis. CNS Drugs 2011;25(2):157–69.

64. Wilens TE, Adler LA, Weiss MD, et al. Atomoxetine treatment of adults with ADHD and comorbid alcohol use disorders. Drug Alcohol Depend 2008;96(1–2): 145–54.

65. Bastiaens L, Scott O, Galus J. Treatment of adult ADHD without stimulants: effectiveness in A dually diagnosed correctional population. Psychiatr Q 2019; 90(1):41–6.

66. Thurstone C, Riggs PD, Salomonsen-Sautel S, et al. Randomized, controlled trial of atomoxetine for attention-deficit/hyperactivity disorder in adolescents with substance use disorder. J Am Acad Child Adolesc Psychiatry 2010;49(6):573–82.

67. Nasser A, Hull JT, Liranso T, et al. The effect of viloxazine extended-release Capsules on functional impairments associated with attention-deficit/hyperactivity disorder (ADHD) in children and adolescents in Four phase 3 placebo-controlled trials. Neuropsychiatr Dis Treat 2021;17:1751–62.

68. Altamura AC, Mauri MC, Girardi T, et al. Alcoholism and depression: a placebo controlled study with viloxazine. Int J Clin Pharmacol Res 1990;10(5):293–8.

69. Konstenius M, Jayaram-Lindstrom N, Guterstam J, et al. Methylphenidate for attention deficit hyperactivity disorder and drug relapse in criminal offenders with substance dependence: a 24-week randomized placebo-controlled trial. Addiction 2014;109(3):440–9.

70. Levin FR, Mariani JJ, Specker S, et al. Extended-release mixed amphetamine salts vs placebo for comorbid adult attention-deficit/hyperactivity disorder and cocaine Use disorder: a randomized clinical trial. JAMA Psychiatry 2015;72(6): 593–602.

71. Cunill R, Castells X, Tobias A, et al. Pharmacological treatment of attention deficit hyperactivity disorder with co-morbid drug dependence. J Psychopharmacol 2015;29(1):15–23.

72. Skoglund C, Brandt L, D'Onofrio B, et al. Methylphenidate doses in Attention Deficit/Hyperactivity Disorder and comorbid substance use disorders. Eur Neuro-psychopharmacol 2017;27(11):1144–52.

73. McKowen JW, Isenberg BM, Carrellas NW, et al. Neuropsychological changes in patients with substance use disorder after completion of a one month intensive outpatient treatment program. Am J Addict 2018;27(8):632–8.

74. Helene Bergly T, Julius Sømhovd M. The relation between ADHD medication and mild cognitive impairment, as assessed by the Montreal cognitive assessment (MoCA), in patients entering substance Use disorder inpatient treatment. J Dual Diagn 2018;14(4):228–36.

75. Adler L, Guida F, Irons S, et al. Open label Pilot study of atomoxetine in adults with ADHD and substance Use disorder. J Dual Diagn 2010;6(3–4):196–207.

76. Barkla XM, McArdle PA, Newbury-Birch D. Are there any potentially dangerous pharmacological effects of combining ADHD medication with alcohol and drugs of abuse? A systematic review of the literature. BMC Psychiatry 2015;15(1):270.

77. Grabowski J, Roache JD, Schmitz JM, et al. Replacement medication for cocaine dependence: Methylphenidate. J Clin Psychopharmacol 1997;17(6):485–8.

78. Wilens T, Kwon A, Tanguay S, et al. Characteristics of adults with attention deficit hyperactivity disorder plus substance use disorder: the role of psychiatric comorbidity. Am J Addict 2005;14(4):319–28.

79. Weyandt LL, Oster DR, Marraccini ME, et al. Pharmacological interventions for adolescents and adults with ADHD: stimulant and nonstimulant medications and misuse of prescription stimulants. Psychol Res Behav Manag 2014;7:223–49.

80. Kilmer JR, Geisner IM, Gasser ML, et al. Normative perceptions of non-medical stimulant use: associations with actual use and hazardous drinking. Addict Behav 2015;42:51–6.

81. Faraone SV, Rostain AL, Montano CB, et al. Systematic review: nonmedical Use of prescription stimulants: risk factors, outcomes, and risk reduction strategies. J Am Acad Child Adolesc Psychiatry 2020;59(1):100–12.

82. Wilens T, Zulauf C, Martelon M, et al. Nonmedical stimulant Use in college students: association with attention-deficit/hyperactivity disorder and other disorders. J Clin Psychiatry 2016;77(7):940–7.

83. Wilens TE, Martelon M, Yule A, et al. Disentangling the social context of nonmedical Use of prescription stimulants in college students. Am J Addict 2020;29(6): 476–84. https://doi.org/10.1111/ajad.13053.

84. Wilens TE, Carrellas NW, Martelon M, et al. Neuropsychological functioning in college students who misuse prescription stimulants. Am J Addict 2017;26(4): 379–87.

85. Colaneri NM, Keim SA, Adesman A. Physician perceptions of ADHD stimulant diversion and misuse. J Atten Disord 2020;24(2):290–300.

86. Wilens TE, Kaminski TA. Editorial: stimulants: Friend or Foe? J Am Acad Child Adolesct Psychiatry 2020;59(1):36–7.

87. Whitaker TM, Oldenhof J, Szeto IW, et al. Abuse-Deterrent properties of a novel formlation of immediate-release dextroamphetamine compared to reference dextroamphetamine immediate-release. J Am Acad Child Adolesc Psychiatry 2020;59(10):S262.

88. McCabe SE, West BT, Teter CJ, et al. Trends in medical use, diversion, and nonmedical use of prescription medications among college students from 2003 to 2013: connecting the dots. Addict Behav 2014;39(7):1176–82.

89. McCabe SE, Veliz P, Wilens TE, et al. Adolescents' prescription stimulant Use and adult functional outcomes: a national prospective study. J Am Acad Child Adolesc Psychiatry 2017;56(3):226–233 e224.

90. Molina BSG, Kipp HL, Joseph HM, et al. Stimulant diversion risk among college students treated for ADHD: primary care provider Prevention Training. Acad Pediatr 2020;20(1):119–27.

91. McGuier EA, Kolko DJ, Joseph HM, et al. Use of stimulant diversion Prevention strategies in Pediatric primary care and associations with provider characteristics. J Adolesc Health 2021;68(4):808–15.

Addressing the Treatment and Service Needs of Young Adults with Attention Deficit Hyperactivity Disorder

Javier Quintero, M.D., Ph.D., Head of Service[a,b,*],
Alberto Rodríguez-Quiroga, M.D., Ph.D.[a,b],
Miguel Ángel Álvarez-Mon, Ph.D, M.D.[a,d,e],
Fernando Mora, M.D., Ph.D.[a,b], Anthony L. Rostain, M.D., M.A.[c]

KEYWORDS

- ADHD • Transition of care • Stimulants • Methylphenidate • Lisdexamfetamine
- Nonstimulants • Atomoxetine • Guanfacine

KEY POINTS

- The transition from adolescence to adulthood is a critical period during which many important changes take place (education, work, independent living, and social relations).
- Transfer of care is defined as "the purposeful, planned movement of adolescents and young adults with chronic physical and medical conditions from child-centered to adult-oriented healthcare systems".
- There are many barriers to achieving a smooth transfer of care from childhood and adolescent mental health services to adult mental health services for people suffering from attention deficit hyperactivity disorder (ADHD).
- Optimal transfer of care must be planned, structured, and coordinated.
- Young people with ADHD benefit from ongoing medical treatment with either psychostimulant or nonstimulant medications and psychosocial interventions such as cognitive behavioral therapy and mindfulness practices.

---

[a] Psychiatry and Mental Health Department, Hospital Universitario Infanta Leonor, Avenida de la Gran Vía del Este 80, Madrid 20830, Spain; [b] Department of Legal Medicine & Psychiatry, Complutense University, Spain; [c] Department of Psychiatry, Cooper Medical School of Rowan University, 401 Broadway, Camden, NJ 08103, USA; [d] Department of Medicine and Medical Specialities, Faculty of Medicine and Health Sciences, University of Alcala, 28801 Alcala de Henares, Spain; [e] Ramon y Cajal Institute of Sanitary Research (IRYCIS), 28034 Madrid, Spain
* Corresponding author.
E-mail address: fjquinterog@yahoo.es

Child Adolesc Psychiatric Clin N Am 31 (2022) 531–551
https://doi.org/10.1016/j.chc.2022.03.007
1056-4993/22/© 2022 Elsevier Inc. All rights reserved.
childpsych.theclinics.com

Abbreviations	
ADHD	Attention Deficit Hyperactivity Disorder
CAMHS	Childhood and Adolescent Mental Health Services
AMHS	Adult Mental Health Services
ASD	Autism Spectrum Disorder
TAY	Transitional Aged Youth
PFC	Prefrontal Cortex
HIV	Human Immunodeficiency Virus
COVID-19	Coronavirus Disease 2019

INTRODUCTION

Attention deficit hyperactivity disorder (ADHD) is a neurodevelopmental disorder characterized by a persistent pattern of inattention and/or hyperactivity-impulsivity that interferes with functioning or development.[1] It usually begins in childhood and persists through adolescence into adulthood in approximately 35% to 50% of individuals diagnosed as children,[2] with an estimated worldwide prevalence of 7.2%.[3] A systematic review and meta-analysis describes childhood factors that predict persistence into adulthood.[4] These include severity of ADHD symptoms, receiving treatment of ADHD, comorbid conduct disorder, and comorbid major depressive disorder.

The transition between adolescence and adulthood is a critical period in which many important changes take place (education, work, independent living, and social relations).[5] Similar to other adolescents with mental disorders, individuals diagnosed with ADHD are at risk of falling between the cracks of different mental health service systems[6] because levels of psychiatric care and educational services provided to youth with ADHD decreases when they move from adolescence to adulthood.[7] Despite the rising incidence of mental illness in adolescents,[8] there are many barriers to achieving a smooth transition childhood and adolescent mental health services (CAMHS) to adult mental health services (AMHS),[9,10] especially in the case of ADHD, one of the most common disorders in youth.[11] Although it is true that continuity of treatment and follow-up has always been a challenge in ADHD, the COVID-19 pandemic has worsened this difficulty.

DISCUSSION
Developmental Risk Factors

ADHD confers ongoing developmental risk throughout the individual's lifetime because it is associated with other mental disorders, educational and occupational failure, accidents, criminality, social disability, and addictions.[12] Unfortunately, discontinuation of treatment during transition between adolescence and adulthood is much higher than at other ages.[13] The proportion of young adults who continue treatment declines at a greater rate than age-related decrease in symptoms and there is a drop-off in levels of ADHD treatment among young adults. This means that people with ADHD do not receive the care they need when they transition to adults.[14,15] Moreover, patients rarely resume the treatment of ADHD after discontinuation.[13] Continuity of care is hampered by a multitude of circumstances and factors, including individual and system variables, which have been described in previous studies. **Table 1** summarizes the different risk factors. Individual factors include sociodemographic and clinical variables. Sociodemographic variables can be classified into age, age of diagnosis, and gender. Younger age is correlated with better use of mental health-care services[16] and being older at the time of discontinuing treatment of ADHD in

Table 1
Risk factors that affect the transition process

Individual Factors		Organizational Factors
Sociodemographic	Clinical Variables	Lack of information
Age	Symptom severity	Different thresholds between CAMHS and AMHS
Age of diagnosis	Comorbidities	Adult service workloads
Gender	Treatment	Variability in service cut-off ages

adolescence made it more likely for patients to resume treatment during young adulthood.[17] Moreover, age of diagnosis is a predictor of treatment continuity because adolescents first diagnosed with ADHD during this period who attended in CAMHS are more likely to continue mental health treatment at AMHS.[18] Finally, regarding gender, girls diagnosed with ADHD in CAMHS continue treatment in AMHS more than boys do.[16]

Clinical variables include symptom severity, comorbidities, and treatment. Severity has been directly related with continuity of ADHD treatment in young adulthood in different studies, as more patients with severe or persistent ADHD symptoms and a greater level of impairment were more likely to be referred to AMHS to continue treatment.[16,19] In general, the presence of comorbidities makes it easier for ADHD patients to continue follow-up and treatment at AMHS. Psychotic and affective disorders, as well as learning disabilities increase the use of AMHS.[17,18] With respect to the presence of autism spectrum disorder (ASD), studies have shown conflicting results. On one hand, ASD may be associated with a more difficult transition to AMHS,[20] and on the other hand, ASD is associated with a lower likelihood of medication cessation.[18] Receiving treatment during adolescence increases the likelihood of continuity of treatment during young adulthood. Specifically, being on pharmacologic treatment or in combined treatment (medication and psychotherapy) increases the probability of attending AMHS.[18,21] Furthermore, taking non-ADHD psychotropic medication is associated with a reduced likelihood of medication cessation and taking an antipsychotic medication is strongly associated with resumption of ADHD treatment after cessation.[17,19] Psychotherapy itself, however, is associated with decreased use of AMHS.[18] Finally, organizational factors also play an important role in the transition process. Lack of clarity on service availability and eligibility criteria, different thresholds between CAMHS and AMHS, adult service workloads, and variability in service cut-off ages have been proposed as broad factors that could hamper transition.[22] In addition, patients and parents have identified several critical factors predicting maintenance of treatment: Clinician qualities and ability to form a treatment relationship, professional roles, responsibility of care, nature and severity of problems, expectations focused in AMHS, uncertainties around transition,[23,24] lack of information on available services, and no help or guidance.[25,26]

Clinicians have described several considerations and recommendations for an optimal transition process. These are summarized in **Box 1**. There must be anticipatory guidance with shared information among clinicians, patients, and parents[25,27] that includes discussions about the changing health needs of adolescents transitioning to adulthood.[24] There must also be an adult community mental health service to refer patients to.[27] Optimally, this process should last between 2 and 6 months, with parallel care and parental involvement during the whole process[24] and should be completed by the age of 18.[25] Of note, parent or caregiver involvement has been reported as a highly significant factor in young people accessing adult services.[28]

> **Box 1**
> **Clinician's recommendations for an optimal transition process**
>
> 1. There must be anticipatory guidance with shared information among clinicians, patients, and parents.
> 2. The changing health needs of adolescents transitioning to adulthood should be discussed.
> 3. There should be an adult community mental health service to refer patients to.
> 4. The transition process should last between 2 and 6 months, with parallel care and parental involvement during the whole process.
> 5. The transition process should be completed by the age of 18.

There has also been a claim from several authors for more education, training and skill development in clinicians supporting adults with ADHD, especially because many patients perceive negative attitudes and skepticism about adult ADHD when they transition to adult services.[28] Finally, functional difficulties associated with the transition from adolescence to adulthood (referred to as transitional aged youth; TAY) also play an important role.[29] Throughout the transition, TAY must face the challenge of being more autonomous and responsible while external structures and family supports decrease. Therefore, ADHD is likely to lead to considerable impairments in multiple settings.[30]

To address these gaps, *transitional care* has arisen as "the purposeful, planned movement of adolescents and young adults with chronic physical and medical conditions from child-centered to adult-oriented healthcare system".[31] To date, there has been relatively little research on the transition of ADHD patients from CAMHS to AMHS, with little information available on the quality of transition experiences and on the variety of organizational arrangements that exist in different countries.[32]

How Is Transition Assessed?

Measuring transition can be extremely challenging. On the one hand, one can assess the ways in which the transition between different health service systems occurs (*situational*). On the other hand, one can examine the changing expectations and skills required in navigating the passage from adolescence to adulthood (*developmental*).[33] The latter has often been assessed using the "big five" social roles of adulthood: educational attainment, employment, partnership, residential independence, and parenthood.[34] However, given recent extensive and rapid social changes, transition into adulthood is no longer a predictable linear sequence but a discontinuous route with multiple paths.[35] The Inventory of the Dimensions of Emerging Adulthood was developed to explore individual differences in self-identification within the processes of emerging adulthood, which is the time of life roughly between ages 18 and 25.[36,37] By contrast, some authors assert that markers of adulthood, which could be useful to assess during this period, are no longer valid indicators.[38] A study comparing how emerging adults with ADHD experienced their transition into adulthood and how they accomplished this transition (depending on the intensity of ADHD symptoms) found that the level of ADHD symptoms was associated with a lower success in the transition into adulthood, with inattention symptoms showing the strongest association with outcome.[39] Considering that the transition between different health-care service systems is complex and multifactorial, studies have used qualitative methodology to assess transition protocols. These include retrospective case note surveys and reviews evaluating transition experiences, electronic monitoring of ADHD medication, surveillance systems and transfer processes, and accounts of users', carers', and professionals' views of transition processes.[22,40–44] These studies conclude that being involved in multiple transitions is a complex and unsettling experience for most people because it is usually poorly planned and poorly executed. The whole experience improves when this happens gradually, and it is tailored to the young person's needs.

Executive Functioning and Self-Monitoring

Children and adolescents with ADHD show significant impairments on measures of response inhibition, working memory, and motivation.[45] Executive functions are the "neurocognitive processes that maintain an appropriate problem-solving set to attain a later goal".[46] Deficits in executive functioning are not specific to ADHD because they can occur in children with other conditions and in children without mental disorders.[45] These deficits are thought to be caused by anomalies in prefrontal striatal brain circuitry, which are insufficiently or inconsistently modulated by the expression of catecholamines.[47,48] During adolescence, significant neurocognitive reorganization and development occur. For instance, the prefrontal cortex (PFC) is the last brain region to mature, continuing to myelinate into early adulthood.[49] The PFC is responsible for highly integrative cognitive functions such as executive control.[46]

The self-monitoring construct refers to interindividual differences in the degree to which people observe, regulate, and control the image of themselves that they display in social situations and in interpersonal relationships.[50] Snyder developed a scale to assess self-monitoring (self-monitoring scale). This scale includes 5 hypothetical components of the self-monitoring construct[51]: concern with the adequacy of one's social behavior or self-presentation, sensitivity to the clues that indicate the situational adequacy of self-presentation, the ability to control and modify self-presentation and expressive behavior, the use of this ability in particular situations, and the degree of situational specificity of expressive behavior and self-presentation. Adolescence is configured as a time in which the individual experiences entry into new social worlds, more complex and changing than those that had constituted their childhood. Such social and interpersonal microworlds are primarily constructed with the establishment of groups and romantic and sexual relationships, both of which shape the identity of the person. This implies a greater concern for the adolescent's social image and greater attention to social information, both of which will allow the adolescent to choose the appropriate self-representations with which to integrate and participate in these new social scenarios.[52] Thus, adolescence is an intermediate phase between child and adult behavior models, in which the adolescent seeks to outline their own identity, an adult identity. This also implies a greater sensitivity to how adults behave, especially those who serve as identity models.[52]

Adolescence is also a highly stress-sensitive period that differs considerably from other stages of development.[53] This increased susceptibility is associated with changes in neuroplasticity in the prefrontal cortex, mainly through the maturation of mesocortical dopaminergic projections. Alterations in this maturation process due to adverse events during adolescence and mediated by an excess of stress hormones, such as glucocorticoids, are the cause of aberrant behavior models in animals, such as deficiencies in information processing, mood control, and hypersensitivity to psychostimulants.[54,55] A large study in the neuroimaging of ADHD, in addition to other mental disorders (Enhancing NeuroImaging Genetics through Meta-Analysis) collected information from 2264 participants with ADHD and 1934 controls from up to 36 sites.[56] Results showed lower total surface area, mainly in frontal, cingulate, and temporal regions, especially in children, and a reduction in bilateral amygdala, striatal, and hippocampal volumes.[56]

Adolescents with ADHD tend to have limited insight into the nature of ADHD, the possible benefits of medication, and the importance of treatment adherence.[57] There is a tendency to believe that the only purpose of ADHD medication is to assist with completion of schoolwork. If this is the case, adolescents transitioning to adulthood might assume that treatment is no longer needed if they are no longer attending school.[56] The stigma associated with mental disorders and the adolescent's perception of peer attitudes might also contribute as factors to withdraw from treatment.[58] Even more, parents can also be reluctant about treatment or even if they are supportive and positive, this might be completely outweighed by peer and/or adolescent's own beliefs.[59]

COVID-19 Impact

As COVID-19 has spread worldwide, there has been growing recognition of the mental health implications of the pandemic, both for people with mental disorders and for the general population.[60] The pandemic seems to worsen ADHD symptoms resulting in increasing emotional disturbance, social disability, and functional impairment because individuals with neurodevelopmental disorders are especially vulnerable to the distress caused by the pandemic's consequences (eg, physical distancing measures).[61] ADHD symptoms need to be adequately treated in view of the broad restrictions imposed by lockdowns and other measures to reduce spread of the coronavirus.[62] Among the factors that may have contributed to worsening ADHD symptoms are the loss of environmental structure and daily routine,[63] the loss of opportunities for educational special needs,[64] and the reduction of physical, academic, and working activities.[62] Individuals with ADHD are generally less tolerant of uncertainty compared with peers. In addition, they may have more difficulties in following instructions and understanding the complexity of the pandemic situation.[65] During the early stages of the pandemic, the European ADHD Guidelines Group recommended avoiding using higher doses of medication to manage crisis or stress, or using antipsychotics to manage disruptive behavior.[61] A survey following children and adolescents from 2017 in England found that those with a probable mental disorder were more likely to say that lockdown had worsened their life (54.1% of 11–16-year-old children, and 59.0% of 17–22-year-old adolescents), compared with those unlikely to have a mental disorder (39.2% and 37.3%, respectively).[66] Emotional and behavioral problems have also been found in a group of children with neurodevelopmental disorders in the United Kingdom, especially conduct problems in the ADHD group.[67] In fact, a recent systematic review and meta-analysis found that children with neurodevelopmental disorders (ADHD and ASD) had a high probability for worsening of their behavioral symptoms.[68] A study based on a survey in the United States described that the most common problems for adolescents and young adults with ADHD were social isolation, difficulties engaging in online learning, motivation problems, and boredom.[69]

Among parents and caregivers, there was an increase in irritability (37.5%), shouting at the child (43.8%), verbal abuse (25%), and use of punishments (27.1%).[70] During the pandemic, and especially during lockdown, parents and other caregivers had to face educational, emotional, and behavioral problems on their own.[71] Diminished family support due to social distancing might have contributed to increased parenting stress and burden, often leading to exacerbations of their children's behavioral problems.[63]

A study of university students in Wuhan, China, found an increase in problematic Internet use in individuals with ADHD.[72] A survey of parents of ADHD youth in Zurich, Switzerland, found higher rates of difficulties concentrating, excessive irritability, or worsening symptoms of ADHD under lockdown for those spending the most time with screen media.[73] A survey study from Shanghai, China, found that during the COVID-19 pandemic, patients with ADHD and problematic Internet use experienced more severe core symptoms, more negative emotions, greater executive function deficits, worsening family relationships, more pressure from life events, and a lower motivation to learn.[74]

By contrast, other findings during the lockdown suggest that there may have been an *improvement* in both the behavior and mood of ADHD children and adolescents.[74] In order to prevent the delay in transition between services, a specific tertiary-level specialist ADHD pathway (ADMiRE) was introduced in South Dublin (Ireland) as a way to provide early access to evidence-based assessment, diagnosis, and intervention for children who were presenting difficulties suggestive of ADHD.[75] Among the challenges this group identified were delays in new assessments, changeover to telemetric evaluation, lack of school feedback, and delays in the start of psychopharmacological treatment as well as in the titration and optimization of ADHD medication. Furthermore, there was a significant decrease in the number of referrals. Another study using qualitative measures to assess the psychosocial and behavioral impact of Japan's lockdown found 5 different themes in adults with ADHD[1]: Terrible feeling caused by frustration, stress, and anger[2]; closeness due to the internal difficulties and conflict[3]; deteriorating ADHD symptoms and executive function related matters[3]; condition is the same as usual; and[5] positive aspects associated with the self-lockdown.[76] Another study performed in Israel, which investigated the rate of ADHD among COVID-19-positive subjects, found that untreated, rather than treated ADHD, could be a risk factor for COVID-19.[77] Even more, ADHD can be associated with increased severity of COVID-19 symptoms.[78] These studies suggest clinicians should proactively discuss COVID-19 prevention with ADHD patients. In a different study from the United Kingdom, the authors found that the pandemic had mild effects on the mental health of treated ADHD adults.[79]

However, a study in the United States found there no correlations among ADHD and population size, and infection and mortality rates from coronavirus. In fact, recovery rates increased with the prevalence of ADHD, leading the authors to hypothesize that ADHD may promote evolutionary advantages.[80] Along similar lines, a French study reported improvements in restlessness and in the length of studying time linked to a decrease of distress created by rhythms imposed by academic activities.[81] According to these authors, the less school-related strain, the more flexible schedules, and the lower exposure of children to school's negative feedback led to an improvement in self-esteem among children and adolescents with ADHD.[81] An Italian survey study of 992 parents corresponding to 528 children and adolescents with ADHD found a significant decreased frequency of mood and behavioral problems but an increase in the frequency of boredom, temper tantrums and little enjoyment, with an increase in sadness for children and an increase in physical aggression for adolescents.[65] In some cases, as reported in a survey conducted in Chandigarh, India, lockdown led parents to increase their praising and the time spent with their children.[70]

Unmet Needs

Given the transition gap between different health-care systems, it is highly probable that adult ADHD remains underrecognized, underdiagnosed, and, therefore, undertreated.[82] Difficulties with service availability and delivery have been previously described,[22–29] with an increasing demand to provide services to both young people and adults with ADHD. Insufficient and/or inadequate clinical education relating to developmental, psychosocial, and even cultural issues associated with ADHD in the transition period can also be a barrier.[57] For some authors, ADHD is yet to be seen as a universal condition that should be managed by AMHS, in multidisciplinary services with specialist expertise.[83] Of even greater concern, some clinicians are still skeptical about the validity of the diagnosis[84] or are reluctant to diagnose young people.[85] Despite these attitudes, many studies have concluded that, although ADHD may manifest in childhood, more than half of cases persist into adult life.[86]

Protocols, practice guidelines, and public health policies available to manage patients with ADHD transitioning to adulthood are limited.[87] A review of the literature surrounding ADHD and transition found that policies related to adult ADHD are sparse; whereas, there are many recommendations regarding transition for young people with ADHD, there is still little research demonstrating how this process can best be implemented.[83] The main policy document identified for children, young people, and adults with ADHD is the National Institute for Health and Clinical Excellence Clinical Guideline 72, published in 2008, which recommends the establishment of multidisciplinary teams with expertise in adult ADHD as well as providing guidance for an adequate transition.[88] In view of the paucity of health services research, Singh recommends documenting unmet service user needs in people with ADHD in the process of transition.[41]

The rate of use of AMHS in the population aged 18 to 19 years is approximately half (18 per 1000 inhabitants) of the rate of use of AMHS in patients aged 16 to 17 years (34 per 1000 inhabitants); and it remains low until 25 years of age.[89] Attrition to follow-up and failure to complete treatment pose a major problem for the successful treatment of transitional age youth with severe mental illness because it is highly associated with major clinical and socio-economic problems.[90] As mentioned before, the factors that may be acting in the process of transition can be divided into patient-dependent factors (ambivalence or denial[91]), disease-related factors (interference with psychosocial functioning[42]), and factors dependent on the treatment system (ie, organization of Health Services). Given that most mental disorders have a chronic course, most people will need psychopharmacological treatments and psychosocial interventions throughout life.[92] Clinical practice guidelines emphasize the importance of long-term supportive therapeutic relationships with health-care professionals to ensure that patients receive individualized care focused on their needs.[93] This is especially important during this phase of life.[94] Several countries have promoted the role of case managers—people in charge of administering and coordinating patient care—to ensure that people with chronic mental illness receive consistent and coordinated care, tailored to their needs.[94,95] The lack of consistent implementation of this type of evidence-based practice is considered one of the treatment-dependent factors leading to suboptimal care.[96] Most patients with severe mental illness who receive elective and continuous care over time have been shown to have fewer relapses, less hospital care, and more medical care related to physical health issues, along with reduced overall costs.[97] Currently, many adolescents and young adults experience poorer control of chronic diseases at the time of transition, such as poorer glycemic control in diabetes,[98] organ rejection problems in transplant recipients,[99] poorer epilepsy control,[100] and poorer HIV control.[101] Adolescents and young adults with mental disorders face similar challenges during the transition to AMHS.

Previous studies have shown that young people transitioning to adult health services experience concern about the loss of known and familiar surroundings, as well as concern about the loss of the bond with the therapist,[102] while they continue to expect health-care providers and professionals meet their needs.[103] Patients have emphasized the importance of relationships with staff, as well as their qualities, that is, their flexibility, their ability to instill hope, to provide support and comfort, without prejudice, or to be a good listener. They also value receiving sufficient preparation (through advance notification of the transition to AMHS) as well as having direct participation in the transition planning itself.[104] Furthermore, a negative emotional experience is preceded by the loss of the clinical relationship and the fear of less support in AMHS.[103] During the transition stage, patients believed that the timing of the transition was arbitrary, and some questioned the need for a transition. In addition, they greatly appreciated those transitions that occurred gradually and were tailored according to their individual needs.[104] Once in AMHS, the lack of information exchange between services forced patients to repeat their personal history to various professionals.[105] The relationship between patients and health-care providers, and specifically, the therapeutic bond, is paramount.[106] For patients with a personal history of trauma or family conflict, the loss of important relationships can contribute to poorer transition experiences that affect overall well-being. Difficulty forming new relationships with AMHS clinicians may also lead to a poorer therapeutic alliance and an increased risk of loss to follow-up.[107]

Knowing that an optimal transition requires adequate planning, good information transfer and joint work between teams, as well as continuity of care after the transition,[31] transfer of care must be planned, structured, and coordinated.[41,91] Transition is a *process* and not simply the moment when care is transferred from the pediatrician to the adult specialist.[31] This process should be referred to as *transfer of care* and should include psychoeducation, opportunities to practice and develop self-management and self-regulation skills, to promote autonomy and independence before transfer. It is also important for the patient to have adequate time to establish a relationship with the new AMHS specialist.[42] Recommendations also include addressing both the farewell to the CAMHS team and the beginning of the new therapeutic bond with the AMHS one.[108] Most studies suggest that transition in ADHD patients has not been successful because it is a particular challenge because of differences in training, thresholds, and focus between children and adolescent and adult services, leaving a proportion of young people without a clear pathway.[109]

Three different clinical trajectories have been identified for adults with ADHD[87]: (1) a transition group, consisting of young adults diagnosed and treated for ADHD in childhood and still in treatment, (2) adults diagnosed in childhood who are currently untreated, and (3) adults presenting for the first time for assessment of ADHD. For patients who have stopped treatment, symptom recurrence or exacerbation tends to occur during a critical time in life, when many changes are taking place (academic, social changes, and so forth) and when the individual's coping resources are overwhelmed.[57] Thus, the transition of youth with ADHD to adult services must involve both systems: pediatric providers and the adult primary care or psychiatric care provider.[57] When this transfer of care is planned, there are better outcomes.[7] A longitudinal study found that most help aimed at meeting needs for adolescents and young adults with ADHD came from friends and family rather than from professional services.[110] Around half of all young people (and two-thirds of all parents) reported a need for more support from professionals in accessing information regarding which services are available when they grow up, how to implement transition plans and where to find someone to talk to about practical as well as emotional needs.[110] Treatment must be optimized to ensure a successful transition,[111] thus strategies should address factors leading adolescents with ADHD to be more vulnerable to poor outcomes.[112] These factors include (but are not limited to) poor insight into one's own functioning and limited capacity for self-reflection, poor decision-making, a tendency to pursue immediate gratification, difficulties in organization and planning, poor time estimation and difficulties with time management, mood dysregulation, poor conflict resolution skills, and a desire to be autonomous and independent coupled with an overestimation of one's own capabilities (positive attribution bias).[113] Buitelaar suggests motivational interviewing as a key method to promote the adolescent's own decision-making and to reduce the ambivalence many adolescents express toward being dependent on medication and being a patient in need of treatment.[111] Emphasizes that a successful transition requires time so as to foster the treatment alliance.[111]

In conclusion, health systems across the globe need to respond to the growing burden of adolescent-onset and early adulthood mental illness by implementing proven and cost-effective interventions.[113] Recent evidence confirms that treatment in the early stages of disease is an efficient strategy with good clinical and economic results and with a reduction in the burden of the disease over the long term. This evidence has given rise to very solid arguments that an early intervention paradigm should apply to *all* childhood and adolescent-onset disorders.[114] Singh directly proposes that, instead of fixing "the broken bridge" between the 2 models of care (CAMHS and AMHS), neither of which has proven to be optimal for patients of transitional age, a radical redesign is required, with a new seamless path within a specialized adolescent-friendly model that also avoids stigmatization.[115] Although prevention should be supported by primary prevention and the promotion of mental health, there is still much room for improvement through the implementation of secondary and tertiary preventive strategies in early ages. The duration of psychiatric disorders in children and adolescents is one of the main predictors of mental disorders in adulthood,[116] highlighting the role of early intervention in promoting mental health throughout life.

Attention Deficit Hyperactivity Disorder Treatment

Currently clinical guidelines recommend the introduction of pharmacologic treatment (both stimulant medication such as methylphenidate, lisdexamfetamine dimesylate, or amphetamines and nonstimulants, such as atomoxetine or guanfacine) for school-age children and adolescents with ADHD, along with the implementation of psychological interventions based on behavioral, cognitive training, and psychopedagogical approaches.[117–119] Psychopharmacological treatment continues to be the fundamental pillar on which therapeutic intervention for patients with ADHD is based.[120] Treatment has proven to be effective in reducing both the symptoms and the functional impairment and improving quality of life.[121] Moreover, ADHD medication is also associated with long-term benefits, such as academic and occupational performance improvement and reduced substance use.[122] A study analyzing the rates of psychopharmacological prescriptions in children and adolescents found that ADHD medications were the most prescribed class of psychotropic drugs (1.5% globally, ranging from 0.19% in Italy to 53% in the United States).[123]

Transition stage is a period in which there is a decline in the prescription and use of ADHD treatment, as different studies have shown.[82,124] Discontinuing treatment of ADHD has been controversial. On the one hand, several clinical guidelines, based on the concerns regarding long-term effects and risks of medication, recommend an agreed cessation for a specified period of time to determine whether medication continues to be necessary for successful functioning.[119] On the other hand, if medications are discontinued, there is a high risk of ADHD symptoms exacerbation.[125] To address this issue, a systematic review and meta-analysis investigated whether discontinuing ADHD medication had an impact on the quality of life of ADHD patients who had responded to treatment.[126] Quality of life is defined by the WHO as "individuals' perceptions of their position in life in the context of the culture and value systems in which they live and in relation to their goals, expectations, standards and concerns".[127] Results showed that discontinuing medications was associated with a significant decrease in quality of life among children and adolescents with ADHD.[126] More research is needed to understand the circumstances under which medication discontinuation can be undertaken without the risk of clinical deterioration.

A recent study explored the reasons given by patients in the transition period for discontinuing ADHD medication. These were classified into different groups: the perceived balance between benefits and adverse effects of medication, perceptions of ADHD as a childhood or educational disorder, life circumstance of the young person, and challenges young people faced in accessing services.[121] A different study assessing treatment nonadherence in the transition stage found that nonwhite race/ethnicity, lower estimated income and male sex were risk factors for nonadherence.[128] Thus, this same study proved that medication adherence was associated with fewer negative outcomes (less unwanted pregnancies in women, less sexually transmitted infections, and lesser emergency department visits).

A systematic review with network meta-analyses of randomized trials evaluated the efficacy and safety of different treatment approaches for children and adolescents with ADHD, including pharmacologic, psychological, complementary, and alternative medicine interventions.[129] Regarding medical treatment, methylphenidate, lisdexamfetamine, amphetamine, atomoxetine, guanfacine, and clonidine were significantly more efficacious than placebo and among them, methylphenidate and amphetamine were most efficacious.[129] Another study comparing lisdexamfetamine dimesylate and methylphenidate showed improvements in pediatric-adolescent and adult patients, although lisdexamfetamine potentially added some benefits controlling ADHD symptoms in children and adults.[130] These same findings have been reported in a recent systematic review and network meta-analysis, which found that all medications, except modafinil in adults, were more efficacious than placebo for the short-term treatment of ADHD.[131] Psychostimulants are highly effective, when compared with other medications[120,130] and to other interventions, such as behavioral therapy and cognitive training.[130] Regarding tolerability, children tolerated worse than placebo amphetamines and guanfacine, whereas adults tolerated worse than placebo methylphenidate, amphetamines, and atomoxetine.[131] In general, methylphenidate and clonidine are better accepted than atomoxetine.[130] A meta-analysis analyzing the efficacy and safety of modafinil concluded that, potentially, it could constitute another treatment option in children and adolescents with ADHD.[132]

Considering other interventions, a systematic review and a meta-analysis found that mindfulness-based interventions were effective in reducing ADHD symptoms.[133,134] Behavioral therapy has proven to be effective, especially in combination with stimulants.[129] Yet, there is lack of evidence for meditation-based therapies, neurofeedback, antidepressants, antipsychotics, dietary therapy, fatty acids, and other complementary and alternative medicine[129,135,136] in the treatment of ADHD in young adults.

SUMMARY

The transition from adolescence to adulthood represents an important flexion point in the human life cycle. On the one hand, maturational changes and societal expectations offer youth new opportunities for autonomy, independence, and self-management. On the other hand, the multiple social-emotional challenges and health risks facing transitional age youth can lead to heightened stress, anxiety, and distress, as well as to the onset of severe mental disorders. Given the neurobiological and psychosocial burdens associated with neurodevelopmental disorders, young adults with ADHD are vulnerable to adverse events and outcomes including worsening core symptoms, impaired social and occupational functioning, and comorbid conditions such as anxiety, mood, and substance use disorders. It is vital for clinicians to be aware of the critical importance of planning for a successful transition of care from child and adolescent to AMHS, and to engage the young adult patient with ADHD in this process. This includes providing in-depth psychoeducation about ADHD and its treatment; establishing a therapeutic alliance to facilitate clinician–patient communication, collaborative problem-solving, and treatment adherence; targeting both medication and psychosocial interventions to the most salient symptoms and impairments; and encouraging the young adult to make sound decisions with respect to self-care and health maintenance. Although a great deal of research is still needed to validate best practices for improving long-term outcomes in young people with ADHD, there is a growing evidence base to justify ongoing medical treatment with either psychostimulant or nonstimulant medications and psychosocial interventions such as cognitive behavioral therapy and mindfulness practices.

CLINICS CARE POINTS

- The transition between adolescence and adulthood is a critical period in which many important changes take place (education, work, independent living, and social relations).
- Despite the rising incidence of mental illness in adolescents there are many barriers to achieving a smooth transition childhood and adolescent mental health services to adult mental health services, especially in the case of attention deficit hyperactivity disorder (ADHD), one of the most common disorders in youth.
- Continuity of care is hampered by a multitude of circumstances and factors, including individual and systems level variables. Individual factors include sociodemographic and clinical variables. Sociodemographic variables can be classified into age, age of diagnosis, and gender. Clinical variables include symptom severity, comorbidities, and treatment.
- Adolescents with ADHD tend to have limited insight into the nature of ADHD, the possible benefits of medication, and the importance of treatment adherence.
- The COVID-19 pandemic has worsened ADHD symptoms resulting in increasing emotional disturbance, social disability, and functional impairment.
- Given the transition gap between different health-care systems, it is highly probable that adult ADHD remains underrecognized, underdiagnosed, and, therefore, undertreated.
- Protocols, practice guidelines, and public health policies available to manage patients with ADHD transitioning to adulthood are limited.
- Young people transitioning to adult health services experience concern about the loss of known and familiar surroundings, as well as concern about the loss of the bond with the therapist, while they continue to expect health-care providers and professionals meet their needs.
- Transition is a process and not simply the moment when care is transferred from the pediatrician to the adult specialist. This process should be referred to as transfer of care and should include psychoeducation, opportunities to practice and develop self-management and self-regulation skills, to promote autonomy and independence before transfer.
- Psychopharmacological treatment continues to be the fundamental pillar on which therapeutic intervention for patients with ADHD.

- Discontinuing medications for ADHD seems to be associated with a significant decrease in the quality of life.

DISCLOSURE STATEMENT AND CONFLICT OF INTEREST

J. Quintero has served as speaker and/or on scientific advisory boards for Takeda, Janssen, and Rubio. A. Rodríguez-Quiroga has received funding from Takeda. F. Mora has served as speaker and/or on scientific advisory boards for Takeda and Janssen. A.L. Rostain has served on the scientific advisory board of Arbor, Supernus, Takeda, and Vallon.

REFERENCES

1. American Psychiatric Association. Diagnostic and statistical manual of mental disorders. Fifth edition. Arlington, VA: American Psychiatric Publishing; 2013.
2. Kessler RC, Adler LA, Barkley R, et al. Patterns and predictors of attention-deficit/hyperactivity disorder persistence into adulthood: results from the National Comorbidity Survey Replication. Biol Psychiatry 2005;57:1442–51.
3. Thomas R, Sanders S, Doust J, et al. Prevalence of attention-deficit/hyperactivity disorder: a systematic review and meta-analysis. Pediatrics 2015;135: e994–1001.
4. Caye A, Spadini AV, Karam RG, et al. Predictors of persistence of ADHD into adulthood: a systematic review of the literature and meta-analysis. Eur Child Adolesc Psychiatry 2016;25(11):1151–9.
5. Paus T, Keshavan M, Giedd JN. Why do many psychiatric disorders emerge during adolescence? Nat Rev Neurosci 2008;9(12):947–57.
6. Singh SP. Transition of care from child to adult mental health services: the great divide. Curr Opin Psychiatry 2009;22(4):386–90.
7. Young S, Murphy CM, Coghill D. Avoiding the 'twilight zone': recommendations for the transition of services from adolescence to adulthood for young people with ADHD. BMC Psychiatry 2011;11(1):174–81.
8. Blomqvist I, Henje Blom E, Hägglöf B, et al. Increase of internalized mental health symptoms among adolescents during the last three decades. Eur J Public Health 2019;29(5):925–31.
9. Singh SP, Evans N, Sireling L, et al. Mind the gap: the interface between child and adult mental health services. Psychiatr Bull 2005;29:292–4.
10. Sikirica V, Flood E, Dietrich CN, et al. Unmet needs associated with attention-deficit/hyperactivity disorder in eight European countries as reported by caregivers and adolescents: results from qualitative research. Patient 2015;8(3): 269–81.
11. Centers for Disease Control and Prevention. Attention-defcit/hyperactivity disorder fact sheet. 2020. Available a. https://www.cdc.gov/ncbddd/adhd/facts.html. Accessed May 6, 2021.
12. Faraone SV, Asherson P, Banaschewski T, et al. Attention-deficit/hyperactivity disorder. Nat Rev Dis Primers 2015;1:15020.
13. Farahbakhshian S, Ayyagari R, Barczak DS, et al. Disruption of pharmacotherapy during the transition from adolescence to early adulthood in patients with attention-deficit/hyperactivity disorder: a claims database analysis across the USA. CNS Drugs 2021;35:575–89.

14. Coghill DR. Organisation of services for managing ADHD. Epidemiol Psychiatr Sci 2017;26(5):453–8.

15. Johansen ME, Matic K, McAlearney AS. Attention deficit hyperactivity disorder medication use among teens and young adults. J Adolesc Health 2015;57(2): 192–7.

16. Eklund H, Cadman T, Findon J, et al. Clinical service use as people with Attention Deficit Hyperactivity Disorder transition into adolescence and adulthood: a prospective longitudinal study. BMC Health Serv Res 2016;16:248.

17. Newlove-Delgado T, Blake S, Ford T, et al. Young people with attention deficit hyperactivity disorder in transition from child to adult services: a qualitative study of the experiences of general practitioners in the UK. BMC Fam Pract 2019;20(1):159.

18. Blasco-Fontecilla H, Carballo JJ, Garcia-Nieto R, et al. Factors contributing to the utilization of adult mental health services in children and adolescents diagnosed with hyperkinetic disorder. ScientificWorldJournal 2012;2012:451205.

19. Newlove-Delgado T, Ford TJ, Hamilton W, et al. Prescribing of medication for attention deficit hyperactivity disorder among young people in the Clinical Practice Research Datalink 2005-2013: analysis of time to cessation. Eur Child Adolesc Psychiatry 2018;27(1):29–35.

20. Tatlow-Golden M, Gavin B, McNamara N, et al. Transitioning from child and adolescent mental health services with attention-deficit hyperactivity disorder in Ireland: case note review. Early Interv Psychiatry 2018;12(3):505–12.

21. McNicholas F, Adamson M, McNamara N, et al. Who is in the transition gap? Transition from CAMHS to AMHS in the Republic of Ireland. Ir J Psychol Med 2015;32(1):61–9.

22. Belling R, McLaren S, Paul M, et al. The effect of organisational resources and eligibility issues on transition from child and adolescent to adult mental health services. J Health Serv Res Policy 2014;19(3):169–76.

23. Swift KD, Hall CL, Marimuttu V, et al. Transition to adult mental health services for young people with attention deficit/hyperactivity disorder (ADHD): a qualitative analysis of their experiences. BMC Psychiatry 2013;13:74.

24. Newlove-Delgado T, Ford TJ, Stein K, et al. 'You're 18 now, goodbye': the experiences of young people with attention deficit hyperactivity disorder of the transition from child to adult services. Emotional Behav Difficulties 2018;23(3): 296–309.

25. Reale L, Frassica S, Gollner A, et al. Transition to adult mental health services for young people with attention deficit hyperactivity disorder in Italy: parents' and clinicians' experiences. Postgrad Med 2015;127(7):671–6.

26. Price A, Newlove-Delgado T, Eke H, et al. In transition with ADHD: the role of information, in facilitating or impeding young people's transition into adult services. BMC Psychiatry 2019;19(1):404.

27. Syverson EP, McCarter R, He J, et al. Adolescents' perceptions of transition importance, readiness, and likelihood of future success: the role of anticipatory guidance. Clin Pediatr (Phila) 2016;55(11):1020–5.

28. Price A, Janssens A, Woodley AL, et al. Review: experiences of healthcare transitions for young people with attention deficit hyperactivity disorder: a systematic review of qualitative research. Child Adolesc Ment Health 2019;24(2): 113–22.

29. Hechtman L, Swanson JM, Sibley MH, et al, MTA Cooperative Group. Functional adult outcomes 16 Years after childhood diagnosis of attention-deficit/

hyperactivity disorder: MTA results. J Am Acad Child Adolesc Psychiatry 2016; 55(11):945–52.

30. Wilens TE, Isenberg BM, Kaminski TA, et al. Attention-deficit/hyperactivity disorder and transitional aged youth. Curr Psychiatry Rep 2018;20(11):100.

31. Blum RW, Garell D, Hodgman CH, et al. Transition from child-centered to adult health-care systems for adolescents with chronic conditions. A position paper of the Society for Adolescent Medicine. J Adolesc Health 1993;14(7):570–6.

32. Singh SP, Tuomainen H, Girolamo G, et al. Protocol for a cohort study of adolescent mental health service users with a nested cluster randomised controlled trial to assess the clinical and cost-effectiveness of managed transition in improving transitions from child to adult mental health services (the MILESTONE study). BMJ Open 2017;7(10):e016055.

33. Singh SP, Paul M, Ford T, et al. Transitions of care from child and adolescent mental health services to adult mental health services (TRACK study): a study of protocols in greater london. BMC Health Serv Res 2008;23(8):135.

34. Settersten RA. The new landscape of adult life: road maps, signposts, and speed lines. Res Hum Dev 2007;4:239–52.

35. Seiffge-Krenke I. She's leaving home . . ." Antecedents, consequences, and cultural patterns in the leaving home process. Emerg Adulthood 2013;1(2):114–24.

36. Reifman A, Arnett JJ, Colwell MJ. Emerging adulthood: theory, assessment, and application. J Youth Dev 2007;2(1).

37. Arnett JJ. Emerging adulthood: the winding road from the late teens through the twenties. New York: Oxford University Press; 2004.

38. Baggio S, Iglesias K, Studer J, et al. An 8-item short form of the inventory of dimensions of emerging adulthood (IDEA) among young Swiss men. Eval Health Prof 2015;38(2):246–54.

39. Baggio S, Studer J, Fructuoso A, et al. Does level of attention deficit-hyperactivity disorder symptoms predicts poor transition into adulthood? Int J Public Health 2019;64(2):165172.

40. Hovish K, Weaver T, Islam Z, et al. Transition experiences of mental health service users, parents, and professionals in the United Kingdom: a qualitative study. Psychiatr Rehabil J 2012;35(3):251–7.

41. Singh SP, Paul M, Ford T, et al. Process, outcome and experience of transition from child to adult mental healthcare: multiperspective study. Br J Psychiatry 2010;197(4):305–12.

42. Paul M, Ford T, Kramer T, et al. Transfers and transitions between child and adult mental health services. Br J Psychiatry Suppl 2013;54:s36–40.

43. Gray WN, Kavookjian J, Shapiro SK, et al. Transition to college and adherence to prescribed attention deficit hyperactivity disorder medication. J Dev Behav Pediatr 2018;39(1):1–9.

44. Eke H, Janssens A, Downs J, et al. How to measure the need for transition to adult services among young people with Attention Deficit Hyperactivity Disorder (ADHD): a comparison of surveillance versus case note review methods. BMC Med Res Methodol 2019;19(1):179.

45. Tripp G, Wickens JR. Neurobiology of ADHD. Neuropharmacology 2009; 57(7–8):579–89.

46. Willcutt EG, Doyle AE, Nigg JT, et al. Validity of the executive function theory of attention-deficit/hyperactivity disorder: a meta-analytic review. Biol Psychiatry 2005;57(11):1336–46.

47. Barkley RA. Behavioral inhibition, sustained attention, and executive functions: constructing a unifying theory of ADHD. Psychol Bull 1997;121(1):65–94.

48. Sonuga-Barke EJ. The dual pathway model of AD/HD: an elaboration of neuro-developmental characteristics. Neurosci Biobehav Rev 2003;27(7):593–604.

49. Giedd JN, Blumenthal J, Jeffries NO, et al. Brain development during childhood and adolescence: a longitudinal MRI study. Nat Neurosci 1999;2(10):861–3.

50. Snyder M. Self-monitoring of expressive behavior. J Pers Soc Psychol 1974; 30(4):526–37.

51. Snyder M. Self-monitoring processes. In: Berkowitz L, editor. Advances in experimental social psychology, 12. New York: Academic Press; 1979.

52. Sanz J, Graña JL. [Auto-observación en adolescentes. Los problemas de la escala de auto-observación de Snyder en poblaciones no adultas]. Anuario de Psicología 1994;60:63–80.

53. Casey BJ, Glatt CE, Lee FS. Treating the developing versus developed brain: translating preclinical mouse and human studies. Neuron 2015;86(6): 1358e1368.

54. Niwa M, Jaaro-Peled H, Tankou S, et al. Adolescent stress-induced epigenetic control of dopaminergic neurons via glucocorticoids. Science 2013;339(6117): 335–9.

55. Lockhart S, Sawa A, Niwa M. Developmental trajectories of brain maturation and behavior: relevance to major mental illnesses. J Pharmacol Sci 2018. pii: S1347-8613(18)30081-1.

56. Thompson PM, Jahanshad N, Ching CRK, et al, ENIGMA Consortium. ENIGMA and global neuroscience: a decade of large-scale studies of the brain in health and disease across more than 40 countries. Transl Psychiatry 2020;10(1):100.

57. Robb A, Findling RL. Challenges in the transition of care for adolescents with attention-deficit/hyperactivity disorder. Postgrad Med 2013;125(4):131–40.

58. Bussing R, Zima BT, Mason DM, et al. Receiving treatment for attention-deficit hyperactivity disorder: do the perspectives of adolescents matter? J Adolesc Health 2011;49(1):7–14.

59. DosReis S, Barksdale CL, Sherman A, et al. Stigmatizing experiences of parents of children with a new diagnosis of ADHD. Psychiatr Serv 2010;61(8):811–6.

60. The Lancet Psychiatry. Send in the therapists? Lancet Psychiatry 2020;7(4):291.

61. The European ADHD Guideline Group (EAGG). ADHD management during the COVID-19 pandemic: guidance from the European ADHD guidelines group. Lancet Child Adolesc Health 2020;4:412–4.

62. Kavoor AR, Mitra S. Managing attention deficit hyperactivity disorder during COVID-19 pandemic. J Neurosci Rural Pract 2021;12(1):1–2.

63. Cortese S, Coghill D, Santosh P, et al, European ADHD Guidelines Group. Starting ADHD medications during the COVID-19 pandemic: recommendations from the European ADHD Guidelines Group. Lancet Child Adolesc Health 2020; 4(6):e15.

64. Zhang J, Shuai L, Yu H, et al. Acute stress, behavioural symptoms and mood states among school-age children with attention-deficit/hyperactive disorder during the COVID-19 outbreak. Asian J Psychiatr 2020;51:102077.

65. Melegari MG, Giallonardo M, Sacco R, et al. Identifying the impact of the confinement of Covid-19 on emotional-mood and behavioural dimensions in children and adolescents with attention deficit hyperactivity disorder (ADHD). Psychiatry Res 2021;296:113692.

66. Lifestyles Team, NHS Digital. Mental health of children and young people in England, 2020: wave 1 follow up to the 2017 survey. NHS Digital, part of the Government Statistical Service. Availble at: https://digital.nhs.uk/data-and-

information/publications/statistical/mental-health-of-children-and-young-people-in-england/2020-wave-1-follow-up/copyright. Accessed July 28, 2021.

67. Nonweiler J, Rattray F, Baulcomb J, et al. Prevalence and associated factors of emotional and behavioural difficulties during COVID-19 pandemic in children with neurodevelopmental disorders. Children (Basel) 2020;7(9):128.

68. Panda PK, Gupta J, Chowdhury SR, et al. Psychological and behavioral impact of lockdown and quarantine measures for COVID-19 pandemic on children, adolescents and caregivers: a systematic review and meta-analysis. J Trop Pediatr 2021;67(1):fmaa122.

69. Sibley MH, Ortiz M, Gaias LM, et al. Top problems of adolescents and young adults with ADHD during the COVID-19 pandemic. J Psychiatr Res 2021;136: 190–7.

70. Shah R, Raju VV, Sharma A, et al. Impact of COVID-19 and lockdown on children with ADHD and their families-an online survey and a continuity care model. J Neurosci Rural Pract 2021;12(1):71–9.

71. Shorey S, Lau LST, Tan JX, et al. Families with children with neurodevelopmental disorders during COVID-19: a scoping review. J Pediatr Psychol 2021; 46(6):729.

72. Zhao Y, Jiang Z, Guo S, et al. Association of symptoms of attention deficit and hyperactivity with problematic internet use among university students in wuhan, China during the COVID-19 pandemic. J Affect Disord 2021;286:220–7.

73. Werling AM, Walitza S, Drechsler R. Impact of the COVID-19 lockdown on screen media use in patients referred for ADHD to child and adolescent psychiatry: an introduction to problematic use of the internet in ADHD and results of a survey. J Neural Transm (Vienna) 2021;22:1–11.

74. Shuai L, He S, Zheng H, et al. Influences of digital media use on children and adolescents with ADHD during COVID-19 pandemic. Glob Health 2021; 17(1):48.

75. McGrath J. ADHD and Covid-19: current roadblocks and future opportunities. Ir J Psychol Med 2020;37(3):204–11.

76. Ando M, Takeda T, Kumagai K. A qualitative study of impacts of the COVID-19 pandemic on lives in adults with attention deficit hyperactive disorder in Japan. Int J Environ Res Public Health 2021;18(4):2090.

77. Merzon E, Manor I, Rotem A, et al. ADHD as a risk factor for infection with covid-19. J Atten Disord 2020;25(13):1783–90.

78. Merzon E, Weiss MD, Cortese S, et al. The association between ADHD and the severity of COVID-19 infection. J Atten Disord 2021;2. 10870547211003659.

79. Adamou M, Fullen T, Galab N, et al. Psychological effects of the COVID-19 imposed lockdown on adults with attention deficit/hyperactivity disorder: cross-sectional survey study. JMIR Form Res 2020;4(12):e24430.

80. Arbel Y, Fialkoff C, Kerner A, et al. Can increased recovery rates from coronavirus be explained by prevalence of ADHD? An analysis at the US statewide level. J Atten Disord 2020;21. 1087054720959707.

81. Bobo E, Lin L, Acquaviva E, et al. Comment les enfants et adolescents avec le trouble déficit d'attention/hyperactivité (TDAH) vivent-ils le confinement durant la pandémie COVID-19 ? [How do children and adolescents with Attention Deficit Hyperactivity Disorder (ADHD) experience lockdown during the COVID-19 outbreak?]. Encephale 2020;46(3S):S85–92.

82. Edwin F, McDonald J. Services for adults with attention-deficit hyperactivity disorder: national survey. Psychiatr Bull 2007;31(8):286–8.

83. Swift KD, Sayal K, Hollis C. ADHD and transitions to adult mental health services: a scoping review. Child Care Health Dev 2014;40(6):775–86.

84. Moncrieff J, Timimi S. Is ADHD a valid diagnosis in adults? No. BMJ 2010;340: c547.

85. Ahmed AA, Cress S, Lovett L. Adult ADHD: the new kid on the block has grown up. Psychiatr Bull 2009;33(1):37.

86. Asherson P, Adamou M, Bolea B, et al. Is ADHD a valid diagnosis in adults? Yes. BMJ 2010;340:c549.

87. Treuer T, Chan KLP, Kim BN, et al. Lost in transition: a review of the unmet need of patients with attention deficit/hyperactivity disorder transitioning to adulthood. Asia Pac Psychiatry 2017;9(2).

88. National Institute for Health and Clinical Excellence. Attention deficit hyperactivity disorder: diagnosis and management of ADHD in children, young people and adults. London: Clinical guideline 72; 2008.

89. Pottick KJ, Bilder S, Vander Stoep A, et al. US patterns of mental health service utilization for transition-age youth and young adults. J Behav Health Serv Res 2008;35(4):373–89.

90. Lehner RK, Dopke CA, Cohen K, et al. Outpatient treatment adherence and serious mental illness: a review of interventions. Am J Psychiatr Rehabil 2007; 10:245–74.

91. Velligan DI, Weiden PJ, Sajatovic M, et al. Assessment of adherence problems in patients with serious and persistent mental illness: recommendations from the Expert Consensus Guidelines. J Psychiatr Pract 2010;16(1):34–45.

92. Viswanath B, Rao NP, Narayanaswamy JC, et al. Discovery biology of neuropsychiatric syndromes (DBNS): a center for integrating clinical medicine and basic science. BMC Psychiatry 2018;18(1):106.

93. National Institute for Health and Care Excellence. Service user experience in adult mental health: improving the experience of care for people using adult NHS mental health services. NICE; 2011. Available at: https://www.nice.org. uk/guidance/cg136.

94. Eldreth D, Hardin MG, Pavletic N, et al. Adolescent transformations of behavioral and neural processes as potential targets for prevention. Prev Sci 2013; 14(3):257–66.

95. Horvitz-Lennon M, Kilbourne AM, Pincus HA. From silos to bridges: meeting the general health care needs of adults with severe mental illnesses. Health Aff 2006;25(3):659–69.

96. Mojtabai R, Olfson M, Sampson NA, et al. Barriers to mental health treatment: results from the national comorbidity survey replication. Psychol Med 2011; 41(8):1751–61.

97. van der Lee A, de Haan L, Beekman A. Schizophrenia in The Netherlands: continuity of care with better quality of care for less medical costs. PLoS One 2016; 11(6):e0157150.

98. Nakhla M, Daneman D, To T, et al. Transition to adult care for youths with diabetes mellitus: findings from a Universal Health Care System. Pediatrics 2009; 124(6):e1134–41.

99. Watson AR. Non-compliance and transfer from paediatric to adult transplant unit. Pediatr Nephrol 2000;14(6):469–72.

100. Andrade DM, Bassett AS, Bercovici E, et al. Epilepsy: transition from pediatric to adult care. Recommendations of the Ontario epilepsy implementation task force. Epilepsia 2017;58(9):1502–17.

101. Sam-Agudu NA, Pharr JR, Bruno T, et al. Adolescent Coordinated Transition (ACT) to improve health outcomes among young people living with HIV in Nigeria: study protocol for a randomized controlled trial. Trials 2017;18(1):595.
102. Fegran L, Hall EO, Uhrenfeldt L, et al. Adolescents' and young adults' transition experiences when transferring from paediatric to adult care: a qualitative meta-synthesis. Int J Nurs Stud 2014;51(1):123–35.
103. Betz CL, Lobo ML, Nehring WM, et al. Voices not heard: a systematic review of adolescents' and emerging adults' perspectives of health care transition. Nurs Outlook 2013;61(5):311–36.
104. Broad KL, Sandhu VK, Sunderji N, et al. Youth experiences of transition from child mental health services to adult mental health services: a qualitative thematic synthesis. BMC Psychiatry 2017;17(1):380.
105. Whitney J, Costa A. One size does not fit all. Psychiatr Rehabil J 2012;35(3): 273–4. Winter.
106. Gilburt H, Rose D, Slade M. The importance of relationships in mental health care: a qualitative study of service users' experiences of psychiatric hospital admission in the UK. BMC Health Serv Res 2008;8:92.
107. Priebe S, Watts J, Chase M, et al. Processes of disengagement and engagement in assertive outreach patients: qualitative study. Br J Psychiatry 2005; 187:438–43.
108. Segura-Frontelo A, Alvarez García R, López de Lerma Borrué V, et al. Transitioning from the child and adolescent to the adult mental health services: an unresolved challenge and an opportunity. Rev Psiquiatr Salud Ment (Engl Ed) 2020; 13(4):180–3.
109. Sayal K, Prasad V, Daley D, et al. ADHD in children and young people: prevalence, care pathways, and service provision. Lancet Psychiatry 2018;5(2): 175–86.
110. Murphy D, Glaser K, Hayward H, et al. Crossing the divide: a longitudinal study of effective treatments for people with autism and attention deficit hyperactivity disorder across the lifespan. Southampton (UK): NIHR Journals Library; 2018.
111. Buitelaar JK. Optimising treatment strategies for ADHD in adolescence to minimise 'lost in transition' to adulthood. Epidemiol Psychiatr Sci 2017;26(5):448–52.
112. Chan E, Fogler JM, Hammerness PG. Treatment of attention-deficit/hyperactivity disorder in adolescents: a systematic review. JAMA 2016;315(18):1997–2008.
113. Whiteford HA, Ferrari AJ, Degenhardt L, et al. Global burden of mental, neurological, and substance use disorders: AnAnalysis from the global burden of disease study 2010. In: Een: Patel V, Chisholm D, Dua T, et al, editors. Mental, neurological, and substance use disorders: disease control priorities, 4, 3rd edition. Washington (DC): The International Bank for Reconstruction and Development/The World Bank; 2016. Cp 2.
114. Birchwood M, Singh SP. Mental health services for young people: matching the service to the need. Br J Psychiatry 2013;202(Suppl.54):s1–2.
115. Singh SP, Tuomainen H. Transition from child to adult mental health services: needs, barriers, experiences and new models of care. World Psychiatry 2015; 14(3):358–61.
116. Patton GC, Coffey C, Romaniuk H, Mackinnon A, Carlin JB, Let al Degenhardt. The prognosis of common mental disorders in adolescents: a 14-year prospective cohort study. Lancet 2014;383(9926):1404–11.
117. National Guideline Centre (UK). Attention deficit hyperactivity disorder: diagnosis and management. London: National Institute for Health and Care Excellence (UK); 2018.

118. JJS Kooij, Bijlenga D, Salerno L, et al. Updated European Consensus Statement on diagnosis and treatment of adult ADHD. Eur Psychiatry 2019;56:14–34.

119. Medina R, Bouhaben J, de Ramón I, et al. Electrophysiological Brain Changes Associated With Cognitive Improvement in a Pediatric Attention Deficit Hyperactivity Disorder Digital Artificial Intelligence-Driven Intervention: Randomized Controlled Trial. J Med Internet Res 2021;23(11):e25466.

120. Caye A, Swanson JM, Coghill D, et al. Treatment strategies for ADHD: an evidence-based guide to select optimal treatment. Mol Psychiatry 2019;24(3): 390–408.

121. Titheradge D, Godfrey J, Eke H, et al. Why young people stop taking their ADHD medication. A thematic analysis of interviews with young people. Child Care Health Dev 2022;1–12.

122. Shaw M, Hodgkins P, Caci H, et al. A systematic review and analysis of long-term outcomes in attention deficit hyperactivity disorder: effects of treatment and non-treatment. BMC Med 2012;10:99.

123. Piovani D, Clavenna A, Bonati M. Prescription prevalence of psychotropic drugs in children and adolescents: an analysis of international data. Eur J Clin Pharmacol 2019;75(10):1333–46.

124. Eke H, Ford T, Newlove-Delgado T, et al. Transition between child and adult services for young people with attention-deficit hyperactivity disorder (ADHD): findings from a British national surveillance study. Br J Psychiatry 2020;217(5): 616–22.

125. MTA Cooperative Group. National Institute of Mental Health Multimodal Treatment Study of ADHD follow-up: 24-month outcomes of treatment strategies for attention-deficit/hyperactivity disorder. Pediatrics 2004;113(4):754–61.

126. Tsuji N, Okada T, Usami M, et al. Effect of continuing and discontinuing medications on quality of life after symptomatic remission in attention-deficit/hyperactivity disorder: a systematic review and meta-analysis. J Clin Psychiatry 2020;81(3):19r13015.

127. The world health organization quality of life assessment (WHOQOL): position paper from the world health organization. Soc Sci Med 1995;41(10):1403–9.

128. Catalá-López F, Hutton B, Núñez-Beltrán A, et al. The pharmacological and non-pharmacological treatment of attention deficit hyperactivity disorder in children and adolescents: a systematic review with network meta-analyses of randomised trials. PLoS One 2017;12(7):e0180355.

129. Gutiérrez-Casares JR, Quintero J, Jorba G, et al. Methods to Develop an in silico Clinical Trial: Computational Head-to-Head Comparison of Lisdexamfetamine and Methylphenidate. Front Psychiatry 2021;12:741170.

130. Cortese S, Adamo N, Del Giovane C, et al. Comparative efficacy and tolerability of medications for attention-deficit hyperactivity disorder in children, adolescents, and adults: a systematic review and network meta-analysis. Lancet Psychiatry 2018;5(9):727–8.

131. Wang SM, Han C, Lee SJ, et al. Modafinil for the treatment of attention-deficit/hyperactivity disorder: a meta-analysis. J Psychiatr Res 2017;84:292–300.

132. Cairncross M, Miller CJ. The effectiveness of mindfulness-based therapies for ADHD: a meta-analytic review. J Atten Disord 2020;24(5):627–43.

133. Xue J, Zhang Y, Huang Y. A meta-analytic investigation of the impact of mindfulness-based interventions on ADHD symptoms. Medicine (Baltimore) 2019;98(23):e15957.

134. Cortese S, Ferrin M, Brandeis D, et al. European ADHD Guidelines Group (EAGG). Cognitive training for attention-deficit/hyperactivity disorder: meta-

analysis of clinical and neuropsychological outcomes from randomized controlled trials. J Am Acad Child Adolesc Psychiatry 2015;54(3):164–74.

135. Zhang J, Díaz-Román A, Cortese S. Meditation-based therapies for attention-deficit/hyperactivity disorder in children, adolescents and adults: a systematic review and meta-analysis. Evid Based Ment Health 2018;21(3):87–94.

136. Cortese S, Ferrin M, Brandeis D, et al. European ADHD Guidelines Group (EAGG). Neurofeedback for attention-deficit/hyperactivity disorder: meta-analysis of clinical and neuropsychological outcomes from randomized controlled trials. J Am Acad Child Adolesc Psychiatry 2016;55(6):444–55.

Updates in Pharmacologic Strategies in Adult Attention-Deficit/Hyperactivity Disorder

Deepti Anbarasan, MD[a,b,*], Gabriella Safyer, MD[b],
Lenard A. Adler, MD[b,c]

KEYWORDS

• Adult ADHD • ADHD medications • Attention • Hyperactivity • ADHD treatment

KEY POINTS

• Adults with attention-deficit/hyperactivity disorder (ADHD) experience worse long-term functional outcomes in several domains of life.
• The armamentarium of therapeutic options for the treatment of adult ADHD has expanded in the past 2 decades.
• Several research trials continue to actively investigate medication options with unique mechanisms of action.

INTRODUCTION

Attention-deficit/hyperactivity disorder (ADHD) constitutes a childhood-onset neurodevelopmental disorder identified in approximately 6% to 10% of children and 4.4% of adults in the United States, suggesting remission for some by adulthood.[1,2] Yet, nearly 60% to 90% of pediatric patients continue to exhibit ADHD symptoms as adults.[3–5] The typical lifelong nature of this disorder possibly compounds its effects. ADHD causes significant functional impairments in adults, including a high prevalence of secondary comorbid psychiatric disorders, accidents causing injuries, academic and professional setbacks, social difficulties, as well as early mortality.[6,7] Clinicians must therefore exercise vigilance in identifying and treating ADHD in adults.

Although the Diagnostic and Statistical Manual of Mental Disorders, fifth edition uses similar criteria to diagnose childhood ADHD and adult ADHD, important

a Department of Neurology, NYU Grossman School of Medicine, One Park Avenue, 8th Floor, New York, NY 10016, USA; b Department of Psychiatry, NYU Grossman School of Medicine, One Park Avenue, 8th Floor, New York, NY 10016, USA; c Department of Child & Adolescent Psychiatry, NYU Grossman School of Medicine, One Park Avenue, 8th Floor, New York, NY 10016, USA
* Corresponding author.
E-mail address: Deepti.Anbarasan@nyulangone.org

Child Adolesc Psychiatric Clin N Am 31 (2022) 553–568
https://doi.org/10.1016/j.chc.2022.03.008
1056-4993/22/© 2022 Elsevier Inc. All rights reserved.

childpsych.theclinics.com

phenotypic distinctions exist in adult ADHD patients.[8] About 70% of adult ADHD patients meet criteria for the combined type of ADHD, 25% meet criteria for primarily inattentive type of ADHD, and less than 5% meet criteria for the primarily hyperactive-impulsive type of ADHD.[7] Symptoms of inattention seem to drive the presentation of adults with ADHD for treatment.[6] Although diagnosis of ADHD in male children surpasses that in female children, this gap seems to close in adulthood with the man to woman prevalence ratio persisting at approximately 1.6:1.[2] Finally, adults with ADHD suffer high comorbidity if not outright increased risk for other psychiatric disorders, suggesting a greater overall burden on quality of life and functioning.[2]

NATURE OF THE PROBLEM

Patients with ADHD experience worse long-term functional outcomes when compared with the non-ADHD population.[9] Young adults in college with ADHD have lower graduation rates than their peers without ADHD.[10] Adults with ADHD encounter greater difficulties professionally with higher levels of unemployment, job-switching, and financial stress.[10] They also experience increased difficulty in maintaining healthy interpersonal relationships, a phenomenon that corresponds with higher rates of separation and divorce.[11] From a broader population-based perspective, the annual costs to society due to ADHD range between estimates of $143 and $266 billion in the United States.[12]

Given the profound negative impacts of ADHD for those both directly and indirectly affected by the disorder, appropriate identification and management of the condition remains imperative. Pharmacologic treatment of ADHD has been shown to improve long-term outcomes, diminishing risks for secondary comorbid mental disorders, academic failures, and accidents.[9] Psychotropic treatment has been associated with improvements in multiple domains including academic and occupational achievement, self-esteem, social functioning outcomes, nonmedicinal drug use and addictive behavior, driving, as well as antisocial behaviors.[12]

Multiple organizations, including the American Academy of Child and Adolescent Psychiatry, the Canadian ADHD Resource Alliance, the European Network Adult ADHD, and the United Kingdom National Institute for Health and Care Excellence, have provided guidelines that describe the phenomenology of ADHD across the life span as well as recommendations for the assessment and treatment of ADHD.[13–16]

Although psychosocial therapy in combination with medications serves as the most widely accepted treatment strategy for ADHD in school-age children and adolescents, pharmacotherapy alone generally remains the first-line treatment of adults with ADHD.[16] This may be in part due to adult patients suffering from lifelong symptoms.[16] Despite advances in establishing the efficacy of psychotropics for adult ADHD, most of this population remains untreated.[2] This article seeks to amend this clinical gap by outlining current treatment standards and innovations that have United States Food and Drug Administration (FDA) indications for the treatment of adult ADHD. We will describe not only the currently available medication options but also review future directions in the pharmacologic treatment of adult ADHD.

THERAPEUTIC OPTIONS

ADHD medications can be categorized into stimulants and nonstimulants. Stimulants are further dichotomized into amphetamine (AMPH) and methylphenidate (MPH) compounds. Although there are multiple nonstimulant options FDA approved for use in children and adolescents, only 2 nonstimulants have been approved for use in

ADHD patients 6 years and older. Patient response or lack thereof to stimulants versus nonstimulants does not predict a positive or negative response to the other psychotropic class.[17] Therefore, in the event of suboptimal symptom control with one class of ADHD medications, subsequent trials with an alternative class should be considered. Clinicians may also consider subsequent trials to optimize patient response based on duration of effect (short, intermediate, long) as determined by medication delivery mechanism. This section on therapeutic options will be categorized by stimulants versus nonstimulants, with further specification for stimulant type and duration of medication effect.

Stimulants

Stimulants, including AMPH and MPH, have historically represented the best-studied and most frequently used psychotropic treatment of ADHD across the life span. Not only do stimulants show significant efficacy in the management of ADHD symptoms, they also lead to improvements in self-esteem, cognition, and interpersonal functioning.[18]

Controlled studies indicate that adults have a wider fluctuation in symptom reduction with stimulants ranging from 25% to 88%, whereas children and adolescents seem to exhibit consistently high response rates of about 70%.[17] It should be noted that large-scale studies demonstrated higher response rates in adults.[19,20] Aside from variability in study size, variability in clinical trial dosing of stimulants may account for the wide range in adult response rates.[17]

It has been generally considered that higher stimulant doses correspond with more compelling response rates in adults.[17] Contrast this tenet with a network meta-analysis of ADHD medication clinical trials published in 2018 by Cortese and colleagues[21] that showed no dose-dependent differences in AMPH efficacy.

AMPH and MPH generally propagate similar side effect profiles, which include decreased appetite, disrupted sleep, abdominal discomfort, headaches, and emotional disturbances including irritability.[22] Schedule II status from the Drug Enforcement Agency (DEA) confers a higher risk of potential misuse or addiction with stimulants.[22] Diligence in assessing for simultaneous substance use is therefore paramount. The FDA cautions clinicians to monitor for psychiatric adverse events such as worsening thought disorder in patients with preexisting psychotic or bipolar affective disorder, emergence of new psychotic or manic symptoms in patients without prior psychotic or bipolar affective illness, and aggression.[23] Other potential negative consequences in adults include seizures, priapism, peripheral vasculopathy, and visual disturbances.[23]

A meta-analysis carried out on 2665 patients observed that stimulants used to treat adult ADHD resulted in a statistically significant increase in resting heart rate by 5.7 beats per minute and an increase in systolic blood pressure by 2.0 mm Hg.[24] No statistical significance was observed in diastolic blood pressure changes.[24] The FDA product labeling for stimulants recommends using these agents with caution in patients with known structural cardiac abnormalities, cardiomyopathy, serious heart rhythm abnormalities, preexisting hypertension, heart failure, or recent myocardial infarction.[25] Even mild increases in heart rate and blood pressure have been associated with increased risk of adverse cardiovascular events.[26–28] Clinicians should monitor both heart rate and blood pressure before initiating the treatment with stimulants and at regular intervals to monitor for changes.[29]

AMPH and MPH promotion of norepinephrine peripherally can account for the autonomic changes described above.[30] Promotion of both norepinephrine and dopamine contribute to the central side effects described above.[31] The centrally acting effects of stimulants ultimately produce their desired effect in the case of ADHD treatment. Improved attention, concentration, and executive functioning may be explained by stimulant enhancement of dopamine and norepinephrine in the dorsolateral prefrontal cortex.[23] Dopamine and norepinephrine enhancement in the medial prefrontal cortex and hypothalamus may lessen fatigue.[23] Finally, the enhancement of dopamine actions in the basal ganglia may ameliorate hyperactivity.[23]

Amphetamine

AMPH treats ADHD by allowing for more noradrenergic and dopaminergic activity in the prefrontal cortex via 2 mechanisms: (1) AMPH blocks the reuptake of norepinephrine and dopamine and (2) AMPH promotes release of dopamine from synaptic vesicles.[23] The AMPH class includes both racemic drugs and D-AMPH drugs. The D-isomer of AMPH may have a more profound action on dopamine than norepinephrine, whereas the L-isomer of AMPH may act on dopamine and norepinephrine in a more balanced manner.[30] No clear clinical significance has been established because of these racemic differences.[30] Although general consensus suggests that the D-isomer may in fact be more potent.[23]

Several AMPH medications have been approved by the FDA specifically for the treatment of ADHD in adults. These options have been developed with extended-release technologies, allowing for their long-acting effects. The short-acting and intermediate AMPH formulations have not been approved for use in adult populations. We will review the formulations that have both FDA approval for adult use and have active clinical studies or data in adult populations.

Long-acting amphetamine

1. Mixed AMPH salts extended-release (MAS XR; brand name *Adderall XR*) is a mixture of D-AMPH and L-AMPH salts by a ratio of 3:1.[32] MAS XR comes in capsule form containing immediate-release beads and beads that require intestinal entry for release due to a pH-dependent coating.[32] This technology allows for once-a-day dosing. The capsules can be opened with the contents sprinkled over applesauce for an alternative route of administration.[32,33] Food does not seem to affect its efficacy, although it may prolong the amount of time that the medication is present at its maximum concentration, especially when taken with fatty foods.[23] MAS XR is dosed between 5 and 30 mg by mouth daily.[32] In adults, the half-life for D-AMPH is 1 hour, whereas that of L-AMPH is 13 hours.[23] The duration of effect is 10.5 to 12 hours with an onset of clinical effect at 1.5 hours.[33] Efficacy was established for the treatment of adult ADHD in a 4-week double-blind, randomized, placebo-controlled, parallel-group study.[34] Trial participants who received MAS XR demonstrated significant improvement in symptoms as measured by the ADHD-rating scale (ADHD-RS).[34]

2. Triple-beaded MAS extended-release (TB-MAS XR; brand name *Mydayis*) offers an additional option for AMPH daily dosing in adults with ADHD. Similar to MAS-XR as described above, TB-MAS XR also contains a 3:1 mixture of D-AMPH to L-AMPH.[35] This formulation boasts 3 types of drug-releasing beads.[22] It contains an immediate-release bead alongside 2 different types of delayed release beads that deliver their contents at a pH of 5.5 and 7.0, respectively.[35] This technology accounts for the medication's particularly long duration of effect of 14 hours, and even sometimes up to 16 hours.[33,35] Therefore, TB-MAS XR should ideally be taken on waking to ward off the potential for insomnia.[22] TB-MAS XR can be taken with or without food.[33] The capsules can also be opened with the contents sprinkled over applesauce for immediate consumption.[33] The onset of clinical effect is 2 hours and

the recommended starting dose in adults is 12.5 mg daily with a maximum daily dose of 50 mg.[33,35] A post hoc responder and remission analyses performed on 2 adult ADHD studies demonstrated that TB-MAS XR was associated with 1.7 to 3.6 times the response rates and with 1.9 to 5.9 times the remission rates as seen with placebo.[36]

3. Lisdexamfetamine dimesylate (LDX; brand name *Vyvanse)* constitutes an additional FDA-approved AMPH option for the treatment of ADHD in adults also with daily dosing. LDX takes advantage of a prodrug mechanism, whereby lisdexamfetamine is converted into D-AMPH and L-lysine via hydrolytic activity of red blood cells after absorption in the intestinal tract.[37] Of note, substantial red blood cell hydrolysis occurs even at low hematocrit levels, allowing for metabolism of lisdexamfetamine even in patients with anemia.[37] This prodrug technology allows for once daily dosing and avoids a rapid increase in D-AMPH levels. LDX comes in both a capsule and chewable tablet.[37] The capsule may be opened with the contents dissolved in water for immediate consumption, whereas the chewable tablet must be chewed thoroughly before swallowing.[33] Its duration of effect is 12 to 14 hours with an onset of clinical effect at 1.5 to 2 hours.[33] The longer duration of action occurs due to the prodrug nature of LDX that leads to the D-AMPH peaking at about 4.4 hours after ingestion and persisting throughout the day.[38] The recommended dose for adults with ADHD ranges from 30 to 70 mg daily.[37] Dose adjustments should be made for patients with severe renal impairment for a maximum dose of 50 mg daily as well as those with end stage renal disease for a maximum dose of 30 mg daily.[22] A systematic review and meta-analysis of 20 studies by Stuhec and colleagues[39] suggests that LDX has the largest effect size in treating adult ADHD when compared with MAS, MPH, and Modafinil, the last of which does not have FDA approval but has been used off-label in the treatment of adult ADHD. In a study by Adler and colleagues,[40] LDX improved not only ADHD symptoms but also executive functioning deficits and self-reported quality of life measures in adults with ADHD. A systematic review and meta-analysis by Fridman and colleagues[41] similarly demonstrated a large treatment effect size of 1.070 for LDX in European adults with ADHD.

4. AMPH extended-release oral suspension (AMPH EROS; brand name Dyanavel XR) serves as yet another daily dosing option with FDA approval for the treatment of ADHD in patients 6 years and older. It contains a combination of D-AMPH and L-AMPH in a 3.2:1 ratio with both immediate and extended-release components.[42] The extended-release component is coated in a pH-independent polymer.[42] Its duration of effect is 13 hours with an onset of clinical effect at only 30 minutes.[43] The efficacy of AMPH EROS was established in a randomized, parallel-group, double-blind, placebo-controlled dose-optimized laboratory classroom study.[44]

5. AMPH extended-release chewable tablets (AMPH ER TAB; brand name Dyanavel XR) gained FDA approval for the treatment of ADHD in patents 6 years and older in November 2021.[45] Similar to the oral suspension formulation, the chewable tablets also contain a combination of D-AMPH and L-AMPH in a 3.2:1 ratio.[46] A crossover study that compared 20 mg of the tablet with 20 mg of the oral suspension showed that both agents demonstrated comparable bioavailability.[46] A double-blind, placebo-controlled, fixed-dose phase 3 study evaluated AMP-ER tablets in adults with ADHD and indicated that the tablets achieved statistically significant improvements in mean Permanent Product Measure of Performance Total (PERMP-T) scores averaged across all postdose time points up to 14 hours when compared with placebo.[45] Although the oral suspension is commercially available, the chewable tablet formulation has not been made available as of March 2022.

Methylphenidate

MPH seems to treat ADHD by increasing noradrenergic and dopaminergic activity in the prefrontal cortex through the inhibition of neurotransmitter reuptake.[30] To be more exact, MPH inhibits the norepinephrine and dopamine transporters, increasing the concentration of these neurotransmitters in the synaptic cleft.[30] In contrast to AMPH, MPH does not promote dopamine release from synaptic vesicles.[22] MPH is a racemic mixture of D-threo and L-threo enantiomers, with the D-threo enantiomer proving to be more pharmacologically active.[22]

A variety of MPH medications has been FDA approved. These medications are differentiated by their stimulant delivery systems and by their duration of action (short-acting, intermediate-acting, or long-acting). The MPH formulations that have both FDA approval for adult use and have active clinical studies or data in adult populations are reviewed below. These medications all share the property of long-acting duration.

Long-acting methylphenidate

1. Osmotic release oral system MPH (OROS MPH; brand name *Concerta)* contains approximately 22% immediate-release and 78% extended-release MPH.[47] OROS MPH HCL capsules possess a unique delivery system. The capsule contains an immediate-release overcoat that is metabolized first.[48] Two drug compartments and a push compartment constitute the extended-release portion of the drug.[22] The OROS technology requires osmotic pressure to activate the push compartment in the capsule so that the 2 extended-release MPH compartments get released through an orifice over time.[22] Dosages in adults start at 18 mg daily and should not exceed 72 mg daily.[48] The duration of action for this drug is 12 hours with an onset of effect of 1 to 2 hours.[33] The minimal effective dose trial by Adler and colleagues[49] established the efficacy and safety of OROS MPH. In association with being a minimal effective dose trial, the effect size of the Adler and colleagues study was smaller than one by Medori and colleagues.[49,50] This latter study by Medori and colleagues,[50] a double-blind, randomized, placebo-controlled, parallel-group, fixed-dose trial at 51 sites, established that OROS-MPH resulted in decreased ADHD symptoms compared with placebo. Larger doses were associated with greater symptom reduction; OROS-MPH at 18, 36, and 72 mg had an effect size of 0.38, 0.43, and 0.62, respectively.[50] A randomized, placebo-controlled trial of OROS MPH demonstrated efficacy in the treatment of adult ADHD via improvements in the clinical global impression-improvement (CGI-I) scale and adult ADHD investigator symptom RS (AISRS) with a clinically significant response rate of 66% of subjects receiving OROS MPH versus 39% of subjects on placebo.[51] A double-blind, placebo-controlled, crossover study of OROS MPH demonstrated efficacy in the treatment of adult ADHD via significant improvements in the Wender-Reimherr adult attention deficit disorder scale (WRAADDS) and ADHD-RS.[52] An uncontrolled, open-label trial primarily investigated the safety and tolerability of OROS MPH had the added benefit of demonstrating improvement in executive functioning among adults with ADHD.[53]

2. Dexmethylphenidate ER (D-MPH ER; brand name *Focalin XR)* is approved for the treatment of ADHD in adults. D-MPH ER uses Spheroidal Oral Drug Absorption System technology, a 2-pulse system, whereby each capsule releases half of its dose as immediate-release beads and the other half as enteric-coated, delayed release beads.[23] D-MPH is often thought to be twice as potent as D,L-MPH, and yet, some studies suggest that the D-isomer is more than twice as effective.[23] Recommended doses range from 10 to 40 mg daily in adults.[54] Taking D-MPH ER with food may

delay its peak actions for 2 to 3 hours, although capsules may be opened with their contents sprinkled on applesauce for immediate consumption.[54] Its duration of effect lasts 12 hours with its onset of effect at 30 minutes.[33] A randomized, controlled, fixed-dose study of D-MPH ER has demonstrated safety and efficacy in the treatment of adult ADHD via improvements in ADHD-RS and CGI-I scores. Effect sizes for improvement in the total score ADHD-RS with D-MPH ER varied from 0.53 to 0.83 in a dose-dependent fashion.[55] A 6-month open-label extension trial, following a 5-week fixed-dose study of D-MPH ER, demonstrated the long-term safety and efficacy of this agent.[56] The mean improvements in ADHD-RS scores were 10.2 points for subjects switched from placebo to D-MPH-ER and 8.4 points for subjects who continued on D-MPH-ER.[56]

3. Multilayer release MPH extended-release capsules (MLR MPH XR; brand name *Adhansia XR*) possess a triple bead delivery system and demonstrate a bimodal plasma concentration peak at 1.5 hours and at 12.5 hours, ensuring continued symptom control for the entire course of the day.[57] This medication has been FDA approved for patients aged 6 years and older. Recommended doses range from 25 to 85 mg once daily in adults.[57] This medication can be taken with or without food.[33] Capsules may be opened and sprinkled onto applesauce or yogurt for consumption within 10 minutes.[33] The duration of effect for MLR MPH XR ranges between 13 and 16 hours with an onset of clinical effect at 1 hour.[33] A randomized, double-blind study of adults with ADHD evaluated the onset and duration of efficacy of MLR MPH XR capsules in a simulated workplace environment. MLR MPH XR-treated adults had greater mean PERMP total scores across all time points compared with placebo ($P = .0064$).[58] A 6-month open-label extension trial, following a 5-week fixed-dose study of MLR MPH XR, demonstrated the long-term safety and efficacy of this agent.[59] In the extension trial, MLR MPH XR-treated subjects experienced greater symptom reduction in ADHD-RS-5 total score from baseline compared with placebo in the double-blind study ($P = .003$).[59]

4. Serdexmethylphenidate and D-MPH (SDX and D-MPH; brand name *Azstarys*) gained FDA approval for the treatment of ADHD in patients 6 years and older in 2021. This is the first drug formulated with 30% immediate-release D-MPH and 70% SDX, a prodrug of D-MPH.[60] SDX is likely converted to D-MPH in the lower gastrointestinal tract; however, the enzymes involved in this metabolism have not been identified.[60] The efficacy of SDX was established via a randomized, double-blind, placebo-controlled, parallel-group, analog classroom study.[61]

Nonstimulants

Currently, the FDA has approved only one nonstimulant medication options for adults with ADHD–atomoxetine (ATMX; brand name *Strattera*); however, viloxazine extended-release (brand name *Qelbree*)[62,63] is currently being considered for adult ADHD by FDA.

ATMX functions as a selective norepinephrine reuptake inhibitor, binding to the norepinephrine transporter, increasing synaptic norepinephrine.[64] ATMX has minimal effects on serotonin reuptake and primarily inhibits presynaptic norepinephrine reuptake to effectively increase synaptic norepinephrine levels and prefrontal cortex dopamine levels.[64]

DEA standards do not label ATMX a controlled substance, given the limited abuse potential of atomoxetine.[65] Accordingly, ATMX is preferred for ADHD patients with active comorbid substance-use disorders. Additionally, ATMX may be preferred over stimulants in patients with comorbid tic disorders.[66]

In adult clinical trials of ATMX, the most common adverse events were constipation, dizziness, xerostomia, anorexia, as well as urinary retention and sexual dysfunction in men.[23] Clinicians need to monitor for emergence of suicidal ideation, emergence of new psychotic or manic symptoms, serious cardiovascular side effects, and severe liver dysfunction.[62] A black box warning describes reports of hepatotoxicity.[67] Dose adjustments should be made for moderate and severe liver impairment. Of note, a study of adults treated with ATMX for ADHD by Adler and colleagues,[68] found no significant differences in hepatic measures among groups stratified by heavy, nonheavy, and no alcohol use.

In adults, FDA label dosing starts around 40 mg daily with a maximum recommended daily dose of 100 mg.[23] However, a retrospective review analysis has shown that real-world dosing patterns of ATMX start lower than 40 mg daily to minimize side effects seen early in the treatment.[69] ATMX possesses a half-life of 5 hours; however, the success of once daily dosing suggests that therapeutic effects persist beyond the pharmacologic effects of ATMX.[22] Although stimulants typically have fast onset of clinical effects, it can take 2 to 3 weeks to see results with ATMX.[65]

The efficacy of ATMX in adults was established in 2 randomized, double-blind, placebo-controlled clinical studies of adult patients, which evaluated for improvements with the Conners' Adult ADHD RS that included adult ADHD prompts.[70] The treatment effect sizes were statistically significant with sizes of 0.35 and 0.40 in each of the 2 studies.[70] According to a 2009 meta-analysis by Mészáros and colleagues,[71] the effect size of atomoxetine is approximately half of the effect size of stimulants.

Viloxazine ER is a multimodal nonstimulant and norepinephrine reuptake inhibitor that increases intrasynaptic serotonin levels by modulating several serotonin receptors.[72] In April 2021, the FDA approved this nonstimulant option for the treatment of ADHD in patients aged 6 to 17 years. A phase 3, randomized, double-blind, placebo-controlled trial was recently completed with 374 adults with ADHD that evaluated the drug's efficacy and safety.[73] With flexible daily doses of up to 600 mg, viloxazine ER was associated with significant improvement of ADHD symptoms in adults, as measured by the AISRS, when compared with placebo and was also well tolerated.[73] The trial's secondary endpoint of improvements in CGI-severity (CGI-S) scores was also met with clinical significance.[73] Given the encouraging results from this phase 3 trial, viloxazine provides an alternative nonstimulant agent for prescribers when stimulants are contraindicated in adult patients with ADHD.

Alternative Considerations

In addition to the FDA-approved medication options for adult ADHD, there are additional pharmacotherapeutic options that the clinician can opt to use with the patient's informed consent that the medication is being prescribed off-label.

Some of these agents are stimulants in the AMPH and MPH classes that have only been approved in the pediatric population to manage ADHD, such as MAS IR and MPH IR.[74,75]

Others are nonstimulant medications that are labeled for conditions different from ADHD but have been shown to have some positive or mixed effects in adults with ADHD, such as some tricyclic antidepressants, bupropion, and modafinil.[76–79] One double-blind trial studying extended-release bupropion in adults achieved statistical significance in a post hoc measure of change in WRAADDS scores compared at the time of screening.[76] A multisite, placebo-controlled, 8-week prospective trial with 162 adults with ADHD showed that 53% of subjects treated with extended-release bupropion had at least a 30% reduction in ADHD-RS scores at week 8 as opposed to 31% of subjects treated with placebo ($P = .004$).[77] Another multisite, placebo-controlled, dose-ranging study demonstrated significant changes in self-assessment scores, although not in AISRS scores, of ADHD symptoms for adults taking higher doses of modafinil.[79] Further investigation of these nonstimulant medications may therefore be warranted.[76–79]

FUTURE DIRECTIONS

In spite of the pharmacologic options available for adult ADHD, a critical need exists for novel agents to treat this condition. Despite the effectiveness of stimulants for adult ADHD, in patients with certain comorbidities such as substance use disorders, anxiety disorders, and tic disorders, there exist either relative or FDA-labeled contraindications for both AMPHs and MPHs. Although ATMX presents as an alternative nonstimulant possibility, there exists many nonresponders to this drug.[23] Both stimulants and ATMX can also be associated with side effects that lead to dose-limiting intolerance or discontinuation of these agents. An additional barrier may be that many clinicians including adult primary care physicians have reported lack of familiarity in identifying and treating adult ADHD when compared with other psychiatric disorders.[80] These providers have also reported a hesitancy to prescribe stimulants.[80]

New stimulants and nonstimulant agents have been developed and several have been evaluated in adult clinical trials with promising results.[81] We will briefly review 5 agents below.

1. CTx-1301 (D-MPH HCl extended-release tablets): CTx-1301 has a trimodal pharmacokinetic profile that offers rapid rate of onset within 30 minutes and entire active-day duration of up to 16 hours.[82] It also has the potential to minimize rebound and crash. CTx-1301 contains 3 separate layers of D-MPH released via its drug-delivery platform technology: IR D-MPH, then delayed sustained-release D-MPH, and then IR D-MPH again.[82] In a single-dose, 4-sequence, 4-period crossover study to evaluate comparative bioavailability and safety of CTx-1301, 45 adult subjects with ADHD were randomized to receive single doses of 2 different CTx-1301 dosages and 2 different Focalin XR doses.[83] When compared with Focalin XR, CTx-1301 exhibited a statistically significant higher plasma concentration between 9 and 16 hours at both low and high doses.[83] Phase 3 trials are being planned to prospectively evaluate efficacy including onset, duration, safety, and additional pharmacodynamic benefits.[83]

2. Mazindol controlled release (MZD-CR): MZD exhibits a multimodal mechanism that includes inhibition of the norepinephrine, dopamine, and serotonin transporters as well as modulation of serotonin, muscarinic, histamine H1, μ-opioid, and orexin-2 receptors. MZD immediate-release was approved in the United States for treatment of obesity in adults but was withdrawn in the early 2000s.[84] NLS Pharmaceutics has recently been reexamining this agent for the treatment of ADHD and narcolepsy in controlled-release and extended-release formulations, respectively.[85] A phase 2, double-blind, placebo-controlled, study using flexible dosing of MZD-CR during 6 weeks was conducted with 85 adults with ADHD aged 18 to 65 years.[85] A significant difference in ADHD-RS-5 scores between MZD-CR and placebo groups were seen starting day 7. MZD-CR was also well tolerated with minimal cardiovascular side effects.[85]

3. Guanfacine extended-release (GXR): GXR recently gained government regulated approval for the treatment of adult ADHD in Japan.[85] A double-blind, placebo-controlled, dose-optimized trial demonstrated the efficacy and safety of GXR in the treatment of adult ADHD.[63] Ten weeks of monotherapy with GXR-improved core ADHD symptoms including executive functioning, physician and patient rated clinical impression, as well as quality of life measures.[63] Although GXR is currently FDA approved for the treatment of ADHD in children in the United States and has

been approved for adult ADHD in Japan, the compound has not been approved for adult ADHD in the United States.[63]

4. Centanafadine sustained release (CTN SR): CTN functions as a monoamine triple reuptake inhibitor, with preferential potency for norepinephrine and dopamine and smaller effects on serotonin.[86] A phase 2 clinical trial completed in 2020 investigated the safety and efficacy of this agent for the treatment of adult ADHD.[87] In one single-blind study with flexible-dosing of up to 500 mg per day, there was a statistically significant improvement in the mean ADHD-RS-IV total score, which improved by 21.41 points during 4 weeks of treatment.[87] The second phase of this clinical trial consisted of a randomized, double-blind, placebo-controlled, crossover investigation with daily doses up to 800 mg of CTN SR. Subjects treated with CTN SR showed a statistically significant improvement in ADHD-RS-IV scores from baseline to week 3 with an effect size of 0.66 when compared with placebo.[87] A recent poster presentation of data from 2 phase 3, randomized, double-blind, multicenter, placebo-controlled trials demonstrated the efficacy of CTN SR at 200 and 400 mg per day in adults with ADHD.[88] CTN SR was associated with significant improvement in ADHD symptoms in adults, as measured by the change in AISRS total score.[88] The secondary endpoint of improvements in CGI-S scores when compared with placebo was also met with clinical significance.[88,89]

SUMMARY

The literature is unequivocal about the effectiveness of pharmacotherapy in the management of adult ADHD with both stimulants and ATMX being available as FDA-approved treatment possibilities. The pharmacotherapy armamentarium has grown as new drug formulations with unique delivery systems have been approved for adult ADHD during the past 2 decades. These options allow clinicians to personalize and optimize the pharmacologic treatment plan for each patient based on their symptomatology and both their psychiatric and medical comorbidities. As our understanding of the neurobiology of ADHD improves, more compounds with novel mechanisms of action are being actively investigated.

CLINICS CARE POINTS

- Stimulants are the most used psychotropics in the treatment of attention-deficit/hyperactivity disorder (ADHD) because they exhibit larger effect sizes than nonstimulants. All stimulant options present with similar adverse side effects and contraindications. The clinician should personalize treatment and choose an agent based on how the individual patient will benefit from the formulation, whereas accounting for medical and psychiatric comorbidities.

- Amphetamines may exhibit higher effect sizes than methylphenidates in adult patients based on large-scale studies, although the choice of medication has to be individualized to the clinical situation.

- ATMX is a valuable nonstimulant option for adult ADHD patients who cannot tolerate stimulants or may have a comorbid substance use disorder or a tic disorder.

- Although patients may self-report symptom relief with initiation of medication, clinicians need to objectively evaluate if the patient's ADHD symptoms have remitted by performing ongoing monitoring via targeted clinical assessment and clinician-rated scales to quantify severity of symptoms and assess for adverse effects of treatment to optimize treatment.

DISCLOSURE

Dr L.A. Adler has received grant and research support from Sunovion Pharmaceuticals, Shire/Takeda Pharmaceuticals, and Otsuka; has served as a consultant to Bracket, Sunovion Pharmaceuticals, Shire/Takeda Pharmaceuticals, Otsuka Pharmaceuticals, SUNY, the National Football League, and Major League Baseball; and has received loyalty payments (as inventor) since 2004 from NYU for license of adult ADHD scales and training materials. Drs D. Anbarasan and G. Safyer have nothing to disclose.

REFERENCES

1. Xu G, Strathearn L, Liu B, et al. Twenty-year trends in diagnosed attention-deficit/hyperactivity disorder among us children and adolescents, 1997-2016. JAMA Netw Open 2018;1(4):e181471.
2. Kessler R, Adler L, Barkley R, et al. The prevalence and correlates of adult ADHD in the United States: results from the national comorbidity survey replication. Am J Psychiatry 2006;163(4):716–23.
3. Goodman D, Lasser R, Babcock T, et al. Managing ADHD across the lifespan in the primary care setting. Postgrad Med 2011;123(5):14–26.
4. Adamis D, Graffeo I, Kumar R, et al. Screening for attention deficit–hyperactivity disorder (ADHD) symptomatology in adult mental health clinics. Ir J Psychol Med 2017;35(3):193–201.
5. Sibley M, Rohde L, Swanson J, et al. Late-Onset ADHD reconsidered with comprehensive repeated assessments between ages 10 and 25. Am J Psychiatry 2018;175(2):140–9.
6. Adler L, Faraone S, Spencer T, et al. The structure of adult ADHD. Int J Methods Psychiatr Res 2017;26(1):e1555.
7. Kessler R, Green J, Adler L, et al. Structure and diagnosis of adult attention-deficit/hyperactivity disorder. Arch Gen Psychiatry 2010;67(11):1168.
8. Diagnostic and statistical manual of mental disorders. 5th ed. Arlington, VA: American Psychiatric Association; 2013.
9. Shaw M, Hodgkins P, Caci H, et al. A systematic review and analysis of long-term outcomes in attention deficit hyperactivity disorder: effects of treatment and non-treatment. BMC Med 2012;10(1).
10. Biederman J, Faraone S, Spencer T, et al. Functional impairments in adults with self-reports of diagnosed ADHD. J Clin Psychiatry 2006;67(04):524–40.
11. Biederman J, DiSalvo M, Fried R, et al. Quantifying the protective effects of stimulants on functional outcomes in attention-deficit/hyperactivity disorder: a focus on number needed to treat statistic and sex effects. J Adolesc Health 2019; 65(6):784–9.
12. Doshi J, Hodgkins P, Kahle J, et al. Economic impact of childhood and adult attention-deficit/hyperactivity disorder in the United States. J Am Acad Child Adolesc Psychiatry 2012;51(10):990–1002.e2.
13. Pliszka S, AACAP Work Group on Quality Issues. Practice parameter for the assessment and treatment of children and adolescents with attention-deficit/hyperactivity disorder. J Am Acad Child Adolesc Psychiatry 2007;46(7):894–921.
14. ADHD Questionnaires | CADDRA. Caddra.ca. 2021. Available at: https://www.caddra.ca/etoolkit-forms/. Accessed October 23, 2021.
15. JJS Kooij, Bijlenga D, Salerno L, et al. Updated European Consensus Statement on diagnosis and treatment of adult ADHD. Eur Psychiatry 2019;56:14–34.

16. Attention deficit hyperactivity disorder: diagnosis and management | Guidance. NICE; 2018. Nice.org.uk. Available at: https://www.nice.org.uk/guidance/ng87. Accessed September 30, 2021.

17. Adler L, Spencer T, Wilens T. Attention-deficit hyperactivity disorder in adults, and children. 1st edition. United Kingdom: Cambridge University Press; 2015.

18. Greenhill L, Pliszka S, Dulcan M. Practice parameter for the use of stimulant medications in the treatment of children, adolescents, and adults. J Am Acad Child Adolesc Psychiatry 2002;41(2):26S–49S.

19. Mattes JA, Boswell L, Oliver H. Methylphenidate effects on symptoms of attention deficit disorder in adults. Arch Gen Psychiatry 1984;41(11):1059–63.

20. Ginsberg L, Katic A, Adeyi B, et al. Long-term treatment outcomes with lisdexamfetamine dimesylate for adults with attention-deficit/hyperactivity disorder stratified by baseline severity. Curr Med Res Opin 2011;27(6):1097–107.

21. Cortese S, Adamo N, Del Giovane C, et al. Comparative efficacy and tolerability of medications for attention-deficit hyperactivity disorder in children, adolescents, and adults: a systematic review and network meta-analysis. Lancet Psychiatry 2018;5(9):727–38.

22. Bulkstein O. Psychostimulants for adult ADHD: formulations, prescribing tips, adverse effects and monitoring. Sheridan (WY): Psychopharmacologyinstitute.com; 2020. Available at: https://psychopharmacologyinstitute.com/section/psychostimulants-for-adult-adhd-formulations-prescribing-tips-adverse-effects-and-monitoring-2510-4923. Accessed September 30, 2021.

23. Stahl S, Grady M, Muntner N. Stahl's essential psychopharmacology. 6th edition. Cambridge, UK: Cambridge University Press; 2017.

24. Mick E, McManus D, Goldberg R. Meta-analysis of increased heart rate and blood pressure associated with CNS stimulant treatment of ADHD in adults. Eur Neuropsychopharmacol 2013;23(6):534–41.

25. Habel L, Cooper W, Sox C, et al. ADHD medications and risk of serious cardiovascular events in young and middle-aged adults. JAMA 2011;306(24):2673.

26. Qureshi A, Suri M, Kirmani J, et al. Is Prehypertension a risk factor for cardiovascular diseases? Stroke 2005;36(9):1859–63.

27. Vasan R, Larson M, Leip E, et al. Impact of high-normal blood pressure on the risk of cardiovascular disease. N Engl J Med 2001;345(18):1291–7.

28. Cooney M, Vartiainen E, Laakitainen T, et al. Elevated resting heart rate is an independent risk factor for cardiovascular disease in healthy men and women. Am Heart J 2010;159(4):612–9.e3.

29. Wilens T, Hammerness P, Biederman J, et al. Blood pressure changes associated with medication treatment of adults with attention-deficit/hyperactivity disorder. J Clin Psychiatry 2005;66(02):253–9.

30. Katzung B, Masters S, Trevor A. Basic & clinical pharmacology. 12th edition. New York: McGraw Hill Lange; 2010.

31. Arnsten A, Pliszka S. Catecholamine influences on prefrontal cortical function: relevance to treatment of attention deficit/hyperactivity disorder and related disorders. Pharmacol Biochem Behav 2011;99(2):211–6.

32. Highlights of prescribing information. Adderall XR label. Accessdata.fda.gov. Available at: https://www.accessdata.fda.gov/drugsatfda_docs/label/2013/021303s026lbl.pdf. Accessed September 30, 2021.

33. Mattingly G, Wilson J, Ugarte L, et al. Individualization of attention-deficit/hyperactivity disorder treatment: pharmacotherapy considerations by age and co-occurring conditions. CNS Spectr 2021;26(3):202–21.

34. Biederman J, Spencer T, Wilens T, et al. Long-term safety and effectiveness of mixed amphetamine salts extended release in adults with ADHD. CNS Spectr 2005;10(S20):16–25.
35. Highlights of prescribing information. Mydayis label. Accessdata.fda.gov. Available at: https://www.accessdata.fda.gov/drugsatfda_docs/label/2017/022063s000lbl.pdf. Accessed September 30, 2021.
36. Adler LA, Robertson B, Chen J, et al. Post hoc responder and remission analyses from two studies of SHP465 mixed amphetamine salts extended-release among adults with attention-deficit/hyperactivity disorder. J Child Adolesc Psychopharmacol 2020;30(7):427–38.
37. Highlights of prescribing information. Vyvanse label. Accessdata.fda.gov. Available at: https://www.accessdata.fda.gov/drugsatfda_docs/label/2017/208510lbl.pdf. Accessed September 30, 2021.
38. Adler L, Alperin S, Leon T, et al. Pharmacokinetic and pharmacodynamic properties of lisdexamfetamine in adults with attention-deficit/hyperactivity disorder. J Child Adolesc Psychopharmacol 2017;27(2):196–9.
39. Stuhec M, Lukić P, Locatelli I. Efficacy, acceptability, and tolerability of lisdexamfetamine, mixed amphetamine salts, methylphenidate, and modafinil in the treatment of attention-deficit hyperactivity disorder in adults: a systematic review and meta-analysis. Ann Pharmacother 2018;53(2):121–33.
40. Adler L, Dirks B, Deas P, et al. Self-Reported quality of life in adults with attention-deficit/hyperactivity disorder and executive function impairment treated with lisdexamfetamine dimesylate: a randomized, double-blind, multicenter, placebo-controlled, parallel-group study. BMC Psychiatry 2013;13(1):253.
41. Fridman M, Hodgkins P, Kahle J, et al. Predicted effect size of lisdexamfetamine treatment of attention deficit/hyperactivity disorder (ADHD) in European adults: estimates based on indirect analysis using a systematic review and meta-regression analysis. Eur Psychiatry 2015;30(4):521–7.
42. Highlights of prescribing information. Dyanavel XR label. Accessdata.fda.gov. Available at: https://www.accessdata.fda.gov/drugsatfda_docs/label/2017/208147s003lbl.pdf. Accessed March 14, 2022.
43. Childress AC, Chow H. Amphetamine extended-release oral suspension for attention-deficit/hyperactivity disorder. Expert Rev Clin Pharmacol 2019;12(10):965–71.
44. Childress AC, Wigal SB, Brams MN, et al. Efficacy and safety of amphetamine extended-release oral suspension in children with attention-deficit/hyperactivity disorder. J Child Adolesc Psychopharmacol 2018;28(5):306–13.
45. Tris Pharma Presents positive results from phase 3 study of amphetamine extended-release tablet in adults with ADHD. BioSpace Available at: https://www.biospace.com/article/releases/tris-pharma-presents-positive-results-from-phase-3-study-of-amphetamine-extended-release-tablet-in-adults-with-adhd/. Accessed March 14, 2022.
46. Herman B, Kando J, King T, et al. 178 single-dose pharmacokinetics of amphetamine extended-release tablet compared with amphetamine extended-release oral suspension. CNS Spectr 2020;25(2):312–3.
47. Katzman M, Sternat T. A review of OROS methylphenidate (Concerta®) in the treatment of attention-deficit/hyperactivity disorder. CNS Drugs 2014;28(11):1005–33.
48. Highlights of prescribing information. Concerta label. Accessdata.fda.gov. Available at: https://www.accessdata.fda.gov/drugsatfda_docs/label/2017/021121s038lbl.pdf. Accessed September 30, 2021.

49. Adler L, Zimmerman B, Starr H, et al. Efficacy and safety of OROS methylphenidate in adults with attention-deficit/hyperactivity disorder. J Clin Psychopharmacol 2009;29(3):239–47.

50. Medori R, Ramos-Quiroga J, Casas M, et al. A randomized, placebo-controlled trial of three fixed dosages of prolonged-release oros methylphenidate in adults with attention-deficit/hyperactivity disorder. Biol Psychiatry 2008;63(10):981–9.

51. Biederman J, Mick E, Surman C, et al. A randomized, placebo-controlled trial of oros methylphenidate in adults with attention-deficit/hyperactivity disorder. Biol Psychiatry 2006;59(9):829–35.

52. Reimherr F, Williams E, Strong R, et al. A double-blind, placebo-controlled, crossover study of osmotic release oral system methylphenidate in adults with ADHD with assessment of oppositional and emotional dimensions of the disorder. J Clin Psychiatry 2007;68(01):93–101.

53. Fallu A, Richard C, Prinzo R, et al. Does OROS-methylphenidate improve core symptoms and deficits in executive function? Results of an open-label trial in adults with attention deficit hyperactivity disorder. Curr Med Res Opin 2006; 22(12):2557–66.

54. Highlights of prescribing information. Focalin XR label. Accessdata.fda.gov. Available at: https://www.accessdata.fda.gov/drugsatfda_docs/label/2017/021802s033lbl.pdf. Accessed September 30, 2021.

55. Spencer T, Adler L, McGough J, et al. Efficacy and safety of dexmethylphenidate extended-release capsules in adults with attention-deficit/hyperactivity disorder. Biol Psychiatry 2007;61(12):1380–7.

56. Adler L, Spencer T, McGough J, et al. Long-term effectiveness and safety of dexmethylphenidate extended-release capsules in adult ADHD. J Atten Disord 2009; 12(5):449–59.

57. Highlights of prescribing information. Adhansia XR label. Accessdata.fda.gov. Available at: https://www.accessdata.fda.gov/drugsatfda_docs/label/2019/212038 Orig1s000lbl.pdf. Accessed September 30, 2021.

58. Wigal SB, Wigal T, Childress A, et al. The Time course of effect of multilayer-release methylphenidate hydrochloride capsules: a randomized, double-blind study of adults with ADHD in a simulated adult workplace environment. J Atten Disord 2020;24(3):373–83.

59. Weiss MD, Childress AC, Donnelly GAE. Efficacy and safety of PRC-063, extended-release multilayer methylphenidate in adults with ADHD including 6-month open-label extension. J Atten Disord 2021;25(10):1417–28.

60. Highlights of prescribing information. Aztaryz label. Accessdata.fda.gov. Available at: https://www.accessdata.fda.gov/drugsatfda_docs/label/2021/212994 s000lbl.pdf. Accessed September 30, 2021.

61. Kollins SH, Braeckman R, Guenther S, et al. A randomized, controlled laboratory classroom study of Serdexmethylphenidate and d-methylphenidate capsules in children with attention-deficit/hyperactivity disorder. J Child Adolesc Psychopharmacol 2021;31(9):597–609.

62. Highlights of prescribing information. Strattera label. Accessdata.fda.gov. Available at: https://www.accessdata.fda.gov/drugsatfda_docs/label/2011/021411s 035lbl.pdf. Accessed September 30, 2021.

63. Bymaster F, Katner J, Nelson D, et al. Atomoxetine increases extracellular levels of norepinephrine and dopamine in prefrontal cortex of rat a potential mechanism for efficacy in attention deficit/hyperactivity disorder. Neuropsychopharmacology 2002;27(5):699–711.

64. Mattingly GW, Young J. A clinician's guide for navigating the world of attention deficit hyperactivity disorder medications. CNS Spectr 2021;26(2):104–14.
65. Upadhyaya H, Desaiah D, Schuh K, et al. A review of the abuse potential assessment of atomoxetine: a nonstimulant medication for attention-deficit/hyperactivity disorder. Psychopharmacology (Berl) 2013;226(2):189–200.
66. Pringsheim T, Steeves T. Pharmacological treatment for Attention Deficit Hyperactivity Disorder (ADHD) in children with comorbid tic disorders. Cochrane Database Syst Rev 2011;13(4):CD007990.
67. Reed V, Buitelaar J, Anand E, et al. The safety of atomoxetine for the treatment of children and adolescents with attention-deficit/hyperactivity disorder: a comprehensive review of over a decade of research. CNS Drugs 2016;30(7):603–28.
68. Adler L, Wilens T, Zhang S, et al. Retrospective safety analysis of atomoxetine in adult ADHD patients with or without comorbid alcohol abuse and dependence. Am J Addict 2009;18(5):393–401.
69. Kabul S, Alatorre C, Montejano L, et al. Real-world dosing patterns of atomoxetine in adults with attention-deficit/hyperactivity disorder. CNS Neurosci Ther 2015;21(12):936–42.
70. Michelson D, Adler L, Spencer T, et al. Atomoxetine in adults with ADHD: two randomized, placebo-controlled studies. Biol Psychiatry 2003;53(2):112–20.
71. Mészáros A, Czobor P, Bálint S, et al. Pharmacotherapy of adult attention deficit hyperactivity disorder (ADHD): a meta-analysis. Int J Neuropsychopharmacol 2009;12(08):1137.
72. Johnson J, Liranso T, Saylor K, et al. A phase II double-blind, placebo-controlled, efficacy and safety study of SPN-812 (Extended-Release viloxazine) in children with ADHD. J Atten Disord 2020;24(2):348–58.
73. Nasser A, Hull J, Liranso T, et al. A phase 3, randomized, double-blind, placebo-controlled trial assessing efficacy and safety of viloxazine extended-release capsules (QelbreeTM) in adults with attention-deficit/hyperactivity disorder. Poster presented at: Psych Congress; Oct 29–Nov 1, 2021; San Antonio, TX.
74. Spencer T, Biederman J, Wilens T, et al. Efficacy of a mixed amphetamine salts compound in adults with attention-deficit/hyperactivity disorder. Arch Gen Psychiatry 2001;58(8):775–82.
75. Spencer T, Biederman J, Wilens T, et al. A large, double-blind, randomized clinical trial of methylphenidate in the treatment of adults with attention-deficit/hyperactivity disorder. Biol Psychiatry 2005;57(5):456–63.
76. Reimherr F, Hedges D, Strong R. Bupropion SR in adults with ADHD: a short-term, placebo-controlled trial. Neuropsychiatr Dis Treat 2005;1:245–51.
77. Spencer T, Biederman J, Wilens T. Nonstimulant treatment of adult attention-deficit/hyperactivity disorder. Psychiatr Clin North Am 2004;27(2):373–83.
78. Wilens TE, Haight BR, Horrigan JP, et al. Bupropion XL in adults with attention-deficit/hyperactivity disorder: a randomized, placebo-controlled study. Biol Psychiatry 2005;57(7):793–801.
79. Arnold V, Feifel D, Earl C, et al. A 9-week, randomized, double-blind, placebo-controlled, parallel-group, dose-finding study to evaluate the efficacy and safety of modafinil as treatment for adults with ADHD. J Atten Disord 2012;18(2):133–44.
80. Adler L, Farahbakhshian S, Romero B, et al. Healthcare provider perspectives on diagnosing and treating adults with attention-deficit/hyperactivity disorder. Postgrad Med 2019;131(7):461–72.
81. Childress A, Beltran N, Supnet C, et al. Reviewing the role of emerging therapies in the ADHD armamentarium. Expert Opin Emerg Drugs 2020;26(1):1–16.

82. Cingulate Technology. 2021. Available at: https://cingulatetherapeutics.com/technology/cingulate-technology/#anchor. Accessed September 30, 2021.

83. Brams M, Silva R. 5.7 comparative bioavailability and safety of a novel trimodal dexmethylphenidate tablet in ADHD patients. J Am Acad Child Adolesc Psychiatry 2020;59(10):S150–1.

84. Wigal T, Newcorn J, Handal N, et al. A double-blind, placebo-controlled, phase II study to determine the efficacy, safety, tolerability and pharmacokinetics of a controlled release (CR) formulation of mazindol in adults with DSM-5 attention-deficit/hyperactivity disorder (ADHD). CNS Drugs 2018;32(3):289–301.

85. NLS Pharmaceutics Announces Notice of Allowance for U.S. Patent application covering its proprietary mazindol formulation | NLS Pharmaceuticals 2021. monsolfoundation.ch Available at: https://nlspharma.com/news/nls-pharmaceutics-announces-notice-of-allowance-for-u-s-patent-application-covering-its-proprietary-mazindol-formulation/. Accessed September 30, 2021.

86. Iwanami A, Saito K, Fujiwara M, et al. Efficacy and safety of guanfacine extended-release in the treatment of attention-deficit/hyperactivity disorder in adults. J Clin Psychiatry 2020;81(3):19m12979.

87. Bymaster F, Golembiowska K, Kowalska M, et al. Pharmacological characterization of the norepinephrine and dopamine reuptake inhibitor EB-1020: implications for treatment of attention-deficit hyperactivity disorder. Synapse 2012;66(6):522–32.

88. Wigal S, Wigal T, Hobart M, et al. Safety and efficacy of centanafadine sustained-release in adults with attention-deficit hyperactivity disorder: results of phase 2 studies. Neuropsychiatr Dis Treat 2020;8(16):1411–26.

89. Adler L, Adams J, Madera J, et al. Efficacy, Safety, and tolerability of centanafadine sustained-release tablets in adults with ADHD: results of two phase 3, randomized, double-blind, multicenter, placebo-controlled trials. Poster presented at: The American Professional Society of ADHD and Related Disorders; January 14–16, 2022; Tuscon, AZ.

A Review of Clinical Practice Guidelines in the Diagnosis and Treatment of Attention-Deficit/Hyperactivity Disorder

Steven R. Pliszka, MD[a],*, Victor Pereira-Sanchez, MD, PhD[b], Barbara Robles-Ramamurthy, MD[a]

KEYWORDS

- Clinical practice guidelines • ADHD • Patient outcomes • Evidence-based medicine

KEY POINTS

- Multiple clinical practice guidelines (CPGs) have been developed by professional societies and governments across the world.
- There is a great deal of consensus among these guidelines in terms of diagnosing and treating attention-deficit/hyperactivity disorder.
- More research is needed as to whether the adoption of the practices in CPGs by providers leads to an improvement in patient outcomes.

INTRODUCTION

How do clinicians adopt the methods and treatments that are most effective in treating disease? Once these techniques are mastered, how do clinicians update their approaches? What sources of knowledge are authoritative and who decides how to interpret them? In a historical overview, Trohler[1] noted that physicians, in ancient times, relied on classic systemic views of nature such as the Theory of Four Humors, which in turn was based on the 4 elements of water, earth, wind, and fire. Physicians were discouraged from relying on experience. According to Trohler,[1] "The quest was for certain knowledge, logically deduced from unquestioned first principles. Debates were about the truthfulness of those principles rather than the effectiveness of the recommendations deduced from them." (pg. 52) This may have led medieval physicians to continue to use methods, such as bloodletting, despite lack of positive results.

[a] Department of Psychiatry and Behavioral Sciences, Joe R and Theresa Long Lozano School of Medicine, 7703 Floyd Curl Drive, MC 7792, San Antonio, TX 78229, USA; [b] Columbia University, 40 Haven Avenue, New York State Psychiatric Institute (NYSPI) - Kolb Annex - Suite 171, New York, NY 10032, USA
* Corresponding author.
E-mail address: pliszka@uthscsa.edu

Child Adolesc Psychiatric Clin N Am 31 (2022) 569–581
https://doi.org/10.1016/j.chc.2022.03.009
1056-4993/22/© 2022 Elsevier Inc. All rights reserved.
childpsych.theclinics.com

Around 300 BCE, there emerged a sect of physicians called the Empirics who based their practices on experience, rather than philosophy (in contrast to Hippocratic methods).[2] The name *empiric* derives from Latin *empiricus,* itself from Greek *empeirikos* (experienced). Nonetheless, it took advances in the physical and biological sciences in the sixteenth century and beyond for physicians to gain meaningful clinical experiences that would lead to better patient outcomes. This eventually led to what Trohler[1] called the "individual-clinical" phase of modern medicine where physicians learned from their mentors and adjusted their practices based on what each individual doctor believed "worked." With the emergence of clinical science (ie, randomized controlled trials [RCTs], epidemiology) in the early to midtwentieth century, a new and more rational systematic basis for defining effectiveness of treatment emerged: the "statistic-analytical" tradition.[1] In 1992, the Journal of the American Medical Association declared,[3]

> *A new paradigm for medical practice is emerging. Evidence-based medicine de-emphasizes intuition, unsystematic clinical experience and pathophysiological rationale as sufficient grounds for clinical decision-making and stresses the examination of evidence from clinical research. (pg. 2420)*

Thus, the era of evidence-based medicine (EBM) was born, of which clinical practice guidelines (CPGs) are a key component. This first involved making a transition from a purely experiential view (learning from an individual mentor) to learning from "leaders in the field." Many early guidelines were produced by experts from professional medical societies, an approach referred to as "Good Old Boys Sitting Around a Table (GOBSAT)[4]; the term GOBSAT has been attributed to James Colquhoun Petri.[5] As noted below, more recent CPGs have incorporated more diverse expert opinions. From 1991 to 2007, The American Academy of Child and Adolescent Psychiatry produced "Practice Parameters" on attention-deficit/hyperactivity disorder (ADHD).[6] These evolved from simple opinion articles to the final 2007 version,[7] which came to resemble modern CPGs by adopting some of the practices that are now considered standard.

DEFINING CLINICAL PRACTICE GUIDELINES

Built into the terms "EBM" and "CPG" are an array of complex issues. What constitutes the Evidence Base? In this regard, evidence in the literature has been graded according to its nature and strength.[8] (**Table 1**). Level A consists of RCTs; increasingly, the field can look to meta-analyses and mega-analyses of multiple RCTs. The field of ADHD now has an advantage in this regard because there are several meta-analyses of both psychopharmacological and psychosocial treatment in ADHD.[9–11] Levels B and C refer to clinical trial data (both RCT and open trials) that have mild-to-moderate limitations, whereas Level D now refers to "GOBSAT," that is, expert opinion by itself. In a nod to Hippocrates, Level D also includes "reasoning from first principles." Any given standard thus lies along this continuum; this needs to be borne in mind whenever a particular diagnostic or therapeutic approach is deemed to be or not to be "evidenced based."

A CPG differs very much from a literature review, which reflects only the specific view of the authors who produced it. In contrast, the Institute of Medicine[12] (IOM) defined CPGs as "systematically developed statements to assist practitioner and patient decisions about appropriate health care for specific clinical circumstances." In 2011, the IOM[13] published detailed standards for CPGs, as shown in **Table 2**. Transparency is vital; the scientific community and the public should know the identity of the

Table 1
Assessing level of evidence and strength of recommendations

Level	Aggregate Evidence Quality	Benefit or Harm Predominates	Benefit or Harm Enhanced
A	Well-designed and conducted RTCs of interventions, Meta-and Mega-Analyses of quality studies	Strong recommendation	Weak recommendation (based on balance of harms and benefits)
B	Controlled trials with minor weaknesses, consistent findings from multiple observational studies	Moderate to strong recommendation	
C	Single or few observational studies, studies with inconsistent findings, studies with major limitations	Moderate to weak recommendation	
D	Case reports, expert opinion, reasoning from first principles	Weak recommendation	No recommendation may be made

members of the specific Guideline Development Group (GDG), as well as the process by which the members developed the guideline. The IOM standards are quite strict in terms of conflict of interest (COI) issues; all COIs must be declared. Members of the GDG should divest themselves of any financial investments and should not participate in marketing activities or advisory boards. Members with COIs should not chair a GDG, nor should a GDG contain a majority of members with conflicts. In the area of ADHD, a large number of researchers in the field have worked with the pharmaceutical industry in the development of agents to treat ADHD. This could potentially reduce the expertise available to GDGs. Moreover, pharmaceutical company ties are not the only potential source of bias. Providers of psychosocial treatments may have a financial interest in having their treatment endorsed by a GDG (which can lead to increased demand from the public or funding by third-party payers). Many psychosocial treatment manuals or methods are copyrighted or patented. Thus, there are many biases to consider. Finally, GDGs should be balanced and include representatives of the public to represent patient interests.

The GDG should commission a systematic review of the evidence meeting the IOM's Committee on Standards for Systematic Reviews of Comparative Effectiveness Research.[14] This can be a complex process, with strict standards on how the literature search is performed and documented. Such reviews may have already been done by an external body or the GDG may request one to be done. In the latter case, it is permissible for the GDG and the Systematic Review team to interact regarding both the review and the guidelines being developed. In the area of ADHD, a source for the American Academy of Pediatrics (AAP) has been a review of the literature from 2011 to 2016 on ADHD done by the Agency for Healthcare Research Quality and Review.[15] The diagnostic category to which a guideline applies should be clearly defined. The CPG should make specific instructions (to the degree the literature permits) on handling each major aspect of diagnosing and treating the disorder, with decisions guided by the strength of the evidence. These instructions generally take the form of "Processes of Care" or "Algorithms" with flow charts indicating the major decision points and resulting clinical actions.

Table 2 Institute of medicine standards for development of trustworthy clinical practice guidelines	
Standard	Description
Establishing transparency	• CPG users should be able "to understand how recommendations were derived and who developed them" • CPG should contain "An explicit statement of how evidence, expertise, and values were weighed by guideline writers helps users to determine the level of confidence they should have in any individual recommendation" • "Transparency also requires statements regarding the development team members' clinical experience and potential COIs, as well as the guideline's funding source(s)."
Management of COI	• Members of the guideline development group (GDG) should declare all interests and activities potentially resulting in COI with the development group activity, by written disclosure to those convening the GDG • Each panel member should explain how his or her COI could influence the CPG development process or specific recommendations • Members of the GDG should divest themselves of financial investments and not participate in marketing activities or advisory boards of entities whose interests could be affected by CPG recommendations • Members with COIs should neither Chair a CDG nor comprise most members
Guideline Development Group Composition	• The GDG should be multidisciplinary and balanced, comprising a variety of experts and clinicians and populations expected to be affected by the CPG • Patients, patient representatives or nonmedical public stakeholders should be included on the CPG
Clinical Practice Guideline–Systematic Review Intersection	• Clinical practice guideline developers should use systematic reviews that meet standards set by the Institute of Medicine's Committee on Standards for Systematic Reviews of Comparative Effectiveness Research • When systematic reviews are conducted specifically to inform particular guidelines, the GDG and systematic review team should interact regarding the scope, approach, and output of both processes
Determining Guideline Scope and Requisite Chain of Logic	• Define the scope of the CPG and develop processes of care or algorithms to guide clinicians

DETERMINING THE QUALITY OF CLINICAL PRACTICE GUIDELINES

The Appraisal of Guidelines for Research and Evaluation II (AGREE-II)[16–18] is a structured instrument that allows researchers to systematically evaluate the quality of CPGs. It consists of 23 items in 6 domains: scope and purpose, stakeholder involvement, rigor of development, clarity of presentation, applicability (barriers to implementation), and editorial independence (including managing COIs). Trained reviewers can independently rate each of these items on a seven-point Likert Scale. Andrade and colleagues[19] rated 22 CPGs published from 2005 to 2015 that focused on ADHD using the AGREE-II. They used scores on the stakeholder involvement, rigor of development and editorial independence scales to classify the CPGs as either minimum or high quality. Only two of the CPG's meet criteria for high quality, while another two meet criteria for minimum quality. This is not surprising given that the IOM guidelines[13] for CPGs were only issued in 2011. Indeed, the American Academy of Child and Adolescent psychiatry paused the production of its "Practice Parameters" (the last one issued on ADHD was in 2007[7]) to adapt to these standards.[6]

OVERVIEW OF CURRENT ATTENTION-DEFICIT/HYPERACTIVITY DISORDER CLINICAL PRACTICE GUIDELINES

Table 3 lists the most recent and prominent CPGs on ADHD, pointing out their commonalities as well as their variations from each other. These CPGs are highly congruent with each other. All of them emphasize the need to screen for ADHD and for a complete clinical history (and standardized rating scales) to diagnose ADHD. All point out that there is no laboratory or psychological test for ADHD; they all discuss medication and behavioral treatments as the most evidence-based interventions. The Canadian ADHD Resource Alliance guidelines are the most complete in terms of coverage of comorbid conditions in both children and adults.[20] The SDBP guidelines also deal with complex ADHD (those with comorbid conditions).

There are differences between the CPGs in terms of their emphasis on the relative role of medication and behavioral treatments. The AAP[21] guidelines recommend behavioral treatment *first* for children aged younger than 5 years, based on the results of the National Institute of Mental Health Preschool ADHD Treatment Study (PATS) study.[22] The AAP guidelines interpret the PATS study as showing improvement in ADHD symptoms after behavior treatment alone (pg.10).[21] If one examines Figure 1 from the PATS study article,[22] it shows that 261 participants were enrolled in behavioral treatment but that only 37 (7%) were viewed as substantially improved at the end of the course of behavioral treatment. One-hundred and eighty-three participants (71%) went on to be enrolled in the methylphenidate trial. Thus, the strength of this particular recommendation is somewhat puzzling, given that the PATS study cited showed such a low-response rate of ADHD symptoms to behavior treatment.

The SDBP guidelines state that, "Psychoeducation about ADHD and its coexisting conditions and evidence-based behavioral and educational interventions are foundational for the treatment of complex ADHD and should be implemented at the outset of treatment whenever possible." (pg S35) In the process of care algorithms that are part of the CPG,[23] detailed guidelines are laid out for the treatment of complex ADHD with a variety of concurrent conditions (anxiety, depression, tics, autism, and so forth). An initial overall algorithm states the treatment should begin with behavior treatment. A decision point is then labeled "continued impairment"; a "Yes" response leads to another decision point as to whether to begin medication or not. Thus, the SBDP CPG states that behavior treatment should always be first, even in complex cases, although the statement "whenever possible" certainly allows an individual clinician sufficient latitude to justify starting medication immediately if they believe it is clinically justified. The SBDP CPG recommendations for medications for concurrent conditions (SSRIs for anxiety/depression, alpha agonists for tics) are consistent with earlier recommendations in this area.[24]

How strong is the evidence base that behavior treatment should have such a prominent role in the treatment of ADHD? The Multimodality Treatment Study of ADHD (MTA)[25,26] randomized children with ADHD to treatment as usual (TAU), medication management, intensive behavior therapy, or combination treatment (medication

Table 3
An overview of the most recent and widely disseminated clinical practice guidelines for attention-deficit/hyperactivity disorder

CPG	Age Range	Deals with Comorbidity?	Commonalities	Specific emphasis/Unique Aspects
AAP CPG on diagnosis, evaluation, and treatment of ADHD in children and adolescents (USA)[21]	Up to18 y	No	• Screening of patients with mental health complaints for ADHD • Assessment for ADHD based on informants and rating scales, complete history • Laboratory, neuroimaging, or psychological testing not required for diagnosis • Screen for comorbidity • Medication and BT the mainstays of treatment • No evidence for alternative therapies (diet, neurofeedback) • Manage as a chronic condition. • Routine ECG prescreening or monitoring not required for those with a clear cardiac history	• Behavior therapy (BT) first for those aged <6 y, either medication and/or BT for those aged >6 y. • Primary care physicians may manage comorbidities if trained (but no advice in CPG on this). • Barriers to care discussed. • Medications approved by the Food Drug Administration for ADHD recommended as first line

CADDRA-Canadian ADHD CPGs (CAP-Guidelines Edition 4.1 (Canada)[20]	Child and Adults	Yes		• Extensive discussion of wide range of comorbid conditions for both:
				  ○ Differential diagnosis
				  ○ Combining other psychotropics with ADHD medications.
				• Long-acting stimulants (any type) recommended as first-line treatment.
				• Atomoxetine and guanfacine second line
				• Clonidine, bupropion, imipramine, and modafinil third line.
				• Medication and psychosocial treatments not rank-ordered or sequenced for any age group
				• Extensive discussion of choice/titration of medication and managing side effects

National Health and Medical Research Council Clinical Practice Points on diagnosis, assessment, and management of ADHD in children and adolescents (Australia)[51]	Up to 18 y	No		• Medication and psychosocial treatments not rank-ordered or sequenced for any age group • Pharmacologic intervention limited to stimulants.

National Institute for Health and Care Excellence ADHD CPG (UK)[52]	Child and Adult	No	• Children younger than 5 y of age should have a trial of ADHD-focused BT. Those not responding to BT should be evaluated by a specialist before starting medication • Methylphenidate recommended as first line • Lisdexamfetamine or dexamphetamine as second line • Atomoxetine or Guanfacine as third3rd line • Detailed information on side effect management
Society for Developmental and Behavioral Pediatrics Clinical Practice Guideline for the Assessment and Treatment of Children and Adolescents with Complex ADHD (USA)[23]	Up to 18 y	Yes	• Focus on multiple comorbidities (Complex ADHD) • States that psychosocial treatments are "foundational." (See text) • Detailed process of care algorithms for each comorbid condition • Algorithms imply that psychosocial interventions should be used first • Stimulants are first-line medication treatments

Abbreviations: ECG, Electrocardiogram; SDBP, Society for Developmental and Behavioral Pediatrics; SSRI, Specific Serotonin Reuptake Inihibtor.

with behavior therapy). In the TAU group, one-third of the children did not receive medication at all. At 14 months, outcome was superior in the medication management and the combined treatment groups relative to behavior therapy and TAU; the latter 2 did not differ from each other. For children with ADHD and anxiety, as well as for those who received public assistance, the combined treatment was superior to medication alone, at least on some measures.[26] An alternative analysis did show a superiority of the combined treatment over medication management but the effect size was quite small (0.28).[27] Once the study ended, the effect of all MTA treatments faded, and the groups were indistinguishable in outcome during the long term.[28] Of note, other studies have not shown a benefit of the combined treatment over medication alone in ADHD.[29,30] Thus, it is an open question as to whether there is sufficient evidence (multiple controlled trials, Level A) to show that the behavior treatment alone can be as effective as medication in treating ADHD. Moreover, it has not been proven that the combined treatment is superior to medication alone if comorbidity is not present. This does not mean the 2 pediatric CPGs are "wrong"; rather, it suggests that the issue of combining behavior and medication treatment is not as settled as these CPGs suggest.

IMPACT OF CLINICAL PRACTICE GUIDELINES ON THE QUALITY OF CARE

Does the publication of CPGs really change the provider behavior and improve the quality of care? There are 2 issues here: CPGs may have no impact on changing the provider behavior or they may change the provider behavior with no subsequent improvement in outcome for patients. Grimshaw and colleagues[31] reviewed 235 studies examining the impact of CPG dissemination and implementation on treatment effectiveness; 86.6% of these studies did show modest to moderated improvements in the quality of care. Only 9 of these studies involved the treatment of psychiatric disorders.

Research on the impact of GPGs in the management of ADHD has mostly focused on figures of adherence to guidelines in primary care health professionals,[32–38] as well as trend changes in clinical practice (including diagnosis and pharmacologic treatment) after the publication of guidelines.[39] There has been less attention to the study of implementation challenges and strategies[40–42] and, most importantly, to the actual impact of guidelines' implementation on the quality of care and patients' outcomes.[43] In terms of assessment of adherence, several studies examined self-reported or chart-reviewed clinical practice in specific domains of compliance with national guidelines (in particular, AAP guidelines were the gold standard in US studies[32,33,35–37] and a reference in some studies in other countries,[38] although adherence to other national and local guidelines has been studied in countries such as Canada,[43] Australia,[38] Germany,[44] and the Netherlands[45]), such as diagnostic and differential diagnostic procedures, treatment choice, and follow-up. Results from these studies show that adherence patterns vary across domains in the guidelines, tending to be higher in terms of psychopathological assessment and treatment selection and lower in terms of the use of unnecessary or unrecommended diagnostic tests and follow-up practices.[32–34,37] They vary across professionals, seeming to be higher among pediatricians than among family doctors[32,33,37,38] and nurse practitioners.[35] Studies in the United States also have demonstrated sociodemographic disparities reflecting a lesser adherence to guidelines in the care of patients in public insurance programs.[36,37] It is important to consider, however, that there is evidence suggesting that clinicians' self-reports of adherence tend to be more positive than the actual performance as assessed by chart review.[46] One particular area that has been examined is the impact of guidelines of prescribing stimulants for preschool ADHD. An examination of a large electronic medical record database found that the prevalence of prescription of stimulants for preschool ADHD plateaued at about 0.4% after the release of the 2011 AAP CPG, blunting a trending of rising prescriptions of stimulants in preschoolers before 2011.[39] A more recent study[37] conducted in 2021 examined the electronic medical records of nearly 30,000 preschoolers and found a prevalence of 0.7%; 80% of these individuals were not prescribed a stimulant medication. The study did not report on the prevalence of any psychosocial intervention. The 2 studies do suggest that the AAP CPG does indeed discourage physicians from prescribing stimulants to preschoolers with ADHD.

CLINICAL PRACTICE GUIDELINES AND THE STANDARD OF CARE

How do professional practice guidelines affect medical liability? Clinical practice is guided by many sources of information, including but not limited to our educational training programs, our professional mentors, textbooks, board examination educational materials, scientific journals, nonpeer reviewed literature, public media, online medical education, continuing medical education, and past personal and clinical experiences. CPGs are an important source of information that clinicians use to guide their patient care and help guide our understanding of professional consensus. As such, they may be reviewed and considered by attorneys and the court when determining if liability issues have occurred.

Although they are closely related, the standard of care, which is a legal definition, is not equivalent to the quality of care, which is a framework used by clinicians to provide the optimal clinical care. The quality of care can be influenced by factors, such as available community resources, third-party payers, and the patient's health care decisions. Quality care implies the physician's responsibility to provide care that "increases the likelihood of desired health outcomes."[47] Legal standards, however, are set at an acceptable minimum, so standard of care does not equate to the use of the most up-to-date treatment with the highest level of evidence proving its efficacy.

Clinicians must consider what the standard of care is for their patient population when determining how to apply professional clinical guidelines. Despite managed care's impact on how we practice medicine, the general legal rule is that the clinicians, not the managed care company, remain responsible for clinical decisions. In Wickline v States (1986),[48] the court affirmed a physician's duty to provide care and suggested a duty to appeal denial of coverage by a managed care company. In a more recent court decision in Wit v United Behavioral Health (UBH),[49] the US District Court for the Northern District of California found UBH liable for breach of its fiduciary duty in 4 states (Illinois, Connecticut, Rhode Island, and Texas), specifically noting that UBH should not refuse a patient substance-use treatment when it is consistent with the generally accepted standard of care. As an additional win to patients and clinicians, the court delineated that UBH's actions were motivated by financial factors, and their care coverage was overfocused on the treatment of "acute" symptoms as opposed to respecting the clinical need for a comprehensive care that addresses underlying conditions. Importantly, the court found that medical society-developed treatment guidelines were reliable sources that reflected the generally accepted standard of care.

FUTURE RESEARCH AND DIRECTIONS

Given the hard work and investment associated with the development and dissemination of GPGs, their promise to improve the quality of care, and the observed large variability in implementation and adherence,[50] it is puzzling to find a lack of literature assessing the impact of guidelines on patient outcomes in the area of ADHD. It also can be argued that, although the development of GPCs is one of the milestones of EBM, we still lack evidence to confirm that these guidelines are fulfilling their goal. Therefore, implementation and outcome-based research should be prioritized to understand systemic and clinician-level barriers to compliance with the guidelines, test solutions to overcome those barriers, and measure the actual benefit of well-implemented guidelines to patient care. There should also be a focus on advancing health equity.

CLINICS CARE POINTS

- Clinicians treating attention-deficit/hyperactivity disorder (ADHD) should be familiar with the major national and international clinical practice guidelines (CPGs) that have been developed during the past decade and be aware of the most recent editions.

- Clinicians should prioritize knowledge of the CPG that is most important for their subspecialty and patient population.

- CPGs are guidelines and not absolute rules for patient management. CPGs cannot cover every patient situation; deviation from a guideline is not ipso facto a sign of substandard care but documentation of the clinical situation should make clear the reason for the variation.

- Clinicians should be aware that there are differences in emphasis of treatment methods for ADHD among the available CPGs, particularly in how they view the role of psychosocial treatment. Future studies are needed to resolve these debates.

DISCLOSURE

Dr S.R. Pliszka has received research support from Otsuka Pharma and has been a consultant for Adlon Pharmaceuticals and Ironshore Pharmaceuticals.

REFERENCES

1. Trohler U. The history of clinical effectiveness. Proc R Coll Physicians Edinby 2001;31(Suppl 9):42–5.
2. Pomata G. A word of the Empirics: the ancient concept of observation and its recovery in early modern medicine. Ann Sci 2011;68(1):1–25.
3. Evidence-Based Medicine Working Group. Evidence-based medicine. A new approach to teaching the practice of medicine. J Am Med Assoc 1992; 268(17):2420–5.
4. Wollersheim H. Beyond the evidence of guidelines. Neth J Med 2009;67(2): 39–40.
5. Anonymous. Obituary James Colquhoun Petri. BMJ 2001;323:626.
6. Bukstein O. Clincal practice guidelines: the AACAP experience 30 years on. The American Professional Society for ADHD and Related Disorders Annuall Meeting. 2021. Virtual Meeting. Available at: https://apsard.org/meetings/past-meetings/. Accessed September 24, 2022.
7. Pliszka S. Practice parameter for the assessment and treatment of children and adolescents with attention-deficit/hyperactivity disorder. J Am Acad Child Adolesc Psychiatry 2007;46(7):894–921.

8. Shiffman RN, Marcuse EK, Moyer VA, et al. Toward transparent clinical policies. Pediatrics 2008;121(3):643–6.

9. Cortese S, Adamo N, Del Giovane C, et al. Comparative efficacy and tolerability of medications for attention-deficit hyperactivity disorder in children, adolescents, and adults: a systematic review and network meta-analysis. Lancet Psychiatry 2018;5(9):727–38.

10. Evans SW, Owens JS, Wymbs BT, et al. Evidence-based psychosocial treatments for children and adolescents with attention deficit/hyperactivity disorder. J Clin Child Adolesc Psychol 2018;47(2):157–98.

11. Pelham WE Jr, Fabiano GA. Evidence-based psychosocial treatments for attention-deficit/hyperactivity disorder. J Clin Child Adolesc Psychol 2008;37(1):184–214.

12. Institute of Medicine. Clinical practice guidelines: directions for a new program. Washington, D.C.: The National Academies Press; 1990.

13. Institute of Medicine. Clinical practice guidelines we can trust. Washington,D.C.: The National Academic Press; 2011.

14. Institute of Medicine. Finding what works in health care: standards for systematic reviews. Washington, D.C.: The National Academies Press; 2011.

15. Kemper A, Maslow G, Hill S, et al. Attention deficit hyperactivity disorder: diagnosis and treatment in children and adolescents. In: Comparative effectiveness review No. 203. Rockville. MD: AHRQ Publication No. 18-EHC005-EF; 2018.

16. Brouwers MC, Kho ME, Browman GP, et al. Agree II: advancing guideline development, reporting and evaluation in health care. CMAJ 2010;182(18):E839–42.

17. Brouwers MC, Kho ME, Browman GP, et al. Development of the AGREE II, part 1: performance, usefulness and areas for improvement. CMAJ 2010;182(10):1045–52.

18. Brouwers MC, Kho ME, Browman GP, et al. Development of the AGREE II, part 2: assessment of validity of items and tools to support application. CMAJ 2010;182(10):E472–8.

19. Andrade BF, Courtney D, Duda S, et al. A systematic review and evaluation of clinical practice guidelines for children and youth with disruptive behavior: rigor of development and recommendations for use. Clin Child Fam Psychol Rev 2019;22(4):527–48.

20. CADDRA-Canadian ADHD Resource Alliance. In: Canadian ADHD practice guidelines, 4, 1 Edition. Toronto, ON: CADDRA; 2020.

21. Wolraich ML, Hagan JF, Allan C, et al. Clinical practice guideline for the diagnosis, evaluation, and treatment of attention-deficit/hyperactivity disorder in children and adolescents. Pediatrics 2019;144(4):e20192528.

22. Greenhill LL, Kollins S, Abikoff H, et al. Efficacy and safety of immediate-release methylphenidate treatment for preschoolers with ADHD. J Am Acad Child Adolesc Psychiatry 2006;45:1284–93.

23. Barbaresi WJ, Campbell L, Diekroger EA, et al. The society for developmental and behavioral pediatrics clinical practice guideline for the assessment and treatment of children and adolescents with complex attention-deficit/hyperactivity disorder: process of care algorithms. J Dev Behav Pediatr 2020;41(Suppl 2S):S58–74.

24. Pliszka SR, Crismon ML, Hughes CW, et al. The Texas Children's Medication Algorithm Project: revision of the algorithm for pharmacotherapy of attention-deficit/hyperactivity disorder. J Am Acad Child Adolesc Psychiatry 2006;45(6):642–57.

25. MTA Cooperative Group. 14 month randomized clinical trial of treatment strategies for children with attention deficit hyperactivity disorder. Arch Gen Psychiatry 1999;56:1073–86.

26. MTA Cooperative Group. Moderators and mediators of treatment response for children with attention deficit hyperactivity disorder: the MTA study. Arch Gen Psychiatry 1999;56:1088–96.

27. Conners CK, Epstein JN, March JS, et al. Multimodal treatment of ADHD in the MTA: an alternative outcome analysis. J Am Acad Child Adolesc Psychiatry 2001;40(2):159–67.

28. Swanson JM, Arnold LE, Molina BSG, et al. Young adult outcomes in the follow-up of the multimodal treatment study of attention-deficit/hyperactivity disorder: symptom persistence, source discrepancy, and height suppression. J Child Psychol Psychiatry 2017;58(6):663–78.

29. Satterfield JH, Faller KJ, Crinella FM, et al. A 30-year prospective follow-up study of hyperactive boys with conduct problems: adult criminality. J Am Acad Child Adolesc Psychiatry 2007;46(5):601–10.

30. Abikoff H, Hechtman L, Klein RG, et al. Symptomatic improvement in children with ADHD treated with long-term methylphenidate and multimodal psychosocial treatment. J Am Acad Child Adolesc Psychiatry 2004;43(7):802–11.

31. Grimshaw JM, Thomas RE, MacLennan G, et al. Effectiveness and efficiency of guideline dissemination and implementation strategies. Health Technol Assess 2004;8(6):1–72, iii-iv.

32. Rushton JL, Fant KE, Clark SJ. Use of practice guidelines in the primary care of children with attention-deficit/hyperactivity disorder. Pediatrics 2004;114(1):e23–8.

33. McElligott JT, Lemay JR, O'Brien ES, et al. Practice patterns and guideline adherence in the management of attention deficit/hyperactivity disorder. Clin Pediatr (Phila) 2014;53(10):960–6.

34. Patel A, Medhekar R, Ochoa-Perez M, et al. Care provision and prescribing practices of physicians treating children and adolescents with ADHD. Psychiatr Serv 2017;68(7):681–8.

35. Jansen M. NPs' use of guidelines to diagnose and treat childhood ADHD. Nurse Pract 2019;44(7):37–42.

36. Moran A, Serban N, Danielson ML, et al. Adherence to recommended care guidelines in the treatment of preschool-age medicaid-enrolled children with a diagnosis of ADHD. Psychiatr Serv 2019;70(1):26–34.

37. Bannett Y, Feldman HM, Gardner RM, et al. Attention-deficit/hyperactivity disorder in 2- to 5-year-olds: a primary care network experience. Acad Pediatr 2021;21(2):280–7.

38. Ellis LA, Blakely B, Hazell P, et al. Guideline adherence in the management of attention deficit hyperactivity disorder in children: an audit of selected medical records in three Australian states. PLoS One 2021;16(2):e0245916.

39. Fiks AG, Ross ME, Mayne SL, et al. Preschool ADHD diagnosis and stimulant use before and after the 2011 AAP practice guideline. Pediatrics 2016;138(6).

40. Leslie LK, Weckerly J, Plemmons D, et al. Implementing the American Academy of Pediatrics attention-deficit/hyperactivity disorder diagnostic guidelines in primary care settings. Pediatrics 2004;114(1):129–40.

41. Olson BG, Rosenbaum PF, Dosa NP, et al. Improving guideline adherence for the diagnosis of ADHD in an ambulatory pediatric setting. Ambul Pediatr 2005;5(3):138–42.

42. Hall CL, Taylor JA, Newell K, et al. The challenges of implementing ADHD clinical guidelines and research best evidence in routine clinical care settings: delphi survey and mixed-methods study. BJPsych Open 2016;2(1):25–31.

43. Wagner DJ, Vallerand IA, McLennan JD. Treatment receipt and outcomes from a clinic employing the attention-deficit/hyperactivity disorder treatment guideline of the children's medication algorithm project. J Child Adolesc Psychopharmacol 2014;24(9):472–80.

44. Mucke K, Pluck J, Steinhauser S, et al. Guideline adherence in German routine care of children and adolescents with ADHD: an observational study. Eur Child Adolesc Psychiatry 2021;30(5):757–68.

45. Levelink B, Walraven L, Dompeling E, et al. Guideline use among different health-care professionals in diagnosing attention deficit hyperactivity disorder in Dutch children; who cares? BMC Psychol 2019;7(1):43.

46. Gordon MK, Baum RA, Gardner W, et al. Comparison of performance on ADHD quality of care indicators: practitioner self-report versus chart review. J Atten Disord 2020;24(10):1457–61.

47. World Health Organization. Fact Sheet: Quality health services. 2020. Available at: https://www.who.int/news-room/fact-sheets/detail/quality-health-services. Accessed September 15, 2021.

48. Wickline v State, 192 Cal App 3d 1630 In:1986. Available at: https://law.justia.com/cases/california/court-of-appeal/3d/192/1630.html. Accessed September 10, 2021.

49. American Medical Association. ARC issue brief: Wit v. United behavioral health. AMA Advocacy Resource Center; 2019. Accessed September 10, 2021.

50. Wolraich ML, Chan E, Froehlich T, et al. ADHD diagnosis and treatment guidelines: a historical perspective. Pediatrics 2019;144(4):e20191682.

51. National Health and Medical Research Council. Clinical practice points on the diagnosis, assessment and management of attention deficit hyperactivity disorder in children and adolescents. Canberra (Australia): Commonwealth of Australia; 2012.

52. National Institute for Health Care Excellence (NICE). Attention deficit hyperactivity disorder: diagnosis and management (NG87). 2018. Available at: www.nice.org.uk/guidance/ng87. Accessed September 4, 2021.

Moving?

Make sure your subscription moves with you!

To notify us of your new address, find your **Clinics Account Number** (located on your mailing label above your name), and contact customer service at:

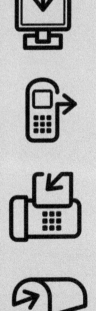

Email: journalscustomerservice-usa@elsevier.com

800-654-2452 (subscribers in the U.S. & Canada)
314-447-8871 (subscribers outside of the U.S. & Canada)

Fax number: 314-447-8029

Elsevier Health Sciences Division
Subscription Customer Service
3251 Riverport Lane
Maryland Heights, MO 63043

*To ensure uninterrupted delivery of your subscription, please notify us at least 4 weeks in advance of move.

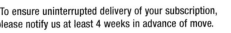